W9-BAG-853

1-15-17

SEEKING THE CURE

———◦◦◦———

A History of Medicine in America

IRA RUTKOW

Scribner

New York   London   Toronto   Sydney

SCRIBNER

A Division of Simon & Schuster, Inc.
1230 Avenue of the Americas
New York, NY 10020

First Scribner hardcover edition April 2010

SCRIBNER and design are registered trademarks of The Gale Group, Inc.,
used under license by Simon & Schuster, Inc., the publisher of this work.

For information about special discounts for bulk purchases,
please contact Simon & Schuster Special Sales at 1-866-506-1949 or
business@simonandschuster.com.

The Simon & Schuster Speakers Bureau can bring authors to your live event.
For more information or to book an event, contact the Simon & Schuster
Speakers Bureau at 1-866-248-3049 or visit our website at
www.simonspeakers.com.

Book design by Ellen R. Sasahara

Manufactured in the United States of America

1   3   5   7   9   10   8   6   4   2

Library of Congress Control Number: 2009049758

ISBN 978-1-4165-3841-7

To my fellow physicians and their patients

CONTENTS

Introduction   *1*

Part I • RISE OF AN INDEPENDENT PROFESSION

One Colonial Medicine   7

Inoculation at Any Cost
Cotton Mather and Smallpox
The Great Inoculator
"Doctor" Benjamin Franklin
Medicine, Just Another Colonial Trade
"I have seen him"
Discourse Upon the Institution of Medical Schools in America
Specialization, a New Style of Practice
Morgan's Fall

Two Democratization of Healing   *31*

America's Hippocrates
Bleed, Blister, Puke, and Purge
Money and Medical Schools
"The people of this state have been bled long enough"
A Time to Organize
Medical Journalism
"The greatest discovery ever made"
"Gentlemen, this is no humbug"

Three Emergence of Modern Medicine   61

"Simply deaf and dumb"
"He does believe in antiseptic surgery"
The Slow Embrace of Listerism
"Doctor, I am a dead man"
"His case is very hopeful"
"Ignorance is bliss"
The Physician Himself
Saving Lives, Millions at a Time

Four Consolidation of Power   90

An Ignorant Fanatic
Lifeless Delusions
"The rectum is the focus of existence"
Science, the Final Arbiter
Irreconcilable Differences
Railroads and Doctors

Part II • COMING OF AGE

Five Scientific Advancement   117

Lehrfreiheit and *Lernfreiheit*
"Popsy"
"If we only had such laboratories in America"
"We are lucky to get in as professors"
Verdeutsched
The Professor and Cocaine
Halsted's Resurrection
Surgeons of the Highest Type
Instruments of Precision
"Hidden Solids Revealed"
"We do not sell Humbug"

Six Professional Authority 147

A Layman's Job
Bulletin Number Four
"Flexnerian" Philanthropy
"Show Me" and "Tell Me"
The Minimum Standard
"Broad and firm foundations"
Ambulance Américaine
Base Hospitals

Seven Challenges of Success 173

Diseases of Deficiency
The Power of Electricity
The Unassuming Appendix
"His appendix was a long affair"
A Higher Price Tag
"Americanism versus Sovietism for the American people"
Bona Fide Specialist or Not
"Handicraft outruns science"

Part III • TRIUMPHS AND TRIALS

Eight Ascendancy 209

Blood for Britain
Charles Drew
The American Red Cross Blood Bank
Drew, Racism, and His Death
An Incentive to Specialize
John Gibbon and His Heart-Lung Machine
Persuasive, Charming, and Indispensable
"Continuously and conspicuously palpable"
Spheres of Influence

Nine Supremacy   *239*

    Organ Transplantation
    Francis Moore and George Thorn
    "This sacred kidney"
    Acquired Tolerance
    Whither the General Practitioner
    The AMA versus National Health Care
    The Battle Over Medicare
    A Prototypical Modern Disease
    "Four-Button Sid"
    The National Cancer Act of 1971

Ten Transformation   *273*

    A Crisis in Manpower
    A Lump of Porridge
    Voyage into the Heart
    The Medical-Industrial Complex
    An Interior View
    A Mainstay of the Surgeon
    Uncontrollable Costs
    Medical Malpractice

    Epilogue   *304*

    Acknowledgments   *309*
    Notes   *311*
    Selected Bibliography   *336*
    Index   *346*

INTRODUCTION

———————

HEALTH CARE AFFECTS the lives of all Americans, yet few understand how the system came to be. The nation certainly was not founded with today's modern arrangement in place—the dizzying network of physicians, hospitals, clinics, insurance companies, and pharmaceutical firms, to name a few. For much of the country's history, doctors were solitary practitioners who followed the untested theories of their mentors, tried to gain respect through professionalization, and vigorously defended themselves against external change. These men (and women, eventually), whose bold innovations helped to meld scientific advancement with clinical care, would expand the possibilities of medical treatment for patients throughout the world. *Seeking the Cure* tells their story. It is a story of medicine, but it is also a story of America.

Fitting this tale into a single, accessible volume has always been difficult. On the one hand, medical history often progresses with discrete breakthroughs, from the introduction of inoculation for smallpox in early-eighteenth-century Boston to the first cardiac surgery using a heart-lung machine two hundred and thirty-two years later in Philadelphia. Each of these discoveries is a story in itself, the tale of a doctor or team of doctors conquering the medical unknown. On the other hand, medical history also moves in gradual, almost imperceptible steps. The growth of medical schools and the ascendance of hospitals, for example, are changes that took centuries to achieve, yet there are few watershed moments that show such evolution. Neither narrative—the discrete or the gradual—is complete without the other.

Seeking the Cure weaves together these two braids of medical history to tell a fascinating chronicle. The steady sociological changes in medicine

1

(the process of professionalization with its side issues of credentialing, education, licensing, standardization, and the rise of the medical-industrial complex) form a backdrop against which astonishing scientific discoveries (transformations in treatments and techniques) are grafted. Thus, the reader is able to understand how the shaping of the profession impacted medical achievements, and vice versa. Such parallels in the science and sociology of medicine appear repeatedly, and this two-pronged discussion best conveys the complexity and richness of the history of medicine in America.

But medicine is not a universe unto itself. It is neither a closed kingdom nor the province of physicians alone. The changes and discoveries within the profession also occurred (and continue to occur) as part of the broader fabric of American life. For example, the fact that the earliest efforts to unite the colonies went hand in hand with the first attempts to unify doctors or that American medicine rose to international preeminence around the same time the nation emerged as a superpower in world affairs was not serendipitous. The evolution of American medicine has often closely mirrored the nation's history. To explain these parallels, *Seeking the Cure* intersperses the story of medicine with the economic, political, and social issues of the country as a whole. Putting medical events in a wider historical context allows readers to better situate themselves within the sweep of the narrative. The doctors are center stage, but the theater in which they are initially performing is America, and later the world.

In this respect, it should be stressed that the book is written for as wide an audience as possible. The work is purposefully free of medical jargon, and when technical terminology is used it is explained in plain English. The hope is that *Seeking the Cure* will be entertaining and educational for the lay reader, the medical professional, and the policy maker, as all three have something to gain by understanding medical history. For the lay reader, the book serves to provide a sophisticated understanding of clinical care that will lessen the anxiety of being a patient. For the physician, it lends perspective to their clinical performance while distinguishing fact from fiction and hero from villain. For the policy maker, it informs the decisions that will shape the future of health care.

At the same time, *Seeking the Cure* is intended to be a work of revelatory history, specifically one about medical practice, its practitioners, and the professionalization of medicine as a discipline, and not brash policy. No book can be entirely free of bias, but I have attempted to limit this distorting lens and to tell medical history as clearly, concisely, and vividly as possible. There are no critiques of current strategies nor suggestions for future ones. Instead, *Seeking the Cure* emphasizes the events of medicine within the full tapestry of the American experience.

To the extent that my own perspective shapes the narrative, it is perhaps most evident in the selection of stories that are featured. It would be wonderful to give lengthy coverage to every medical discovery, every research breakthrough, every professional development, but that would require a multivolume tome. And such a work would be less accessible. For example, late-twentieth-century medicine, which chapters 9 and 10 address broadly, becomes so complex that no sweeping work of American medical history can give adequate treatment to all its facets. The book, consequently, makes little reference to essential, but particularized, phenomena, such as the rise of human experimentation, the right-to-die debate, bioethics, AIDS, other potentially fatal infectious diseases, and the growth of patient activism. Similarly, at times there were multiple events that convey important developments in American medicine, but to tell them all would become distracting. Chapter 8, for instance, which considers racism and segregation in medicine, might have substituted the World War II era tale of Charles Drew, a renowned African-American physician whose medical research led to innovations in the use of blood, with the story of the Tuskegee syphilis study, when doctors intentionally permitted impoverished African-American sharecroppers to suffer from the disease even though by the mid-1940s it was known that penicillin was a cheap and effective cure. Some might argue that my approach results in cursory summarizations or exclusions, but *Seeking the Cure* is not aimed to cover every significant event in America's medical past, nor praise all famous physicians, nor relate the history of each specialty. The personalities and advances that are highlighted are the ones that struck me as most illustrative, important, or, occasionally, simply fascinating. Collectively, they provide a captivating story, even if certain details are spared.

I will, however, confess to having a bias toward events in surgery. After all, I am a general surgeon. But in my defense, I offer the words of Henry Bigelow. He was a faculty member at Harvard's medical school over a century ago and speculated on the differing interest in the progress of surgery versus medicine. "Why is the amphitheater crowded to the roof on the occasion of some great operation, while the silent working of some drug excites little comment? Mark the hushed breath, the fearful intensity of silence, when the blade pierces the tissues, and the blood wells up to the surface. Animal sense is always fascinated by the presence of animal suffering."

I have devoted my professional life to medicine, both as a physician and an author. I hope that my dual perspective on the subject (the combining of contemporary historical scholarship with a doctor's skills at the bedside and in the operating room) proves useful in the retelling. Traditional historians when tackling the material, often quite ably, are still hampered by their outsider status.

Medicine is a quasi-religious, mystical craft that almost no one can avoid encountering over the course of a life. The nonphysician often wants to peer into this mysterious realm, but must do so through closed fingers. It is to better understand medicine's ability to provoke fascination and fear, to serve as a mirror into our lives, that *Seeking the Cure* looks behind medicine's closed curtain and, I hope, provides the reader with a fundamental grasp of its history in America.

Part I

RISE OF AN INDEPENDENT

PROFESSION

❧ One ❧

COLONIAL MEDICINE

Inoculation at Any Cost

ZABDIEL BOYLSTON, ONE of Boston's most distinguished physicians, cowered in a hidden passageway inside his home. Outside, a rabble of angry townspeople demanded that he be lynched. They had gathered there after searching for the doctor throughout the city for several days and nights while flaunting a hangman's noose as their flag. It was mid-summer 1721 and Boston, a city of almost twelve thousand people, was suffering a devastating smallpox epidemic. Nearly half of the city's inhabitants would contract the illness and one in fourteen would die.

The mob had targeted Boylston for attempting the medical unknown. He had taken pus and scabs from the pocks of a patient with active smallpox and placed the putrid material beneath a small cut in the skin of healthy individuals, including several family slaves and his six-year-old son. Boylston intended to induce a mild form of smallpox in these patients, who would, he hoped, recover and be protected against the more severe attacks and possible death that resulted from contracting the illness naturally. "I resolv'd to carry it on for the saving of Lives," he would later write, "not regarding any, or all the Menaces and Opposition that were made against it."[1] This rudimentary inoculation was untried and risky, even without the mob's threats.

The physician and his family feared for their lives with good reason. Boylston's neighbors believed that he was a killer who would expand the disease's toll. "To spread a mortal Contagion, What is it but to cast abroad

Arrows and Death?" stated one outraged citizen. "If a man should will-fully bring infection from a person sick of a deadly and contagious Dis-ease, into a place of Health; is not the mischief as great?"[2] Secreted for fourteen days, the doctor and his kin survived not only the mob's intimi-dations but a dud hand grenade thrown into the house's parlor. So terri-fied was Boylston that for several weeks after the mob attack subsided he visited his patients only at night and in wigged disguise.

Boylston could do little to calm the raging fears but wait for the passage of time to prove his medical claims. The city's selectmen scolded him, his fellow physicians labeled him unscrupulous, and vituperative journalists described him as a mass murderer. A weak-willed man might not have persevered, but the forty-one-year-old Boylston was no ordinary doctor, nor easily bullied. His earliest biographer said he possessed "a strong and reflecting mind, and acute discernment," leading a life of "unimpeached integrity."[3] Unlike other practitioners who were less educated and poorly trained, the bold and stubborn Boylston never shied away from under-taking difficult medical cases. He had a reputation for performing vir-tuoso feats of surgery long before the inoculation crisis—in 1707, he had extracted an egg-sized stone from the urinary bladder of a thirteen-year-old boy, and a decade later, in the presence of clergy and other specta-tors, Boylston had removed a woman's breast for the "repeated bleeding, growth & stench"[4] of cancer.

Cotton Mather and Smallpox

Smallpox and other epidemics, such as diphtheria, dysentery, influenza, measles, scarlet fever, and yellow fever, were the colonialists' persistent nightmare. Medical anthropologists believe that the small pox (or vari-ola)—differentiated from the large pox (or syphilis)—was introduced into Europe around AD 500 by nomadic Saracen tribes from the east. Euro-peans subsequently brought it to the new world, where it ravaged native populations. Smallpox first reached New England in the early 1600s and continued to plague the colonialists every dozen or so years. The disease easily provoked panic due to its gruesome sequelae: "Purple spots, convul-sion fits, bloody urine, violent inflammations in the eyes, throat, and other parts," according to Boylston. "In some, the pock runs into blisters, and the skin stripping off, leaves the flesh raw, like creatures flea'd [flayed]. Some have a burning, others a smarting pain, as if in the fire, or scalded with boiling water."[5]

With no knowledge of virology or pharmacology (smallpox is caused by the double-stranded, DNA-rich variola virus), the colonials could only curb smallpox's spread with strict isolation procedures. A Massachusetts statute even stipulated that all smallpox sufferers should be separated from the healthy population in designated "pox" houses.

As the 1721 smallpox epidemic wore on, news of Boylston's radical smallpox experiments panicked Bostonians, convinced that isolation was the only solution and that other approaches, especially inoculation, would worsen the plague. Then, the city's renowned firebrand preacher, Cotton Mather, publicly declared his support of Boylston's efforts, something few had anticipated.

The fifty-eight-year-old, Harvard-educated Mather, the controversial pastor of the city's original Congregationalist North Church, was a prominent public figure and Boston's "keeper of the Puritan conscience."[6] Mather influenced both spiritual and secular matters, from his youthful persecution of witches to a middle-aged enthusiasm for medical and public health improvements. He advocated Bible societies, the education of slaves, religious missionary work, and temperance. He also helped organize a college in New Haven, Connecticut, and suggested that it be named after the major benefactor, Elihu Yale. In addition to all of this, Mather was, according to one historian, "the most original medical thinker in the colonial period."[7] He was, among other things, one of the first to realize the cyclical nature of smallpox epidemics.

While Mather's curiosity and intellect were rare, his interest in medicine was fairly common for a clergyman in the colonies. Minister-physicians, as they were known, continued a clerical tradition common to England and compounded by a paucity of decent healers in the new world. America's preachers, the colonies' best-educated and most well-read individuals, found that their book knowledge of medicine provided an effective way to establish rapport with congregants and the general public. Since religion and medicine had been interwoven for centuries, especially through the view that illness was the work of the devil and punishment for religious transgressions, it was de rigueur for colonial clergymen to attend to their flocks' medical needs as part of pastoral care.

During the early 1720s, Mather had read a series of articles in the Royal Society of London's *Philosophical Transactions* detailing a little-known Asian and Middle Eastern folk medicine practice of inoculation for smallpox. It appeared from eyewitness accounts that when a person acquired smallpox through inoculation, the resulting illness was less deadly than a natural case. In fact, inoculation, the eighteenth-century version of modern vaccination (there was no word for immunization or immunity in that era's scientific lexicon), caused a case of genuine smallpox, but one considerably milder than smallpox contracted at random. Those who received inoculation were as resistant to subsequent smallpox outbreaks as those who had acquired it naturally, despite the attenuated nature of the induced illness.

The commonsense medical approach of this technique intrigued Mather, who, realizing the severity of the current smallpox epidemic, decided to recommend the immediate use of inoculation to Boston's physicians. "The practice of conveying and suffering the Small-pox by Inoculation, has never been used in America, nor indeed in our nation," Mather wrote in his diary. "But how many Lives might be saved by it, if it were practised?"[8]

The reaction of Boston's approximately dozen physicians was contemptuous at best. Two of them united in violent opposition to the proposal, denouncing it as similar to introducing the plague in Europe. They declared that any attempt to put inoculation into effect would be "no less criminal than murder."[9] Dozens of pamphlets and broadsides were published in a back-and-forth war of words. The dispute became a cause célèbre as the newspapers of the day teemed with accusations and character attacks.

Mather made a personal plea to Boylston, the one physician who he believed would support his radical idea. "You are many ways endeared to me," wrote the preacher, "but by nothing more than the very much good which a gracious God employs you and honors you to do to a miserable world."[10] Mather argued that, with an ongoing epidemic, inoculation should start as soon as possible. An unhesitant Boylston, whose face bore the undulating scars of a childhood case of smallpox, agreed. Two days later, inoculation, and threats to Boylston's life, commenced.

The Great Inoculator

By mid-July, Boylston had successfully treated ten individuals and announced his results in the *Boston Gazette* (colonial newspapers functioned as modern medical journals and were filled with the latest clinical reports as well as advertisements for physicians' services, textbooks, and drugs). He cautioned his critics that he was not afraid of their rage. "I have patiently born with abundance of Clamour and Ralary [raillery], for beginning a new Practice here (for the Good of the Publick), which comes well Recommended, from Gentlemen of Figure & Learning, and which well agrees to Reason,"[11] insisted a determined Boylston. He was so intent that he inoculated an additional seventeen people in August, thirty-one in September, eighteen in October, and in November, at the height of the epidemic, one hundred and three. Shuttling between Boston, Cambridge, and Roxbury, performing up to a dozen inoculations a day, Boylston found that the better-educated townspeople sought his help while the uninformed masses, as well as most of the city's physicians, feared it.

Boylston pleaded with the other doctors to visit his patients and judge his results. Rather than accepting this offer, Boylston's critics only intensified their scolding, accusing him of malpractice and murder. The incensed physicians spread their invective in the *New England Courant,* a newspaper published by James Franklin and his teenaged apprentice, his brother Benjamin. They argued that Boylston's action was imprudent. It would widen the spread of smallpox and worsen the social upheavals brought about by the current epidemic. Commerce and daily business would be halted, and Boston would be an unlivable city under medical siege with no food or other necessities brought in.

The hullabaloo intensified, and as physicians realized the resolve of Mather and Boylston, they appealed directly to the town authorities to stop the inoculation madness. These local selectmen reprimanded and legally threatened Boylston, who was repeatedly summoned before their public tribunals. Out of blind fear, they attacked and abused Mather as well. "They rave, they rail, they blaspheme; they talk not only like Idiots but also like Franticks," observed Mather. "I am an object of their Fury; their furious Obloquies and Invectives."[12]

In November, popular resentment, simmering since the attempted lynching of Boylston in the summer, came to a head again when someone tried to assassinate Mather. The attacker threw a bomb through Mather's window, but it failed to explode. The assailant had tied a chilling message around the device: "COTTON MATHER, You Dog, Dam you: I'll inoculate you with this, with a Pox to you."[13] The attempted murder became the talk of the town and the courts offered a large monetary reward to find the perpetrator, but the case was never solved.

By winter 1721–22, the smallpox scourge had ended and confirmed the assumptions of Boylston and Mather. Of the approximately 5,800 Bostonians who contracted the disease naturally, about 850 died, a death rate of almost 15 percent. The remainder of the city's 6,200 citizens had been presumably exposed to smallpox in prior outbreaks and survived unscathed. Of the 247 people that Boylston inoculated, only six died, a death rate of less than 3 percent. Not only were deaths reduced, but the artificial smallpox attack was mild in character. "They found ease and sweetness, and lay praising God on their beds, or rather sat up in their chairs to do so," said one contemporary observer about Boylston's patients. "Their tongues were filled with laughter, and ours with thanksgiving on their account when we went to see 'em. We saw them recover fast."[14] To deliberately permit oneself to be infected with smallpox, however, was a terrifying decision plagued by the possibility of death or disfigurement. And in the eighteenth century, there was no obvious reason (nor has one been found in the twenty-first century) as to why smallpox acquired through inoculation should somehow be different from the disease that was contracted by chance. Yet the inexplicable worked!

Unique circumstances and a fair bit of luck—if such a thing can be found during a smallpox epidemic—facilitated Boylston's success. There is little doubt that inoculation, contrasted with present-day vaccinations, could have further spread an epidemic. His critics were correct when they demanded that inoculated patients, despite having only the mild form of smallpox, be isolated. Boylston's good fortune was that the epidemic of 1721 was so severe and spread so quickly that the overwhelming number of individuals who naturally contracted the disease left few for the inoculated to cross-infect. Boylston again aroused public apprehension when, in the absence of an ongoing epidemic, he resumed his experiments in spring 1722. Once more, Boston authorities demanded that the newly inoculated be secluded from other citizens or Boylston's experiments would be stopped.

In view of the continuing controversies, it almost seemed expected and welcomed when a year later, in mid-1723, Boylston suddenly uprooted his family and left for London. Members of the Royal Society of London had invited him to present his experience with inoculation. London's physicians were eager to hear about his therapeutic encounters, as he was billed as the inoculator with the largest individual know-how in the Western world. He received numerous honors, including a lectureship before the Royal College of Physicians and membership in the Royal Society. But there was a more intriguing reason behind his visit. Boylston family lore suggested that England's King George I ordered the invitation with the intent that the colonial physician inoculate the royals. Boylston quickly became a medical celebrity in London who, according to a contemporary account, "received the most flattering attentions and friendship of some of the most distinguished characters of the nation."[15]

While abroad, Boylston also authored a small volume that became the chief American contribution to the world of medicine prior to the mid-nineteenth century, *An Historical Account of the Small-Pox Inoculated in New England, Upon All Sorts of Persons, Whites, Blacks, and of All Ages and Constitutions*. The book, an explication of Boylston's inoculation technique and clinical records, meticulously described patients and offered technical explanations and detailed statistical tables. He dedicated it to George I's daughter-in-law, Caroline, the Princess of Wales and wife of the soon-to-be George II: "The countenance which your royal highness hath given to the practice of inoculation, is a noble instance of your royal highness's superior judgment and parental tenderness; and the success with which it hath been attended in your royal family, is alone sufficient to recommend it to the world."[16]

With his business completed, Boylston departed London a wealthy man, supposedly remunerated one thousand gold guineas by the king. Boylston's biographer was careful to note that "he returned home with ample funds to enable him to retire from professional business."[17] Accorded acclaim upon his arrival back in Boston, Boylston was given the epithet "The Great Inoculator." He enjoyed the role of a well-to-do colonial physician and gentleman farmer for the remaining forty years of his life, celebrated by English followers and grudgingly admired by American adversaries. Although it took time for Boylston to earn his peers' admiration, his career and accomplishments were defined by a willingness to challenge conventional wisdom, a go-it-alone mind-set that appears repeatedly in moments of discovery and innovation throughout the history of American medicine.

"Doctor" Benjamin Franklin

Despite lower death rates for the inoculated versus the naturally infected, the practice of inoculation remained restricted and unpopular in the colonies. It would take several decades to spread from New England to New York, Philadelphia, Baltimore, and Charleston. The idea of inoculation was vigorously debated during these years, with one unexpected advocate taking a central role in the discussions, the up-and-coming Benjamin Franklin.

To the well-known image of Franklin as philanthropist, politician, scientist, statesman, writer, and womanizer should be added the honorary title of physician. He invented spectacles, devised a urinary catheter, observed that exposure to lead caused sickness, explored the use of electricity as medical therapy, and advised vigorous daily exercise to maintain one's health. Franklin's friends recognized his lifelong interest in medical problems by frequently referring to him as "doctor."

Franklin was involved in the inoculation fracas at a relatively early age and became a staunch advocate of the practice. In the spring of 1730, while still in his midtwenties, he informed readers of his *Pennsylvania Gazette* about the virtues of the procedure (this was in direct contrast to his older brother, who continued as an anti-inoculationist) and how it could mitigate the consequences of a smallpox epidemic. In 1736, when Franklin's son died from naturally acquired smallpox (the infant had not been inoculated due to his age), Franklin immediately published a public letter in the *Gazette* to dispel rumors that the child succumbed to an inoculation gone awry. A decade later, Franklin made certain that his daughter was preventively inoculated as early in her life as possible. When Franklin was sent to London in 1757 as an official representative of the Pennsylvania Assembly, he campaigned vigorously for inoculations in Europe, particularly for the poor, and even wrote the preface for a physician friend's widely distributed pro-inoculation pamphlet. He then dispatched fifteen hundred copies of the leaflet to American doctors and leading public officials.

But there were other, personal reasons for Franklin's commitment. As a young man, he had met Boylston while living in London and working as a compositor in a printer's shop. Franklin had been, in his words, "reduced to the greatest distress, a youth without money, friends, or counsel." He turned to Boylston, the most lauded of American celebrities in the city, who acted as a surrogate parent. Boylston provided monetary support and fatherly advice. "I was saved from the abyss of destruction,"[18] Franklin told a grandnephew. Later on, Franklin, who admired and believed in Boylston's use of medical statistics, sent the numbers to friends and family members, expecting them to spread the word. He rarely revealed to these individuals the personal gratitude he owed Boylston.

Franklin's unparalleled renown bolstered support for inoculation in a way that no doctor, even one as famous as Boylston, could. His enthusiasm had wide-ranging consequences, from the construction in 1762 in Philadelphia of a specialized inoculation hospital to the increased willingness of wealthy individuals, especially politicians, to undergo the treatment. Franklin's influence in this arena among the intellectual elite and politically powerful altered the course of history in America more than once.

George Washington, the most prominent founding father and general of the Continental Army, heeded Franklin's counsel on inoculation and by doing so changed the outcome of the Revolutionary War. Washington's pockmarked face betrayed a teenage familiarity with smallpox. He understood that the most important deterrent to vulnerability to the disease was prior exposure. In March 1776, rumors abounded that British troops in Boston were attempting to spread smallpox by placing blankets previously used by infected soldiers in various neighborhoods. Fearing the disease would decimate his mostly unexposed troops—upward of one hundred soldiers per week were already dying of smallpox—Washington decided not to mount an attack against the Redcoats. The next winter, Washington, in the face of public skepticism and a stalled war effort, yielded to the wishes of Franklin and others and had mass inoculations performed on veteran troops in Morristown and Philadelphia and new recruits from New England, the middle Atlantic colonies, and Virginia. Inoculation was carried out at Valley Forge a year later. As the grand experiment progressed, it became obvious that Washington was correct in opting for prevention over serendipity. The decision to have the Continental Army inoculated against smallpox was one of the greatest strategic and medical decisions ever conceived by a wartime general. It changed the outcome of the conflict and secured the beginnings of a new country by improving the health of the soldiers.

Less dramatic but equally important was Franklin's insistence that delegates to the Continental Congress get inoculated. When the First Continental Congress met in Philadelphia in fall 1774, the arriving politicians convinced local physicians to halt inoculations because several of the delegates had never been exposed to smallpox. They argued that this pause in inoculations reduced the risk of infection of vulnerable delegates, but Franklin understood the folly of the decision. When the Second Continental Congress began its deliberations in May 1775, Franklin strongly advised susceptible individuals to submit to prophylactic inoculation in view of the pox-plagued environment. Several members, including Josiah Bartlett of New Hampshire and Virginia's Patrick Henry, acted on his recommendation. How many other at-risk delegates paid attention to Franklin's counsel is unknown. At least one individual, Samuel Ward of Rhode Island (his great-granddaughter was Julia Ward Howe, composer of the "Battle Hymn of the Republic"), ignored Franklin's admonitions and succumbed to smallpox when the assembly was in session.

Medicine, Just Another Colonial Trade

In the colonial period, medical care was not a prized commodity, which is why the increasingly successful use of inoculation stands out as such a triumph. With no expectation to reliably help the sick, medicine ranked below the law and the ministry in both its social standing and the intellectual qualities required of its practitioners. There was little of true therapeutic value to offer. No health care provider could conceive of diseases and treatments in anything resembling modern scientific terms. The dominance of ancient remedies and rituals, empiricism, and speculative systems of medical thought meant that filth, sickness, and medical dilettantes ruled the colonialists' day. "Few physicians amongst us are eminent for their skill," wrote one contemporary observer. "Quacks abound like locusts in Egypt, and too many have recommended themselves to a full practice and profitable subsistence."[19]

Few doctors had any level of formal medical education and training. They attended no lectures, performed no laboratory experiments, and never dissected a cadaver. They titled themselves "doctor" not because they had received a diploma, but for the simple reason that they were doing what men with university medical degrees usually did: they took care of patients.

Medicine was more of a trade, a means to secure the scraps of a livelihood. Most colonial physicians were poorly paid and supplemented their income by farming, managing a small business, or owning an apothecary shop, like Boylston, who did all three. There were no licensing authorities, no qualifying examinations, no medical schools, no professional societies, no hospitals, and no medical literature. Health care workers plied their trade without regulations and there was little societal interest in the acquisition or dissemination of medical knowledge.

Medical practice merely followed the teachings from prior centuries with few new clinical discoveries, and most "discoveries" were based on pure speculation. "Bleeding, vomiting, blistering, purging, anodyne, &c" was what one American physician described as acceptable everyday care. "If the illness continued, there was *repetendi* and finally *murderandi*."[20] The most educated and sensible of medical practitioners provided comforting words, but without scientific backing this cant had no effect on diseases and their often fatal outcomes. Physicians could claim little in the way of useful therapeutic actions beyond quarantine schemes during epidemics (and now inoculation). In the middle of a scourge, doctors advised healthy individuals to plug their nostrils with tobacco leaves, light street fires to burn away bad air, hang camphor from their necks, fire their muskets to fill the sky with supposedly healthy gunpowder smoke, or, as a last resort, flee the city. "It is better to let nature under a proper regimen take her course (*naturae morborum curatrices*)," quipped one critic, "than to trust to the honesty and sagacity of the practitioner."[21]

The apprenticeship system was the principal method of medical education and training available in the colonies (Boylston, for example, served as an apprentice to both his physician father and other eminent Boston-based physicians). It emphasized clinical common sense and practical medical, along with surgical, experience, but since individual preceptors established their own standards of schooling, the quality and quantity of apprenticeship instruction varied greatly, and even in the best circumstances the information conveyed was more superstition than science. It was not uncommon for a doctor to treat his apprentice like an indentured servant rather than as a trainee in the art of healing. The teenager was just as likely to look after the physician's horse and saddlebags or serve the evening's meal as he was to prepare medicines, bleed and blister patients, and read the doctor's medical books. The end product of the apprentice system, the generalist doctor—distinctions between physicians and surgeons did not exist—would dominate the American medical scene until specialists arose in the final years of the nineteenth century.

In the mid-eighteenth century medical education first began to expand beyond the apprenticeship system with the advent of private anatomy courses, an early step in the process of professionalization. Although these endeavors were nothing more than nondescript lectures and anatomical demonstrations to groups of eager students, they represented the earliest attempts to provide some manner of formal medical education. Doctors-to-be paid a fee, and they received a signed document at the course's conclusion attesting to their faithful attendance. Instructors soon supplemented these anatomical courses with lecture series in chemistry, which, in turn, led to the organization of the earliest medical schools.

It was also during these years that sons of wealthy colonial families first began to pursue medical education abroad, particularly in the schools of Edinburgh and London. Once resettled in their colonial home cities, they were regarded as physicians in the European sense—that is, as practitioners of privilege with a snobbish university degree. Though poorly trained doctors and various quacks continued to flourish in North America, their presence was increasingly challenged by a vocal cadre of these American-born but British-educated young men. As the better-educated doctors thrived and grew politically stronger, medicine came to rely on their English medical traditions, especially when it concerned a physician's education, training, and practice routines.

Medical organizations, another important symbol of the colonial doctor's emerging professional awareness, first came into existence around this time as well. In 1755, for example, physicians in Charleston, South Carolina, announced in the city's newspaper that they were banding together to protect their financial interests. "We are often called out under the greatest inclemencies of the weather, sometimes merely to gratify the Patient," they complained, "and are often slowly and seldom sufficiently paid."[22] To settle the issue, the physicians announced that they would go on strike unless a reasonable fee was paid at every consultation.

Medical care and medical education in the late colonial period grew and developed alongside broader cultural and economic progress. The population had enlarged noticeably due to a self-sustaining increase in the number of original settlers and their families plus a surge in immigration—estimates for the year 1760 place 1,695,000 individuals in the colonies (approximately 310,000 were African Americans). Outside the urban areas, however, communication remained slow. One stagecoach every few days was the sole connection between the few cities; otherwise contact depended on private conveyance, usually canoe, flatboat, or horseback.

Colonial towns grew in size as a newfound prosperity transformed the continent. A moneyed class emerged with well-fed and well-housed families demanding more of the social and educational amenities of life. Artisan and mechanic classes arose with demands for political power, separate from the claims of the wealthy. By the mid-eighteenth century eight of the colonies had their own private colleges and a public library movement was under way. Weekly newspapers and monthly magazines were available in most major cities. Music was cultivated and larger towns supported their own orchestras.

"I have seen him"

Philadelphia was the second-largest city (behind London) in the British Empire, with twenty-five thousand inhabitants. The town served as the North American colonies' cultural center, home to both the celebrated, science-oriented American Philosophical Society and the influential, literary-minded *American Magazine and Monthly Chronicle*. Of Philadelphia's many learned citizens, few were like John Morgan the physician. A biographer labeled him as "deservedly styled the founder of American medicine,"[23] but he was more than that: Morgan was medicine's main attraction. He was handsome and by all accounts a dandy who wore the latest in colonial haute couture and scandalously twirled a silk parasol. People rushed to the windows when he passed and closely followed him on the streets. It was deemed a privilege to be able to say, "I have seen him."[24]

Born to wealth, Morgan received a bachelor of arts from the College of Philadelphia (now the University of Pennsylvania) in 1757. He concurrently completed a medical apprenticeship, which included a twelve-month term as apothecary to the Pennsylvania Hospital. Four years of service as a physician/surgeon in the Pennsylvania Provisional forces during the French and Indian Wars rounded out his medical training in America. By this time, Morgan's élan was difficult to miss. "So great was his diligence and humanity in attending the sick and wounded," wrote one acquaintance, "that if it were possible for any man to merit heaven by his good works, Dr. Morgan would deserve it for his faithful attendance upon his patients."[25]

Morgan moved to Europe following his stint in the army and studied with some of the most illustrious physicians of the era. He received a medical diploma from the University of Edinburgh, considered the most prestigious British medical school. During this time Morgan also befriended Benjamin Franklin, who opened the doors to the leading homes in London and Paris, such that Morgan became European chic. "I interest myself in what relates to him [Morgan], I cannot but wish him the advantage of your conversation and instructions," Franklin wrote to one European intellectual. "I wish it also for the sake of my country, where he is to reside, and where I am persuaded he will be not a little useful."[26] Morgan's graduation from Edinburgh in 1763 was said to spark the celebration of "an éclat almost unknown before."[27] He spent another two years traipsing through France, Holland, and Italy where he interviewed physicians, inspected hospitals, and met with the leading men of letters. In his time abroad he had become a licentiate of the Royal Colleges of Physicians at Edinburgh and London, fellow of the Royal Society of London, member of the Arcadian Belles Lettres Society at Rome, and correspondent of the

Royal Academy of Surgery at Paris. He had also gained a sinister side that was aloof, arrogant, and conniving—James Boswell, the famous biographer, had traveled with Morgan in Holland and called him "a conceited fool."[28]

Morgan returned to Philadelphia in the spring of 1765. In terms of learning and experience he was now the best medical man in the colonies, and hoped to use his knowledge to transform the country's system of medical education and clinical traditions. Morgan felt that both the apprenticeship system and the supplemental lecture series in anatomy and chemistry had definite sociocultural limitations despite their success in producing clinical practitioners. They failed to provide professional status, which in Europe belonged only to men with university medical degrees. A diploma from a university-affiliated school of medicine was more than just a credential of know-how; it was a warrant of academic authority, something the apprenticeship system's certificate of proficiency did not provide. A university education also inculcated the demeanor and manners expected of a physician if he was to receive the respect due him as a professional person.

Having canvassed Europe's leading university-educated and -trained doctors, he intended to introduce old-world educational and practice standards into a new-world setting. Formal university education along with legally respected medical diplomas would be necessary to transform American medicine into a learned profession. Morgan's enthusiasm was typical of top-tier colonial medical students who had studied in Edinburgh (sixty-three Americans received medical diplomas from that city's university between 1758 and 1788). These British-educated elite physicians understood that their long-term socioeconomic interests benefited from a well-regulated and organized profession. Morgan led the crusade and aimed to lead by example. "I am now preparing for America to see whether, after fourteen years' devotion to medicine, I can get my living without turning apothecary or practicing surgery," he wrote to a British mentor.[29]

Morgan had set forth his proposal for an American academic medical school in a short manuscript that he intended to publish once back in Philadelphia, and his plans were strengthened with a letter of support from Thomas Penn, the sole proprietor of the Pennsylvania colony by royal fiat. Morgan asked Penn to persuade the trustees of the College of Philadelphia to appoint professors for the study of medicine and surgery, thus establishing the colonies' first school of medicine. "Gentlemen," wrote Penn, "his [Morgan's] scheme will give reputation and strength to the institution, and though it may for some time occasion a small expense, yet after a little while it will gradually support itself, and even make considerable additions to the Academy funds."[30] The trustees received the missive in early May 1765, and less than four weeks later, Morgan was standing on the rostrum, dressed in professorial robes (the trustees chose him to be professor of the theory and practice of medicine), as he delivered the public commencement address for the College of Philadelphia.

Discourse Upon the Institution of Medical Schools in America

Morgan had a great deal to declare and took two days to deliver it. His appeal was electrifying to those in attendance. "The perspicuity with which it was written and spoken drew the close attention of the audience, and particularly of the gentlemen of the Faculty of Physic," wrote Franklin in his *Pennsylvania Gazette*.[31] Morgan's *Discourse Upon the Institution of Medical Schools in America* was forceful, logical, and prescient. He took on the apprenticeship system by attacking the majority of American physicians as incapable of acquiring up-to-date medical information. These men "remain in a pitiful state of ignorance without any prospect or opportunity of correcting their errors, or greatly improving their knowledge," proclaimed Morgan.[32] He accused doctors of creating medical havoc and "laying whole families desolate."[33] Condemning apprenticeship as an unsound educational system, Morgan noted that nothing less than a medical school's direct relationship with a university could provide academic prestige, legal authority, and administrative stability. "He had torn American medicine to pieces and offered to rebuild it in a new pattern," wrote James Flexner, a well-known medical historian.[34]

To the surprise of his audience, Morgan insisted that Philadelphia's new medical school should only accept students who first pursued premedical studies as part of an undergraduate degree. Complaining that anyone could proclaim himself a doctor after hanging around a physician's office, Morgan demanded that, in addition to an apprenticeship, admitted students be proficient in Greek, Latin, French, mathematics, and natural philosophy. "Destitute of that general knowledge," he contended, "we cannot penetrate into those truths, that form the rules by which we ought to conduct ourselves, in the cure of diseases."[35] Once matriculated, the doctor-to-be was to study anatomy, botany, chemistry, clinical medicine, materia medica (drugs and other remedial substances), physiology, and pathology.

While Morgan drew many ideas on medical education from European models, he broke from the Continental archetype, especially as concerned hospitals. Morgan based the concepts in his *Discourse* on a style of medical education where the school was affiliated with a university; the more common European and English approach organized medical schools alongside hospital wards as an extension of academic bedside teaching. Morgan could have allied his Philadelphia school with the Pennsylvania Hospital, a thriving health care facility and America's first permanent hospital for the care of needy sick, but he decided against it. This was surprising since Franklin, one of Morgan's main counselors, cofounded the hospital.

Many colonialists in Morgan's day probably knew about hospitals, but only a small minority had intimate knowledge of one. America's hospitals were few in number, poorly managed, and unable to provide administrative support to an affiliated medical school. Aside from almshouses, inoculation buildings, and pest houses, only two general institutions, the Pennsylvania Hospital and the Charity Hospital in New Orleans, were functioning at the end of the Revolution. They were facilities of last resort, ignominious places to receive medical care. These institutions were no more than shelters for those who could not afford treatment at home, had no family to provide nursing needs, or lived in such adverse conditions that there was no space in their house for the sick or dying.

Although Morgan shunned the Pennsylvania Hospital as a formal partner in medical education, he suggested that students spend time there and observe patients. "Nothing can contribute more than a course of clinical practice and clinical lectures by physicians of knowledge and experience," advised Morgan.[36] He was recommending something Franklin had established as hospital policy during its fund-raising campaign of 1751:

one of the stated functions for the new institution was the provision of training facilities for medical students. Physicians who staffed the hospital grew accustomed to taking their young apprentices on the wards. This became so fashionable that even doctors in training, whose mentors were not on staff at the Pennsylvania Hospital, requested similar opportunities. In mid-1763 the administrators of the facility honored this appeal by charging such students "six pistoles [gold coins] as a gratuity for that privilege."[37]

Morgan's scheme of a university-affiliated medical school, augmented with hospital-based instruction, quickly became an accepted blueprint for the future development of American medical education. "It had been shown how," according to Henry Sigerist, one of the renowned medical historians of the mid-twentieth century, "without great ostentation or expense, and using existing equipment, it was possible to give medical instruction an academic form."[38] Medical teaching in this country developed over the next century and a quarter tied to educational institutions, whereas most European countries, including England, organized medical education around hospitals.

Morgan had developed a sophisticated model for schooling the colonies' doctors, an important step in the march toward medicine's becoming a profession. "The historian who shall hereafter relate the progress of medical science in America," cautioned Morgan's earliest biographer, "will be deficient in candor and justice, if he does not connect the name of Dr. Morgan with that auspicious era, in which medicine was first taught and studied as a science in this country."[39] Two years after the school opened, the first students graduated, and by 1774 thirty-four medical degrees had been conferred. Morgan's accomplishment prompted physicians in New York City to establish a medical school in affiliation with King's College (later Columbia University), patterned after the Philadelphia institution. Both of these schools soon discontinued the M.B. and only awarded the M.D., a degree which, thereafter, became customary for American medical students. At the least, the Philadelphia and New York City schools offered a reasonable alternative to traveling to Europe for a medical education.

Specialization, a New Style of Practice

Morgan's dialogue did not stop with medical education. He dared to recommend specialization at a time when every American doctor was a combination physician, surgeon, and apothecary. Morgan, an elitist in both his personal and professional life, prized the social exclusivity then implicit in the concept of a university-educated physician. His new-style colonial physician was not expected to work with his hands, and certainly not to wield a surgeon's knife or to use a mortar and pestle to compound drugs. Morgan analogized physicians to the army general who "should be acquainted with every part of military science . . . but there is no need that he should act as a pioneer and dig in a trench."[40]

Morgan also demanded that doctors' fees be increased. "Were they [physicians] born slaves to the public," asked Morgan, "or, for such a voluntary surrender of their liberty and ease as is necessary to practice conscientiously, are they to have no compensation?"[41] Higher standards in education should lead to higher fees for advice. Morgan may have been explicitly asking for the guarantee of higher income, but he was implicitly also pressing for doctors to assume control of the practice of medicine. The increase of socioeconomic worth and the development of a nascent professional identity go hand in hand.

Morgan wanted to take physicians, who were often divided over clinical questions and financially insecure, and create a united and prosperous profession. Relying on Philadelphia's role as the colonies' social and economic magnet, Morgan hoped to found an august "College of Physicians," based on the British brand, which would administer examinations and license doctors on an intercolonial basis. "Societies form a kind of magazine [warehouse], which collects together all the knowledge of the learned, and consecrates it to public utility," according to Morgan.[42] His mantra was that his society would assist physicians to govern themselves, thus promoting professional unity and socioeconomic strength.

Morgan understood that for professionalization to occur, cultural authority needed to be established and a series of complex economic, political, and sociological transformations required within American medicine and society. For professionals to enjoy special power and prestige, substantial numbers of individuals had to be united in seeking technical competence, standardized education and training, job autonomy, monopoly over practice, and a philosophy of public service. Social and economic stature would follow once these conditions were fulfilled.

Such changes did not come easily. The passage from a preindustrial, largely rural, and tradition-based society to one in which American physicians regarded themselves as a distinct class of upwardly mobile professionals would not be completed until the turn of the twentieth century. But Morgan's preparatory steps signaled the beginnings of the struggle for professional identity and medical distinctiveness.

Unlike his medical school initiative, Morgan's scheme for a centralized medical licensing authority shortly met with opposition. The College of Philadelphia's administrators feared that if a certifying body were created, even a dignified College of Physicians, it would interfere with the functions of their new medical institute. Penn, the colony's proprietor and a Morgan devotee, agreed and refused entreaties to grant a charter. "I think it very early for such an establishment"[43] were his final words on the subject.

Morgan failed in this aspect of his plan to professionalize American medicine, but nascent licensing efforts had already begun in other colonies. In 1760, New York City officials enacted a law stipulating that no one should practice medicine or surgery unless he had taken an examination for licensure. Nine years later Samuel Bard, a well-known physician in the city, reemphasized the need for licensure when he spoke on the expected professional conduct of a physician at the first commencement ceremonies of the King's College medical department. Bard's *Discourse Upon the Duties of a Physician*, published several days later, became the earliest American writing on medical ethics.

Across the Hudson River a group of physicians in 1766 formed a New Jersey medical society, the only state or county medical association that would survive the American Revolution. These physicians requested that the provincial government establish a licensing system and set fines for those who disobeyed the law. And, in a nod to patients' rights, it was mandated that bills be written "in plain English Words."[44] The membership, concerned with raising practice standards as well as income levels, also insisted on publishing a uniform fee table (a simple visit by a doctor cost ten shillings, a nighttime consult necessitated an additional five shillings, removal of a cataract ran three pounds).

But neither the New York nor New Jersey statutes gained much traction initially. The growing political crisis with England diverted attention from them, and they were never vigorously enforced. Most colonials resisted the idea of medical licensure because of the peril it posed to their customary independence in choosing from among a wide variety of health care practitioners. Some resented licensure attempts for imposing European-style class distinctions underscored by educational superiority. Others took exception to the caustic manner in which physicians discredited their peers as charlatans. "No body of men are less in concert, or seem less influenced by the *esprit de corps*, than physicians," remarked one observer. "The quarrels of physicians are proverbially frequent and bitter, and their hatred, in intensity and duration, seems to exceed that of other men."[45]

The public stood in the way not only of Morgan's and others' advocacy of licensing, but also their pleas for the most basic of all health studies, human dissection. Understanding the workings of the human body was central to medicine's future growth, particularly the evolving discipline of pathologic anatomy, which was already well accepted in Europe. But such investigatory work hardly existed in colonial America. Public hostility toward anatomic studies exploded during the 1788 "Doctors' Mob" riot in New York City, when a group of vigilantes tried to lynch doctors teaching human dissection. The rioters refused to disperse despite the pleas of several luminaries, including Alexander Hamilton, John Jay, and Baron von Steuben, the Prussian army officer who served as inspector general of the Continental Army during the Revolutionary War. Militiamen were summoned and the confrontation ended with shots fired and eight demonstrators dead. For three days, in a frenzy of retribution, bands of vigilantes terrorized the medical profession, threatening, according to one account, "a general Hegira of physicians."[46] Medical students were secretly stowed in carriages and evacuated to the countryside as doctors hid wherever possible.

Morgan's Fall

Following two days of oratory, Morgan made a stunning closing announcement to the assembled Philadelphia throng. Not only had he recommended the separation of surgery and pharmacy from medicine, but he was going to practice what he preached. He told the startled crowd (among those present was the colony's governor) that he had imported a fully trained surgeon/apothecary from England, the first ever seen in America. Henceforth, Morgan would refuse all surgical cases and the dispensing of medicines. He insisted that any of his future patients in need of surgical care or pharmaceuticals would have to avail themselves of his colleague. "What I expect from them [patients] is a proper compensation for my advice and attendance as a physician," contended Morgan.[47] He claimed that when a patient received a bill for treatment, the individual did not know what portion of the cost was for drugs versus medical expertise. This demeaned a physician's services and was unworthy of someone who deserved to be compensated as a university-educated scholar, not as a mere maker of pills and potions. And as an expensively schooled physician, Morgan expected to be paid more than other practitioners of his day.

Unfortunately for Morgan, when he stepped off the rostrum his medical career had just reached its zenith. Morgan would sit in his office at Second and Spruce Streets waiting in vain for patients to appear. He was probably the only physician in Philadelphia, if not all thirteen colonies, who refused surgical cases and did not dispense drugs. With the sick slow to appear at his doorway, Morgan was eventually forced to become what he most detested, a colonial physician who had no economic choice but to push pills. What happened to his partner, the English surgeon/apothecary, remains a historical question mark.

Morgan's enduring political contacts soon led him in other directions. With the onset of the Revolution, Congress appointed him director general of hospitals and physician in chief for the Revolutionary army. The Continental Army early on was an amateurish outfit, and the medical organization was even more slapdash. The ever-effete Morgan was intolerant of the situation and went about curtly changing things. From asking physicians to take a competency examination to scolding soldiers he believed to be malingering, Morgan worried little about tact or the enemies he might be making.

Stories soon spread of Morgan's inhumanity and how he ruled by absolute fiat. Physicians told of worsening conditions in military hospitals, so horrendous that to send sick soldiers to them was tantamount to murder. These were the same apprentice-trained, mostly country practitioners who, just a few years ago, Morgan publicly criticized as representing the underbelly of American medicine. The political infighting against Morgan grew and brought about his downfall just fourteen months into his appointment. Back in Philadelphia, a resentful Morgan fussed and fumed and wrote a scurrilous pamphlet in his own defense. He was later vindicated, but few cared.

Morgan's final years were spent largely in solitude. In 1787 he became peripherally involved in establishing the College of Physicians of Philadelphia, but despite his prior recommendation, the institution's charter did not include a provision for licensing as he had hoped. His earlier optimism that such an organization would spur America's doctors to perform sophisticated scientific investigations, thus leading to justifiable claims of professional superiority and widening the sociocultural gap between them and quacks, soon faded. The College of Physicians did contain one of the country's first medical libraries, but the building was more of a social gathering place for Philadelphia's physician elite than a scientific research institute. Morgan's last days were spent in a small hovel, on a filthy bed, forgotten by most Philadelphians. His funeral was attended by several leftover friends. There were few tributes and no tombstone ever marked Morgan's final resting place.

American medicine had passed Morgan by in the end, but many of its developments had resulted directly from his zeal. A cadre of elite physicians had arrived and would provide the basis for future professional growth. More important, the new, albeit few, quasi-university-affiliated medical schools would serve as the foundation for many of these changes. Clearly, Morgan was farsighted, especially in the realm of medical education—a more comprehensive scheme for its reform would only be offered in the 1890s with the opening of The Johns Hopkins Hospital and its affiliated School of Medicine in Baltimore. Unfortunately, he was also a vainglorious and stubborn man who was at his worst when it came to managing sensitive issues.

In hindsight, Morgan's efforts to professionalize medicine were premature and ill served by his abrasive demeanor and absolutism. Despite his endeavors, colonial doctors continued to practice a combination of medicine, surgery, pharmacy, and midwifery without undergoing a licensing examination. Physicians needed one voice to advance their status and improve medical care, but for self-educated and self-determined men, left on their farms and in small-town habitats, this remained impossible to achieve even though Morgan had already articulated many of the vital ideas.

The main eulogy during Morgan's memorial service at the College of Philadelphia was delivered by Benjamin Rush, a rising star on the city's medical scene and a Morgan protégé. He movingly told of his mentor's "uncommon capacity for acquiring knowledge" and how Morgan "advanced in every part of Europe the honour of the American name."[48] Rush had learned much from Morgan, but the most important trait he acquired was the ability to stand out from among his peers. Highly regarded for the intensity of his clinical convictions as well as a domineering style of interpersonal relationships, Rush (and his Morganesque personality) would shortly fashion the earliest well-recognized American style of medical practice.

❧ Two ❧

DEMOCRATIZATION OF HEALING

America's Hippocrates

S ERVANTS POKED AND stirred a fire, they prepared a warm footbath, and placed brandy and wine whey on a table. Their ailing master complained of feeling cold, then of fever and chills, and later of arm and chest pains. His breathing was labored, his pulse was weak, and he hardly ate. The sixty-eight-year-old man asked to be placed close to the fire, then he wanted to be moved to a warm bed; there he tossed and turned all night. Anxiously, he awaited the sunrise when medical help would arrive. It all seemed so ordinary, but it was 1813 and this was Benjamin Rush, the nation's greatest physician, and he was not about to have an ordinary death.

In the morning, as sunlight filtered into the room, Rush extended his forearm and allowed the visiting doctor to inspect his veins. The physician was there to perform a bloodletting, the era's most common medical therapy, the very treatment that Rush had popularized so brilliantly. With a few swift cuts along Rush's arm, the doctor opened the veins like spigots and collected ten ounces of blood. Rush grew faint and fell asleep. Several hours later a barely arousable Rush insisted that the treatment was working and asked to be bled again. The doctor demurred. "I objected on account of the weak state of his pulse," he wrote in his medical notes.

Rush cautioned everyone in the room that unless the therapy continued, "the disease will take hold of my lungs, and I shall go off in a consumption [tuberculosis]." A second physician was consulted and agreed

31

that further bleeding was risky. Rush, however, was so adamant in his demands that the doctors acquiesced. They removed three more ounces of blood. The patient insisted that he felt fine, then fainted again.

This time the doctors believed that Rush had entered, in their words, a "refreshing sleep."[1] In fact, with exiguous knowledge of human physiology or even the freshman basics of fluid therapy, Rush's physicians had put their already weakened patient into irreversible circulatory shock. A comatose Rush, minus approximately 10 percent of his blood supply, soon died. The irony was that Rush hastened his own death by unwavering commitment to the doctrine he was convinced would heal him.

Several decades before he died, Rush had stated the defining clinical principle of his era—the post-Revolutionary era—in one sentence: "There is but one exciting cause of fever [illness] and that is *stimulus,* and that consists in a morbid excitement and irregular action of the blood vessels."[2] He argued that congested arteries and veins and swollen tissues were the mainstays of sickness. To treat these troubles, he and tens of thousands of his acolytes promoted the elimination of blood and other bodily fluids as the sole means to decrease congestion and return a patient to health. Rush pushed his idea—labeled "heroic therapy" for the potency of its action— to the extreme, and bloodletting and forced intestinal evacuation rapidly spread throughout the nation.

This "bleed, blister, puke, and purge" gambit had a several-millennia-long history of therapeutic use, but Rush's reconsideration and reexplanation of the clinical issues represented advanced thinking for the times. Whether cardiac failure, cirrhosis, colitis, epilepsy, leukemia, osteoporosis, rheumatism, or sickle cell anemia (in this medically unsophisticated age, doctors were unable to distinguish between such "internal" diseases), the presence of an ailment was reason enough to remove the body's vital humors, especially its blood.

The use of heroic therapies (also termed "depletion treatments") quickly encompassed all aspects of medical care. Even when an "external" or surgical disease was present, some form of bloodletting or fluid depleting served as a therapeutic adjunct. Physicians in this era, who knew nothing of infection or anesthesia and little of surgical anatomy, invoked heroic therapies as a precursor to performing amputations, setting simple dislocations and fractures, draining superficial abscesses, and removing the occasional bladder stone. Stories abound of bleeding sessions preceding hernia surgery. "I directed leeches to be applied to the tumor [hernia]," stated one physician. "The leech-bites bled freely, and the hernial protrusion retired within the abdomen."[3] Heroic therapy enthusiasts bled and depleted children with as much fervor as adults. "As a general rule we need not be afraid of vomiting the youngest child," wrote one advocate of pediatric heroic therapy. "The mere act of vomiting is attended with no great danger, while the remedial agency of an emetic is one of great power and value."[4]

The rapid ascent of heroic therapy and its conquest of all aspects of clinical care in American medicine was due almost entirely to Benjamin Rush, slight-framed, dome-foreheaded, hook-nosed, censorious. "He was a physician of no common cast," wrote an obsequious biographer, "for he was minutely acquainted with the histories of disease of all ages, countries and occupations."[5] Abolitionist, advocate for the mentally ill, anti–death penalty activist, environmentalist, founder of the Philadelphia Bible Society, prison reformer, protector of Tories, and treasurer of the United States Mint—Rush was a visionary. He was also more than capable of being wrongheaded and equally strongheaded, something his critics enjoyed pointing out. Detractors furthermore demeaned Rush's much ballyhooed social fervor as nothing more than a self-serving ploy to increase the size and financial recompense of his medical practice. "Rush is remarkable for insinuating manners," declared a critic, "and for that smoothness and softness of tongue, which the mock-quality call *politeness,* but which the profane vulgar call *blarny.*"[6] Still, to the vast majority of his contemporaries, Rush was a powerful person, a medical saint, America's Hippocrates.

This future friend of presidents and foe of kings received his undergraduate degree in 1760, at the age of fifteen, from the College of New Jersey (now Princeton University). He spent the next six years as an apprentice to Philadelphia's eminent physician, John Redman. Rush decided to complete his medical schooling in Edinburgh at the urging of both his supervisor and John Morgan, the city's newest medical luminary. He returned three years later not only as a university-educated physician, but imbued with a radicalized political and social conscience. "Three great political subjects, for the time being, engrossed his whole soul," related an acquaintance, "the independence of his country; the establish-ment of good constitutions for the United States, and for his own particu-lar state; [and] to enlighten the public mind and to diffuse correct ideas."[7] Appointed a member of the Continental Congress from Pennsylvania, Rush was among the fifty-six signers (there were four other physician sig-natories) of the Declaration of Independence.

Rush, Morgan's most dazzling charge, was soon named the College of Philadelphia's professor of chemistry. He became the youngest mem-ber of the medical faculty at the age of twenty-three. A steady stream of publications punctuated Rush's first years of practice and teaching. "His medical works are so original, and so well adapted to our local situation," remarked an admirer, "that they should be carefully perused by every medical student."[8]

With the start of the Revolutionary War, Rush was appointed a physician-general in the Continental Army, but his time in the military and any future political aspirations ended in shambles. During the harsh winter of 1777–78 at Valley Forge, he participated in an ill-fated conspir-acy to bring about George Washington's dismissal as commander in chief. Rush's involvement in a separate plot to instigate the resignation of the Continental Army's physician in chief further undermined his standing. Rush had unjustly accused the physician in chief of financial irregularities regarding the procurement of wartime medical supplies. Rush secretly coveted the position and hoped to bring about his own style of military medical reform. "Patience! Patience! Patience!" cautioned Rush's friend John Adams. "The first, the last, and the middle virtues of a politician."[9] The impetuous Rush paid little heed to Adams's advice. Allegations were aired and as one of Rush's contemporaries bluntly noted, he had the "strongest marks of an unprincipled man" and was "capable of LYING in the WORST SENSE of that opprobrious WORD."[10]

Following these repeated military follies, a disgraced Rush resigned from the army and reluctantly resumed his medical life in Philadelphia. "Medicine is my wife; science is my mistress; books are my companions," he told a younger colleague. "My study is my grave. There I lie buried, the world 'forgetting, by the world forgot.' "[11] But he was not to be forgotten. Instead, Rush was forgiven and soon named physician to the Pennsylva-nia Hospital, closely followed by his widely publicized appointment as professor of medicine at the University of Pennsylvania. Rush's celebrity attracted droves of students, who traveled at length to listen to his lectures and learn his clinical methods. He became an effective teacher and proved a mesmerizing speaker, who used his lectern as a bully pulpit. Moreover, an inflexible resolve concerning his clinical convictions, combined with the volume and vigor of his writings, shortly made Rush the most revered of American physicians. "To many obligations I am already under to Dr. Rush," wrote a fawning former student, "I shall take the liberty of adding one more, 'Of making use of his name on all occasions.' It shall be my *Abracadabra* in all difficulties."[12]

Rush decided to risk his revitalized reputation to change the way the country's physicians practiced medicine. "His prescriptions were not confined to doses of medicine," wrote a coworker, "but to the regulation of the diet, air, dress, exercise and mental actions of his patient."[13] Empowered by a growing adulation, the always self-confident Rush dominated his charges as few physicians could. In turn, with a medical degree in hand, these students "extended the blessings of his instructions and improvement in the theory and practice of medicine, over the United States, and in a few instances to South America, the West Indies, and the eastern continent [Europe]."[14] Doctors and laymen idolized him and constantly sought his advice concerning his "American system of medicine."[15] The answer was always a simple, declarative demand: bleed, blister, puke, and purge each and every patient.

Rush's authority over American medicine was all the more pervasive because, during this era, the University of Pennsylvania's medical department graduated a larger number of men than all the other schools in the country combined. He lectured to more than 2,250 doctors-to-be during the course of his professorial career.

As a result of Rush's influence, American clinical customs separated from European ways. "The same hand which subscribed the declaration of the political independence of these states," claimed a contemporary observer of Rush's skills, "accomplished their emancipation from medical systems formed in foreign countries, and wholly unsuitable to the state of diseases in America."[16]

Unfortunately, Rush's system of therapeutics was as speculative and empirical as all the rest of that era's medical thinking. Doctors lacked useful scientific knowledge. The concept of bacteria and viruses as the causes of infection did not exist. There was neither medical instrumentation nor investigative tests. The art of diagnosing diseases was limited to observing a patient's symptoms. The absence of accumulated and accurate medical wisdom was one reason why physicians mistakenly grouped different illnesses together simply due to the similarity of their presenting signs. Skin irritations were regarded as one type of disease category (a rash from lupus received the same treatment as a meningitis-induced epidermal eruption), fevers another, coughs an additional group, and so on. As a result of inaccurate diagnoses, physicians were unable to test the effects of therapies in a methodical and scientific manner. Instead, they were left with a hodgepodge of ineffective treatments.

Nevertheless, America's doctors wanted to believe in an American way of practicing medicine. They considered the Philadelphian's opinions authoritative and state of the art. Patients, too, sought physicians who maintained a self-confident manner about themselves and their therapies. A medical historian described the behavior this way: "A Svengali who could hypnotize himself, his patients, and above all his colleagues into believing he was right was certain to be regarded as a great scientist. Rush was such a man."[17] Although some of Rush's contemporaries found his fondness for the bleeder's lancet unconscionable, and they disagreed with other aspects of heroic therapy, none ever developed a more widely accepted scheme of clinical therapeutics. In truth, Rush was such a well-recognized patriot and social reformer, such an authoritative and enthusiastic person, such a productive author and motivating lecturer, his influence inevitably became far-reaching.

Bleed, Blister, Puke, and Purge

Rush, like generations of physicians before him, turned to ancient healers to lend credence to or justify misgivings about medical opinions. References to Aristotle, Asclepiades, Celsus, Galen, and Hippocrates fill the pages of his and other pre-nineteenth-century medical texts just as citations to current research appear in modern publications. Not until the development of scientifically based medical inquiry (a product of the industrial and scientific revolutions of the last half of the nineteenth century) would the study of history lose its role as medicine's sole source of therapeutic authority. By focusing on the body's fluids, Rush provided an eighteenth-century update to a Greco-Roman formula that related health and sickness to a supposed imbalance among four elemental, personality-altering humors: black bile (melancholy), blood (sanguine), phlegm (phlegmatic), and yellow bile (choleric). An abnormal change of one fluid over the other was thought to be the underlying cause of illness.

Physicians had long regarded blood as the most important humor, since it was the one fluid largely associated with life itself. The fact that blood could be lost without bringing about death—the prime examples being menstrual bleeding and hemorrhage from injuries—partially explains the Greek and Roman belief that diseases were due to an excess of blood and that bloodletting could reestablish health.

Rush encouraged this antediluvian practice through his lectures and writings, and came to be regarded as medicine's premier interventionist. He carried bleeding further than had ever been done before. "It is believed that no man understood the human pulse better than Dr. Rush,"[18] wrote one follower.

Citizens suffered needlessly as a result of Rush's egotism and lack of scientific methodologies. In an age when no one understood what it meant to measure blood pressure and body temperature, and physicians were first determining the importance of heart and breathing rates, America's doctors had no parameters to prevent them from harming patients. The paramount need to reduce bodily excitement determined the extent of treatment. Practitioners often ordered bleeding to continue until swooning or unconsciousness occurred. Regrettably, for some patients, fainting was more a psychological than a physiological response. Simply seeing a bleeder's lancet had the same effect as siphoning off cups, pints, or even quarts of blood. Rush refused to take such an obvious observational difference into account.

The astonishing thing from a modern medical viewpoint is not that bloodletting, also termed "phlebotomy" or "venesection," achieved wide appeal, but that an individual's life force could be withdrawn repeatedly in massive quantities over brief periods of time. Doctors bled some patients sixteen ounces a day up to fourteen days in succession (the average male human body contains one hundred seventy-five ounces of blood). Present-day blood donors, by comparison, are allowed to give one pint (sixteen ounces) per session, with a minimum of two months between each donation.

Nineteenth-century physicians bragged about the totality of their bleeding triumphs as if it were a career-defining statistic. "He verily believed he had drawn more than one hundred barrels of blood during his medical career," one physician wrote about another's claim, "and had yet to see the first instance in which he had drawn blood to the injury of the patient."[19]

The regard for bloodletting was so deep-seated that even the frequent complications and outright failures to cure did not negate the sway of Rush's work. Any clinical catastrophes only emphasized bleeding's limitations in a world full of imperfections. In the end, physicians rationalized bloodletting fiascos as a natural consequence of God's way to maintain order on the new continent.

When bloodletting alone failed to heal, Rush's scheme required further depletive therapy through gastrointestinal catharsis, specifically vomiting and laxation. The preparation of choice for cleansing the upper and lower gastrointestinal tracts was an ivory-colored, tasteless powder called calomel. Considered a wonder remedy and an all-around panacea for mankind's medical miseries, this drug degraded in the gut into highly poisonous and irritative components that brought about volcanic vomiting and explosive evacuation of the bowels. This odious medication of mercurous chloride was also distinguished by its latent side effects. Repeated doses of calomel caused mercury to accumulate in the body, resulting in toxic aftereffects, from extreme salivation to rotting teeth to gangrene of the facial tissues. Yet the ever-haughty Rush was so taken with calomel that he named it the Samson of drugs. His critics agreed with the nom de guerre, but not for its superior qualities; in the battle for health, they said, calomel "has slain its thousands."[20] A white-powdered mixture of antimony and potassium known as tartar emetic (modern toxicology classifies this compound as a lethal poison) supplemented calomel's checkered performance. In small doses this all-purpose depletive produced vomiting. In larger quantities tartar emetic reduced heart activity to critically low levels.

Blistering and cupping were the final ingredients in a physician's heroic therapy armamentarium after bleeding and drugging. Doctors used a mustard plaster or some other form of irritant to excoriate the skin and raise a blister. The outpouring of fluid from the punctured blister was considered a welcome exodus of harmful matter. To prolong the process physicians further inflamed blisters to create a painful ulceration that assured a longer-lasting flow. In cupping, blood was drawn to the body's surface by application of a small glass vessel that was heated to produce a vacuum. The skin was then incised to release blood and fluids. Blistering and cupping, like other aspects of heroic therapy, were thought to do little harm. Whether they helped was a matter of personal perception.

Armed with just a bleeding lancet, a few drugs, and various herbal and mineral concoctions, the country's ill-prepared and poorly educated doctors considered themselves competent to treat almost any condition. Heroic therapy offered genuine psychological relief to the young nation's physicians—the appellation "Rush's system" evoked a sense of American medical pride. It represented the latest and, to many minds, the greatest in late-eighteenth- and early-nineteenth-century medicine.

Rush's heroic therapy produced a long-lived impression upon American health care that, in times of illness, intensive medical intervention was almost always required. After all, anyone, from physicians to patients' families to outside observers, could see that draining off "exciting" fluids from a sick individual produced a calmer state, often culminating in a faint. And when a doctor further recommended rest and quiet augmented by rudimentary sedatives, no one could doubt the ability of physicians to control patients and their clinical situations. Rush and his disciples failed to recognize, or perhaps refused to acknowledge, that a decrease in consciousness represented nothing more than a normal physiologic response to the physical assault of bleeding, blistering, puking, and purging. In no way did these changes in a patient's condition provide a lasting cure.

Rush's point of view so blinded physicians that they readily believed that illnesses would certainly worsen and lead to death without heroic therapy. Rush's smug advice became even more disconcerting when he rejected reliance upon Mother Nature as part of the healing process. It no longer mattered that sick patients were often known to get well by themselves. Healing, in his estimation, could occur only through the heavy-handedness of physicians and their heroic therapies. To think otherwise was considered medical tomfoolery and a breach of professional conduct for a doctor.

The disordered state of American medicine also explained physicians' acceptance of heroic therapy. "The great mass of the profession," according to one contemporary observer, "were alike unsocial and ungoverned by ethical laws, and, consequently, without harmony of action or true dignity of professional character."[21] It was a time of medical anarchy, in which physicians pursued their own individualistic style of practice prescribing unregulated and untested doses of Rush's depletive therapies. If a doctor did not believe in heroic medicine, then he formulated his own clinical scheme while vilifying his competitors along with Rush.

Money and Medical Schools

The homegrown brand of medical apprenticeships that persisted throughout the country ensured the continuation of clinical chaos. Medical students learned the clinical style of their teacher and passed it on to the next generation of healers. While a semester at one of the country's fledgling medical schools sometimes supplemented this education, the apprenticeship system inexorably produced practitioners with little regard for clinical guidelines and professional standards. The system was also inefficient from a financial perspective since doctors could only collect fees one apprentice at a time.

As a reaction to these economic shortcomings in apprenticeships, a novel type of medical college began to dot the American landscape in the 1820s. Proprietary medical schools were independently organized, financially autonomous, profit-making facilities legally authorized to grant doctor of medicine degrees. Three major factors accounted for this rapid growth of schools: the vast size of the country, the entrepreneurial spirit of physicians, and the lack of legislative control over the practice of medicine.

They first appeared in the states and territories west of the Appalachians, with faculties composed of a half dozen or so local practitioners. The population was quickly moving beyond the frontier's edges, and future physicians found the journey to a northeastern educational center burdensome. The only medical schools in existence were located in

Philadelphia (University of Pennsylvania, 1765); New York City (King's College, now Columbia, 1767); Boston (Harvard, 1782); Hanover, New Hampshire (Dartmouth, 1797); and Baltimore (University of Maryland, 1807). The difficulty of travel intersected with physicians' steadfast conviction that diseases were geographically determined, such that weather and topography directly influenced health. These beliefs heightened the desire for schooling in the region where a matriculant wished to practice. "We are compelled to resort to what would be considered by northern practitioners," explained a Charleston-based student discussing sectional medical differences, "enormous doses of calomel, without which, we would be continually foiled in our attempts to cure the biliary disorders of the South."[22]

As the number of medical students in rural locales increased, doctors realized that it was inefficient to continue imparting knowledge on a time-consuming one-to-one or apprenticeship basis. Instead, healers united by renting a room or two for academic lectures, laboratory demonstrations, and the rare anatomical dissection. Since faculty salaries came directly from student fees, physicians, who generally did not have large incomes, were eager to organize new schools with expanding enrollments. These so-called proprietary medical schools were an appealing financial venture with low start-up costs and a high rate of return on investment. No equipment was required other than simple teaching aids, like skeletons and apparatuses for conducting basic chemistry experiments. There was no need for other costly paraphernalia since scientific research did not exist. With few legislative restraints on the educational system, an entrepreneurial spirit engulfed American medicine. Business pursuits pushed clinical concerns aside. The medical apprenticeship, despite its clinical experience, quickly became more a voluntary but necessary supplement to an academic program than the essence of medical education.

As cultural and economic forces encouraged proprietary medical school development, new but poorly managed medical schools inevitably began to form, particularly on the western and southern frontiers. "The [proprietary school] movement was as irresistible as an avalanche," wrote the medical historian Henry Sigerist. "Medical schools shot up like mushrooms after a night of rain."[23] The mania for college-making became so robust that between 1810 and 1865 over fifty schools were founded. From

Brunswick, Maine, and Castleton, Vermont, to La Porte, Indiana, and Lexington, Kentucky, doctors wanted to partake in the personal economic boom that a medical facility would bring.

These physician-owned schools also appeared in virtually every major city. Competing institutions opened down the street from one another as monetary considerations trumped entrance requirements and academic standards. By the late 1850s, Baltimore, Chicago, Cincinnati, Louisville, Nashville, New Orleans, New York, Philadelphia, Savannah, St. Louis, and Washington each had two schools. "If a student applies for admission into one of our colleges six weeks after the commencement of the term," wrote a contemporary observer, "the faculty dare not refuse him, lest he turn on his heel and walk directly into the halls of some rival institution."[24]

Competition forced the schools to search for innovative ways to increase the number of matriculants. The physician-owners were so greedy that they bestowed honorary degrees on countless physicians as an enticement to enroll their apprentices and other youngsters. The nation was flooded with professors of anatomy, medicine, midwifery, materia medica (an archaic term for pharmacology), and surgery, with the title holder having no academic qualifications, just a pecuniary interest in a particular institution. "Every professional man who became ambitious of distinction as a teacher, sought a professorship in some college as the only position in which that ambition could be gratified," explained Nathan Smith Davis, founder of the American Medical Association (AMA). "And as there are always more such men than there are places for them to fill, the constant and inevitable tendency is to the creation of more places."[25]

The proprietary medical schools gained political strength as their numbers grew. Across the nation, their owners directed legislative lobbying efforts to weaken any semblance of licensing requirements. These endeavors resulted in new statutes, stipulating that a diploma from a physician-owned institution was the equivalent of a license granted by a county or state medical society or a university-affiliated medical school. The less stringent licensure laws meant that poorly educated and inadequately trained medical school graduates were free to roam the American countryside and practice medicine however and wherever they chose. "Each roll of parchment endorses its possessor as 'vir ornatissimus' [a man of distinction]," declared one contemporary observer, "and he goes forth amid the sound of martial music and rich bouquets showered upon him by the hands of fair ones, an accredited agent for life or death, endowed with all the paraphernalia of a 'Doctor of Medicine,' but destitute of the brains."[26]

The situation was so confused by mid-century that a number of state legislatures simply repudiated medical licensure as a form of class discrimination. With the coming of the Civil War and the glaring absence of professional hegemony, no effective medical licensing existed in the nation. The country was inundated with physicians by the end of the 1860s (6,849 students graduated during the 1830s, 11,828 individuals in the 1840s, 17,213 throughout the 1850s, and 16,717 for the period of the 1860s).[27] Since medical school admission required neither literacy, prior academic achievements, nor good moral standing (the matriculation fee often supplanted all of this), it was not uncommon for the riffraff in many communities to comprise a large number of medical practitioners. The increasing supply of ill-prepared medical graduates diluted the quality of the nation's physicians while strengthening the political clout of the schools' owners.

The financial autonomy and lobbying power of the proprietary medical schools meant that government officials and leaders of the profession were unable to exert much influence over the goings-on of the institutions or of medicine as a whole. Medical education was in such shambles that even requirements for what constituted a complete course of study did not exist. Some students left after only one year, having earned a bachelor of medicine, while others returned for a second year of repeat lectures to receive a doctor of medicine degree. Sitting uncomfortably upright in a cramped and darkened room, the future doctors endured eight hours of monotonous lectures per day. There were no patients for clinical examination (apprenticeships were supposed to provide that experience), and practitioners-cum-pedagogues gave lecture upon laborious lecture. Antidissection laws and continued public opposition to human dissection meant that anatomy was rarely taught using cadavers. Instead, schools substituted inaccurate papier-mâché models as teaching aids.

"The people of this state have been
bled long enough"

When Rush succumbed in 1813 to his own treatment, his critics were quick to point out the problems with heroic therapy. "Of the effects of his system," wrote a cynic, "the people of America have heard and felt enough." Depletion therapy, sassed this detractor, was one of those "great discoveries ... which have contributed to the depopulation of the earth."[28] By the 1850s heroic therapy was no longer considered the gold standard for medical treatment, although elements of Rush's system remained for several more decades through most of the proprietary medical school boom. "I have no doubt that this remedy has been greatly abused ... and productive of very great evils," wrote the chairman of a conference on the effects of phlebotomy, "but I am well satisfied that [bloodletting] is a remedy of real value."[29] Doctors, especially in this era, were slow to abandon clinical practices for reasons of tradition alone, even when the evidence favored a different conclusion.

Much of the discontent with heroic therapies started when France replaced Great Britain as the educational mecca for ambitious and well-heeled American medical students. Animosity against the British, inflamed by the War of 1812, was one factor that compelled doctors to abandon Edinburgh and London. Growing social and political admiration for the French, initially attributable to their aversion toward the English, intensified in 1824 when the Revolutionary War hero and citizen of Paris, Marquis de Lafayette, made a triumphant tour of the United States. Ten years later, the publication of Alexis de Tocqueville's *Democracy in America,* a widely read and highly positive and optimistic account of American government and society, augmented this approbation for all things Gallic.

As more American doctors visited France, they increasingly realized that Parisian hospitals afforded greater clinical training, especially anatomical studies, than those in Scotland and England. "It may be asserted that in no part of the world can the same practical experience be acquired by the attentive student as in the French capital,"[30] gushed one young American medical scholar in Paris. Over seven hundred American doctors spent time in France from 1820 to 1860. Some condemned French medicine as too fussy—the Parisians practiced medicine in ways antithetical to Rush's inelegant and harsh style—but American physicians soon emulated the customs, such as correlating clinical observations with research findings. This manner of practice facilitated efforts to accurately identify and categorize diseases, an emerging discipline now called pathology. In addition, statistics and instruments became important tools in the diagnosis of illnesses—a Parisian physician invented the stethoscope in 1816 and, several years later, a French practitioner pioneered the use of a watch to measure the pulse rate.

French education imbued many American physicians with a skepticism toward heroic therapy that slowly permeated the country's practice of medicine. These recently returned physicians viewed the nation's doctors as too aggressive in therapy and too feckless at cure. They argued that Rush's policy of active interference must give way to one of caution and moderation.

Criticism of Rush's scheme became part of daily conversation in urbane American medical circles, which espoused a kinder and gentler style of therapeutics. Rush's detractors shunned the rote prescribing of laxatives and purgatives. Acknowledgment of a physician's limited clinical abilities led to renewed respect for nature's healing power. A full day's work, a night of restful sleep, and a hearty diet were more important to an individual's health than a physician's coarse interventions. It seemed as if an underlying philosophy of medical care in mid-nineteenth-century America was that for the public to remain healthy they should avoid doctors.

The precepts of self-help medicine returned egalitarianism to the art of healing, and this coincided with the ascent of President Andrew Jackson's populist embrace of the common man. Medical autonomy, noninterventionist care, and home doctoring were part of Jackson's call for self-determination in one's life. "Completely sincere" was a historian's assessment of Jackson. "He believed in democracy to an extent that no other President had yet done."[31] The eight years of Jackson's administration (1829–37) produced a steady improvement in the country's socioeconomic conditions, while a laissez-faire acceptance of differing styles of medical treatment colored the public's perception of the art of healing. "Our country, by its free institutions brings every question, as it ought, before the tribunal of public opinion," wrote a noted contemporary journalist. "Masonry has submitted to it—Mormonism, Agrarianism, Abolitionism, must all come to this at last, and medicine, like every useful science, should be thrown open to the observation and study of all."[32]

Increasing numbers of self-help medical volumes were published as a result. Different sections of the nation had their favorite authorities. James Ewell's *The Planter's and Mariner's Medical Companion* enjoyed considerable popularity in the southern states and went through numerous editions. The chief home health aid in the West (Kentucky, Ohio, and Tennessee) was John Gunn's *Domestic Medicine, or Poor Man's Friend.* By its eleventh edition in 1840, the author boldly proclaimed that one hundred thousand copies of his over-nine-hundred-page tome were in circulation. Gunn denounced the elitism of doctors and offered his manual as a safe alternative to doctors' visits. "By its limited use, and depending much on the simple, yet efficient directions I have here recommended," suggested the author, "you will have but little use for physicians or their prescriptions."[33]

The vehemence of lay opposition to Rush's schemes sparked a therapeutic reform movement. "The people of this state have been bled long enough in their bodies and pockets," warned a politician from New York, and "it was time they should do as the men of the Revolution did; resolve to sit down and enjoy the freedom for which they bled."[34] And many did just that. They refused to subject themselves to any form of heroic therapy.

This same public sentiment created openings for new medical practitioners. Various medical miscreants rushed into this therapeutic vacuum and practiced what became known as unorthodox medicine. Their theories, which promised cures by gentler methods at odds with bleeding, blistering, puking, and purging, proved appealing to the lay public.

These nontraditional practitioners (also known as cultists, irregulars, unorthodox, and sectarians) were clinical opportunists who championed their own idiosyncratic and hollow theories of disease causation, prevention, and treatment. They were also savvy promoters who quietly organized their own schools and awarded medical degrees indistinguishable from those given to orthodox doctors.

At first there was Thomsonianism, a botanically based movement whose practitioners claimed that most maladies were due to an excess of cold in the body. Thomsonians treated the sick with hot baths while employing a vegetable-based remedy to induce perspiration. By the mid-1840s, Thomsonian physicians were squabbling with one another over issues of therapeutic dogma that caused them to fracture into several competing botanical groups. The eclectics and the physiomedicalists emerged from the fray. The eclectics distinguished themselves with an unwavering reliance on botanical drugs and abhorrence of bloodletting. The physiomedicalists rejected any and everything to do with Benjamin Rush. Then came the hydropathic, or water cure, physicians and their use of Adam's ale externally as a steam bath and internally as an intestinal lavage.

Sylvester Graham, a dietary reformer, and his followers championed vegetarianism as the basis for healing and maintaining good health. Grahamites insisted that a change in dietary habits would also curb unhealthy sexual urges, specifically masturbation and pre- and extramarital relations. This nutritional regimen centered around the ingestion of a whole-wheat flour biscuit. Adherents claimed that steady use of these "Graham crackers" not only controlled onanism but could cure indigestion, inadequate circulation, and insanity, among other things. The Grahamism message of "if it feels good then don't do it" was widely copied and led to the establishment of other demanding alternative healing sects. For instance, homeopathic doctors, the group that eventually posed the gravest financial and professional threat to orthodox medicine, strictly prescribed infinitesimally small doses of botanically based drugs in an effort to rejuvenate an individual's mental and physical vital spirit.

A Time to Organize

As time passed, the differing messages of the unorthodox sects had a profound impact on the nation's medical psyche. The positive reception of these avant-garde therapies forced regular physicians, for the first time, to confront a serious challenge to their clinical authority. These mainstream doctors organized the AMA, hoping to create a unified profession to counter the sectarians' threat.

Since the founding of the country, physicians had been reluctant to form such a national society, fearing it would be regarded as elitist and monopolistic. However, competition from the irregulars was having serious economic repercussions and was affecting physicians' sense of clinical pride. "The profession is environed by difficulties and dangers, arising mainly from the too ready admixture into it of individuals unworthy of the association,"[35] lamented the AMA's president. Moreover, in 1844, the rapidly expanding homeopathic sect was clever enough to establish the American Institute of Homeopathy, the first nationwide medical organization. Sectarians further confused the situation by adopting the title of "doctor." With unorthodox physicians organizing medical colleges, granting degrees, and demanding admitting privileges to city and state hospitals, regulars and irregulars began to appear as equals in the court of public opinion.

Orthodox physicians believed that one way to set themselves apart from unorthodox practitioners was through membership in an American medical association. To ensure this goal of separation, the AMA promulgated a code of ethics forbidding doctors to use public advertisements, private cards, or handbills, and disallowing the prescription of patent or secret medicines. The Association also prevented its members from consulting with sectarian practitioners or treating any individual under a nonorthodox doctor's care. "No one can be considered as a regular practitioner or a fit associate in consultation," explained the new policy, "whose practice is based on an exclusive dogma, to the rejection of the accumulated experience of the profession, and of the aids actually furnished by anatomy, physiology, pathology, and organic chemistry."[36]

Unfortunately for its members, the AMA was fractious from its outset. Fits of anger echoed through the hallways during tumultuous meetings, while actual voting sessions ended in rebellions of factionalism endemic to the era. These internecine divisions sabotaged an early effort to use membership in the organization as a replacement for licensing practitioners, eliminating the demeaned doctor of medicine degree. This proposal barely gained a listening because lobbyists for the proprietary medical schools never allowed serious consideration of the plan. The physician-owners were not about to shut down their moneymaking operations or tighten academic standards.

While the divisive atmosphere precluded overall reform and national medical unity, AMA members at least expected to further segregate themselves from the sectarians. Orthodox physicians hoped that by agreeing to a code of ethics they would keep the irregulars away from patients, weaken public confidence in these clinical adversaries, and better define the therapeutic differences between the groups. In truth, regulars would have to renounce Rush's heroic therapies, shed their own unscientific past, and invoke more formalized education and scientific inquiry as the only acceptable approach to the practice of medicine if they wished to set themselves apart from nontraditional practitioners. This could not occur, however, until the waning years of the nineteenth century, when the principles of bacteriology, immunology, pathology, and physiology became known, as well as other important qualities of modern medical thought, including a scientific attitude, the willingness to question authority, a desire to learn from clinical experience, and the drive to modify therapeutic practices accordingly.

The mid-century leaders of the AMA were left with a meaningless and misguided strategy. They had taken a firm stand against the irregulars (passionate battles between the two groups would continue for over fifty years), but this posturing did little to lessen the public's dislike for the regulars' continued use of heroic therapies. Even more damning was the AMA's profound failure to protect the public from the tens of thousands of orthodox doctors who were poorly educated and clearly incompetent. With so much internal dissent and unable to clean its own house, this democratically designed, national organization of America's doctors had no real power and remained largely ineffective.

The founding of the AMA, however, despite its early disappointments, was an important signpost in the professionalization of American medicine. It was the next step in a progression that included Morgan's efforts to found a state-chartered medical school, the proprietary medical school movement, and the flourishing of state and local medical societies. Physicians were slowly forging a national medical identity, and one of its earliest manifestations came through weekly and monthly medical journals.

Medical Journalism

Medical journals, like schools and societies, served as a timely source of authority as well as a gauge of professionalism within the community. "Journalism, is an American—a republican—propensity," declared a physician, "and it would be remarkable, indeed if it did not display itself beyond the limits of business, politics, religions, popular education, and polite literature."[37] Most of these publications were ephemeral and survived only a few years, but their large numbers and wide circulation brought about the dispersal of scientific know-how.

The first medical journal, *The Medical Repository,* was published in New York in 1797. By the mid-1860s there were twenty-eight periodicals available for orthodox physicians, eleven homeopathic journals, and three intended for eclectic doctors. "[Journals] call forth communications from neighboring physicians, who would never be aroused or emboldened to write for distant, and perhaps more distinguished periodicals," said a doctor in Cincinnati. "Thus our science received many contributions of facts, which otherwise would perish with those who observed them, while the writers themselves are by the very efforts stimulated to improvement."[38] With journals distributed in every section of the country, physicians were more aware of professional happenings and the sense of professionalism that came with this knowledge.

Most of the publications were devoted to medicine in general and presented lengthy articles accompanied by an occasional engraving, case reports, summary accounts of the progress of medicine, and translations from the foreign literature. Medical gossip and long-winded editorials also filled the pages. The major contributions contained little scientific research. Instead, they provided details of a renowned practitioner's recent clinical triumphs. Advertising was nothing more than extravagant assertions that would have no place in a modern scientific journal.

Despite these faults, the nation's early medical journals served an extremely useful function in the development of American medicine. Even the AMA joined the journalism trend. Its leaders ensured that reports from its committees on education, literature, practical medicine, obstetrics, and surgery, as well as extraordinary scientific events, were included in the inaugural volumes of the *Transactions of the American*

Medical Association. They had already distributed two hundred copies of the proceedings of the 1846 and 1847 foundational meetings to editors of domestic and foreign medical journals, public libraries, and learned societies.

Volume 1 of the *Transactions* also contained a series of articles describing the discovery of anesthesia. "The medical press of the country," wrote the editors, "although not unanimous in its favor (so far at least as its general application is concerned), teems with cases and results."[39] The *Transactions* was filled with page after page of descriptions of operations performed under anesthesia at Massachusetts General Hospital, New York Hospital, and the Philadelphia-based clinics of the University of Pennsylvania and Jefferson Medical College. Medical journalism championed and chronicled the new breakthrough, the most important in the history of American medicine so far.

"The greatest discovery ever made"

William Thomas Green Morton, an entrepreneurial, self-taught dentist, was more a bottom-line businessman than a budding medical researcher at the age of twenty-seven. But he was also the man who, on October 16, 1846, first publicly demonstrated the effectiveness of ether in relieving the pain of surgery. The suddenness of this leap in medical knowledge was shocking. One evening surgical anesthesia did not exist and the following morning news of its discovery spread throughout the land. "No single announcement ever created so great and general an excitement in so short a time," wrote an eyewitness. "Surgeons, sufferers, scientific men, everybody, united in simultaneous demonstrations of heartfelt mutual congratulation."[40] Although anesthesia immediately transformed medicine, claims regarding its discovery produced a rancorous battle enveloping much of American medicine, the U.S. Congress, and the French Académie des Sciences.

Ether was first produced in the sixteenth century, but it did not enter the medical lexicon until the mid-1700s. From euphoria through lethargy and finally sleep, the consequences of inhaling the vapors of this aromatic, colorless, highly inflammable liquid were powerful. Physicians used it initially to treat headaches, gastric distress, and respiratory difficulties, but by the 1830s its inebriating effects also provided a form of social enter-tainment. Private ether frolics for the well-to-do young became the rage, with soused partygoers losing all inhibition. Users of ether and similar substances (nitrous oxide, or laughing gas, was a common substitute), however, rarely pushed themselves to the point of unconsciousness. Many feared that an ether-induced sleep would lead to breathing distress and death. As a result, any temptation to use ether to bring about total insensi-bility for medical purposes was strictly shunned. No one recognized that ether's intoxicating charm would lead to one of medicine's holy grails, sur-gical anesthesia.

In an era when the public lecture was part of America's democrati-zation of knowledge, itinerant "professors" of chemistry traveled from town to town speaking on ether and nitrous oxide and their exhilarating features. Eager citizens lined up to have a sniff or two for a few pennies, hoping to achieve a high as their friends laughed in amazement. One such enterprising ballyhoo-talking man showed up in Hartford, Connecticut, in early December 1844 and announced that an evening lecture and grand exhibition of laughing gas would be held at Union Hall. The advertise-ment in the *Courant* promised forty gallons of the substance and eight strong men sitting in front-row seats to prevent injury to any of the par-ticipants. "The entertainment is *scientific* to those who *make* it scientific," promised the lecturer. "I believe I can make you laugh more than you have for six months previous."[41]

Among the throng who purchased a twenty-five-cent ticket was Hor-ace Wells, a twenty-nine-year-old dentist. Painfully serious and slightly depressive, he watched as one of the inebriated audience members wildly jumped about the stage, at one point plowing knee-first into a large wooden bench. The young partaker was injured enough to bleed, but was unaware of the skin slash until the effects of the nitrous oxide had worn off. The incident did not go unnoticed by Wells, who deduced that a tooth might be painlessly pulled while a patient was under the similar effects of laughing gas. Wells arranged to have the "professor" visit his offices the following morning and administer the nitrous oxide to the den-tist himself. After Wells took a few whiffs, one of his dental friends used forceps to extract a long-bothersome molar. Wells awoke within minutes and, tasting blood in his mouth and feeling the space where the tooth once lived, supposedly exclaimed, "A new era in tooth-pulling! It is the greatest discovery ever made! I didn't feel it as much as the prick of a pin!"[42]

One month and about a dozen patients later, Wells was satisfied that nitrous oxide could be used safely. He wanted fame and fortune from his finding. Wells had always been a nervous man who, according to a biographer, was easily "distracted by his nagging sense of ambition" and "spent much of his free time tinkering with inventions and ideas that excited his imagination."[43] He traveled to Boston in January 1845 to reveal his findings to Morton, his former student and practice partner. Wells hoped that Morton's familiarity with the city's medical elite—Boston was one of the principal centers of scientific thinking in America with a medical school, a hospital, and a medical press—would lead to a public demonstration of painless tooth-pulling.

Morton had a successful dental practice and a checkered past. His peers had become wary after repeatedly hearing about unpaid debts, a drinking problem, and a rumor that he had been circumcised in a failed attempt to marry a wealthy Jewish woman and had welched on the physician's seventy-five-dollar fee. Aware of this talk, Morton decided to attend lecture courses at Harvard Medical School to improve his dental skills and upgrade his educational and professional qualifications. This was not unusual; for much of the nineteenth century dentistry was considered part of a physician's overall work. Those individuals who practiced dentistry but were not medical doctors had neither legal nor social standing, and most were viewed as ignorant tradesmen. "Personality, effrontery, chicanery, adroitness, and cunning," according to one medical historian, "were the qualities that enabled dentists to push to the front and win public favor."[44]

Morton improved his professional and social standing through amiability and industry. While at Harvard he met several members of the surgical staff at Massachusetts General Hospital, in particular the sober professor of surgery, John Collins Warren, one of the country's leading physicians. As a founder of the AMA and author of the country's first textbook on surgical oncology, Warren represented a trusted name in the chaotic world of 1840s medicine.

But Morton was never able to avoid trouble and found it in Charles Jackson, an odd but highly regarded geologist and mineralogist who was an 1829 graduate of Harvard Medical School. Morton befriended Jackson after hiring him as a private tutor for supplemental medical chemistry instruction. Jackson was best described as a mad scientist, a quick-tempered, litigious man known to claim the discoveries of others for himself. His lawsuits were legendary, including a nasty disagreement with Samuel Morse over the origins of the telegraph and an ongoing dispute with a Swiss-German chemist about his discovery of the explosive substance guncotton.

Jackson even forced his unreasonableness into William Beaumont's renowned research on the process of digestion, an investigation that some considered almost on a par with the discovery of anesthesia itself. Beaumont, a U.S. Army doctor, began his studies at an isolated military post in the old-growth forests of Michigan's Mackinac Island. He spent years painstakingly analyzing the gastric fluids that flowed from a French-Canadian trapper's unhealed abdominal gunshot wound. The doctor, afforded this window on the man's insides, went on to make groundbreaking observations about digestion. Once, on leave in Boston, Beaumont asked Jackson to perform a sophisticated chemical analysis of the trapper's gastric juices. Jackson hoped to share the kudos that were beginning to surround Beaumont's efforts. Therefore, he attempted to prevent Beaumont's reassignment to a new military posting in St. Louis. Keeping Beaumont in Boston would give Jackson greater access to the doctor's patient and his research findings.

Jackson covered this ruse by saying it was a matter of national medical importance: "credit may be conferred on the medical science of our country and important benefits accrue to humanity." He even circulated a petition to the secretary of war carrying the signatures of more than two hundred members of Congress. The appeal urged that Beaumont be reassigned to "Boston, or in the vicinity, for the term of four months, or longer if necessary."[45] Beaumont, who had not spoken to Jackson about the plans, had no intention of remaining in Boston, and the secretary rejected the chemist's request as inconvenient and meddlesome. Jackson's actions in the Beaumont affair hinted at what was to come with the discovery of anesthesia.

Shortly after arriving from Hartford with news of his successful extraction, Wells met with Morton and Jackson and presented his concept of painless dentistry. "I conversed with [them] upon the subject, both of whom admitted it to be entirely new to them," Wells would later claim. "Dr. Jackson expressed much surprise that severe operations could be performed without pain."[46] After mulling over the situation, Morton introduced Wells to Warren, who invited the dentist to demonstrate his discovery before a class of Harvard medical students.

It was to be an exciting day for the future physicians and one of the young men even volunteered to have a tooth pulled. Wells gave his patient the gas, picked up forceps, and grasped the tooth. Suddenly, the anesthetized student screamed out in pain. Some eyewitness accounts described it as a bleat or groan or muted shout, but the meaning was clear. Pandemonium ensued. Spectators erupted into waves of catcalls and laughter. The disgraced Wells fled the room. In his anxiety he had not administered enough nitrous oxide. Several bystanders hollered that the entire spectacle was "a humbug affair."[47] For the hapless Wells it was too much to bear. He returned to Hartford not as a victorious discoverer but as a defeated adventurer. His house and dental practice were up for sale within months as his depression deepened.

"Gentlemen, this is no humbug"

Morton realized the potential of Wells's idea despite the initial debacle and took up the cause of painless dentistry. Uncertain about the reliability of nitrous oxide, he began to experiment with ether. Jackson had previously suggested that Morton use the compound in its liquid form as a local application to decrease a tooth's sensitivity. The chemist also described the stupefying effects of inhaling sulfuric ether's vapor (there were several forms of ether, notably chlorine, nitric, and sulfuric, but in the manufacturing process, sulfuric ether was always the purest), though he advised combining it with atmospheric air to lessen the chance of any deadly consequences. Armed with this counsel, Morton spent 1846 perfecting his inhalation techniques and learning more about the nature of the substance. He added oil of orange to mask ether's distinctive scent, and devised an expensive glass-and-metal contraption to administer the vapors.

He was not simply discovering painless dentistry but the larger prize of pain-free surgery. By October, Morton was ready to announce the results of his experiments to the world, and Warren offered him a public venue. Two days later, with the seats of Massachusetts General Hospital's operating amphitheater filled to capacity, a nervous Morton, having anesthetized a twenty-year-old man, turned to Warren and informed him that all was ready. The crowd held silent, with all eyes fixed upon the crusty Warren's every move.

The dark and dank operating room had steeply banked rows of seats looking over a small stage. On one side of the proscenium was a dangling skeleton and across the way was an Egyptian mummy with a scarabaeus on the end of its nose—the mummy, a gift to Harvard from a Dutch trader, had been dissected by Warren in 1824. Ebony-handled scalpels and saws along with towels and basins of water were lined up and ready for use. It was like an opening night as the smell of orange-scented ether filled the room and a throng of doctors filled the acting area, crowding around the patient. The rapt audience craned their heads forward not knowing what to expect.

Warren grabbed a knife and made a three-inch incision through the skin of the neck. For twenty-five minutes the spectators watched in stunned disbelief as Warren performed pain-free surgery. The young patient did not budge as the older surgeon cut away an annoying tangle of fragile blood vessels (in Warren's words, the operation required "a protracted dissection among important nerves and blood-vessels").[48]

Whether the men in the room realized they had just witnessed one of the most important moments in medical history is unknown. Warren, however, looked over his audience and slowly uttered five of the most famous words in American medicine: "Gentlemen, this is no humbug."[49] There was a pause and then the slightest of murmurs. No one knew what to say or do. Warren turned to the awakening patient and repeatedly asked him whether he felt anything. The answer was, No! Nothing at all. Perhaps a slight sensation, like the scraping of a blunt instrument against the skin, but no pain. There are few moments in the history of medicine where time slows down and in a single second you can see everything change. This was one.

Morton realized that the only way he could secure some financial recompense for his efforts was through a government-issued patent. At this period in the nation's history neither federal nor private patronage for scientific investigators existed. Precisely because his demonstration was an unqualified triumph, Morton refused to disclose the exact nature of the anesthetic agent until he obtained a patent. When a solicitor of patents assured Morton that rights were available, the dentist looked to strengthen the application through association with a well-known person. He chose Jackson, and, in mid-November 1846, the federal government issued Patent No. 4848 to both Morton and Jackson, with the latter receiving ten percent of the profits. Within days, Morton was assigning national sales territories to businessmen, physicians, and dentists wishing to cash in on the expected boom in painless surgery.

The temperamental Jackson grew jealous and sparked a race for official recognition. During these years, when the French dominated medicine and science, any investigator hoping to establish priority in a discovery used the Académie des Sciences in Paris to arbitrate such issues. The chemist sent a letter to friends in France claiming to be the sole originator of anesthesia. A discouraged Wells also decided to seek his claim to anesthesia fame with the French authorities at the same time that Jackson sent his communiqué. When Morton realized that Wells and Jackson were courting the all-important French recognition, he issued a sixty-page treatise that was translated into French, outlining his justifications for rights to the discovery. Writing with both verve and resentment, Morton pleaded his case on a point-by-point basis. He concluded: "I believe I am the only person in the world to whom this discovery has, so far, been a pecuniary loss."[50]

The French were flummoxed, for the contentiousness that characterized U.S. medicine appeared to have been exported to Paris. In a Solomonic compromise the French Académie des Sciences awarded a joint Maximum Monthyon prize for discovery to both Morton and Jackson: Jackson for his "observations and experiments on the anesthetic effects produced by the inhalation of ether," and Morton for "having introduced this method into surgical practice in conformity to the instructions [*d'après les indications*] of Dr. Jackson."[51] Wells was never in the running.

The split decision only heightened animosities and caused Morton and Jackson and their supporters to seek a more definitive answer from the U.S. Congress. Unfortunately, Congress would be neither decisive nor expeditious. American physicians themselves remained uncertain about the importance of anesthesia and the validity of anyone's claims to the invention. "We have not considered it, by any means, as established that the prevention of pain in surgery is so vital a desideratum, as many seem to suppose," wrote an editor of the *New York Journal of Medicine*.[52]

Morton's life devolved into an endless and fruitless cycle of lobbying one congressman after another, year after year, for a decade and a half. He was seeking recompense for the government's failure to protect his fiduciary rights. Once it became known that Morton's anesthetic agent was not a novel substance but common ether mixed with perfume, attempts to enforce the patent proved difficult. Morton's obsession consumed him. He abandoned his dental practice, became destitute, and lived off the largess of friends. Jackson, who grew increasingly unreasonable, countered Morton's arguments with uncompromising antagonism while revealing salacious stories about the dentist's past.

Congress reached a compromise at one point, but cries on the House floor of "A bargain! A bargain!"[53] squelched the settlement. Each side accused the other of backroom political shenanigans that negotiated away potential profits. During another congressional session, a House committee decided that Morton deserved the credit for discovering surgical anesthesia and awarded him $100,000. The Senate disagreed and referred the anesthesia question back for another round of inconclusive hearings. And so it went, on and on through countless committee reports and thousands of pages of sworn testimony. Congress never determined whether it was Morton, Jackson, or even Wells who discovered surgical anesthesia.

Wells was the first of the three to stop fighting. He succumbed to his worsening depression after the Académie des Sciences rejected his claim. Wells had become a traveling salesman, wandering throughout the Northeast selling pet animals and sundry household goods. He eventually abandoned his family and headed to New York City, where he tangled with prostitutes and ended up in the infamous Tombs Prison. Wells's existence came to a dismal end in January 1848, three days after his thirty-third birthday. The originator of nitrous oxide anesthesia stuffed a silk handkerchief doused with chloroform into his mouth to anesthetize himself and slit an artery in his thigh with a razor. Wells's death, similar to Rush's demise from bloodletting, was aided by his own discovery. The

dentist's widow received a letter shortly after her husband's burial inform-
ing her that another French medical organization, the Paris Medical Society, had declared him the father of painless surgery.

Morton and Jackson's feud extended past Wells's death. Officials from
Massachusetts General Hospital attempted to clear up the confusion. In an
elaborate public report, they announced that Morton was the rightful discoverer of inhalational anesthesia. "He was determined to discover all that
could be discovered," wrote the officers, "and succeeded in demonstrating
all that he hoped and even more than he imagined."[54] Jackson only grew
increasingly incensed while Morton launched renewed efforts to clear his
name and gain what he believed to be his rightful financial windfall.

As late as 1858, a lengthy editorial in the *New York Times* noted that
"the old triangular [anesthesia] war, from every corner, is waged with
more vigor and bitterness than ever." Despite all that had been said, wrote
the editor, "the public has never yet agreed to which of the three several
claimants thanks are due."[55] The members of the AMA adopted a resolution six years later condemning Morton for what they considered egre-
gious public conduct as well as a violation of their Code of Ethics with
regard to patentable rights for anesthesia.

Morton and Jackson became long-term victims of their unresolved
obsession. A despondent and paranoid Morton died of a stroke in 1868.
Five years later a mentally unbalanced Jackson was committed to Massachusetts's McLean Insane Asylum, where he lived out the final seven years
of his life.

The discovery and promotion of anesthesia, regardless of its true
father, also demonstrated the difficulties of pursuing medical research
in mid-nineteenth-century America. An indifference to basic investigatory work permeated clinical practice. Most physicians, affected by poor
education and training and their own financial shortcomings, sought in
medicine only the immediate means to solve a patient's problem. To think
beyond the current crisis was rarely possible. Even a research discovery
as significant as anesthesia continued to meet with profound skepticism.
"I think anesthesia is of the devil, and I cannot give my sanction to any
Satanic influence which deprives a man of the capacity to recognize the
law," wrote one physician several years later. "I wish there were no such
thing as anesthesia! I do not think men should be prevented from pass-

ing through what God intended them to endure."[56] There were still no American research centers, no American research hospitals, and, without patronage, there were few Americans with research careers.

Despite gains in medical and surgical experience, the prestige of the profession was scarcely high at the midpoint of the nineteenth century. Forces, however, were at work to remedy this circumstance. The social and economic influences of sectarians with their dislike of heroic therapies, the impact of the French clinical school, advances in the medical sciences, as well as efforts to organize the nation's doctors were impacting the delivery of and philosophy behind medical care.

Physicians sensed these changes, but first they had to face the most devastating medical event of their times, the Civil War. This bloody, fratricidal conflict would cause more casualties than any other military action in the nation's history. Over 600,000 soldiers died from accidents, diseases, or wounds. A similar number were left with disabling injuries and chronic illnesses. The war led to an unprecedented involvement in medical matters by the government. Most important, it transformed the daily lives of physicians and provided them a depth of clinical experience that they could never have received in peacetime.

⁂ Three ⁂

EMERGENCE OF MODERN
MEDICINE

"Simply deaf and dumb"

IN JUNE 1862, William Goodell, a private in the Sixth Vermont Infantry, was fighting at White Oak Swamp in Virginia when a mortar shell exploded and knocked him unconscious. The blast tattered his knapsack and uniform but caused the soldier no visible injuries. However, when army doctors examined him several hours later, Goodell could neither hear nor speak.

They diagnosed him as "simply deaf and dumb." The symptoms suggested a brain injury and his confident physicians (this was before the words "neurology" and "neurosurgery" appeared in any medical dictionary) quickly determined how to treat the problem. They placed ice on Goodell's head, lanced neck veins, prescribed purgatives, and blistered his skin. This regimen, they assumed, would allow "poisonous" body fluids to escape and reduce the "congestion" in Goodell's head.

The private remained "deaf and dumb" despite several weeks of old-fashioned heroic therapy. His baffled caregivers then began subjecting him to increasingly speculative medical procedures. First, consultant doctors suggested that Goodell might be feigning his illness. They decided to lightly anesthetize him and test his senses in a less guarded state. Dripping ether onto a sponge held at Goodell's nose, a physician repeatedly questioned him as he drifted toward insensibility. The satisfied doctor reported that "the operation only confirmed the reality of the symptoms."[1]

Several days later, the doctors, hoping to undo the "excitement" in Goodell's body, subjected him to an up-and-coming medical fad: electric shock therapy. Using the recently discovered concept of electromagnetic induction, doctors could generate a low-voltage electric current and pass it through a patient. The Civil War provided physicians with unlimited opportunities to experiment with this new procedure. Goodell's doctors placed an electrode to his head, cranked up the machine, and zapped him. The electric shock therapy sapped Goodell's strength, but achieved nothing else.

Goodell continued to deteriorate and six months after the initial injury, the thirty-seven-year-old suffered a catastrophic paralyzing stroke. His doctors, unable to offer any further treatments or rehabilitation services, finally sent him home. There he communicated with his family through a writing slate. The long-suffering soldier did not have visiting nurses, physical therapists, or disability experts to aid in his recovery, and was soon totally incapacitated, his existence reduced to an endless routine of being moved from bed to chair and back as an attendant cared for his basic needs.

Goodell, like countless other soldiers, suffered tremendously due to the backward state of clinical medicine during the Civil War. It did not matter that medicine stood on the cusp of a major scientific revolution, to be heralded within a decade by the likes of Claude Bernard, Louis Pasteur, and Joseph Lister. Nor did it matter that looming advances in technology would soon change the way doctors diagnosed and treated diseases. Civil War–era physicians and combatants remained in the grip of heroic therapy's last act, and if patients were not being bled and blistered to exhaustion they were at the mercy of alternative practitioners whose theories were equally unsound. The physical horror that constituted Civil War medicine—the gangrenous amputations, the dirt-laden surgical procedures, the chaos of camp-site practice—was in many ways the cruel fate of mistiming for a war that arrived little more than a decade ahead of the medical care it required.

Unlike in more modern wars that have seen great technological and medical innovation, during the Civil War doctors made no astounding medical breakthroughs. No one introduced ingenious therapies to counteract field injuries. Even as the shrapnel wounds and splintered bones piled up, no surgeon could claim an enthralling victory; surgical techniques remained crude and wound infections spread unchecked. Communicable diseases ran rampant in unsanitary field camps. Soldiers recovered from severe illness more from serendipity than possibility.

Still, America's physicians obtained a profound depth of clinical and organizational experience in treating millions of sick and injured. Doctors learned about diseases and their clinical manifestations (much of which they were unfamiliar with) on a scale never before witnessed. Physicians who had minimal background in treating complex illnesses such as cardiac failure, cirrhosis of the liver, or respiratory calamities, experienced a lifetime of practice in several years of camping and marching. The war created surgeons from physicians who previously had minimal operating experience; this extensive hands-on training hastened specialization in American medicine. And doctors also acquired administrative skills not possible in antebellum America. For the first time the nation's physicians organized ambulance corps, assembled hospital trains, served on draft boards, resolved questions of medical manpower, and designed, staffed, and managed vast general hospitals. Doctors came to understand that patient well-being depended on adequate cleanliness, controlled sanitation, sound nutrition, and natural ventilation. Similarly, physicians recognized mental health as a vital adjunct to physical health.

As important, with almost thirteen thousand doctors—a cross section of American medicine, ranging from very capable individuals to implicit quacks—providing some level of military medical care, the profession's dedication to a single military medical objective imposed much-needed comradeship and discipline. "The constant mingling of men of high medical culture with the less educated had value," wrote one contemporary observer, "and the general influence of the war on our art was, in this and other ways, of great service."[2] Physicians not only familiarized themselves with disease and injury on an individual level, but the profession of medicine became more cohesive and national in outlook and scope.

The Civil War, while not a turning point in American medicine, ultimately laid the foundations for the remarkable advances that followed in the succeeding generation. The ascendancy of scientific medicine in the 1870s would be the final component to complement the trio of wartime shifts in American medicine: unprecedented clinical experience, improved administration, and the strengthening of medicine's professional status through greater national uniformity.

"He does believe in antiseptic surgery"

A decade after the Civil War had ended, American doctors, for the first time, began to perceive themselves as central players in world medicine, on a par with their European counterparts. No event showcased this new self-assurance as well as the International Medical Congress at the 1876 Centennial Exhibition in Philadelphia. While the Congress was only one part of the much larger Centennial Exhibition, it was the single largest gathering of American physicians to date and the most ambitious.

Five hundred healers gathered from throughout the globe. They came to hear of America's clinical successes and debate the status of these achievements in the world of medicine. "The [medical] profession of the United States has earned for itself an enviable reputation, and it is fully abreast of all the other pursuits that adorn the human mind," the president of the Congress's organizing committee assured the assembled. "We have passed the stage of medical provincialism and stand upon a lofty platform."[3] The Congress focused on nine areas of generalized medical interest (biology, dermatology and syphilography, medicine, mental diseases, obstetrics, ophthalmology, otology, sanitary science, and surgery). Thomas Eakins's masterpiece, *The Gross Clinic,* with its depiction of a bloody surgical operation, lorded over the medical proceedings in the Exposition's United States Hospital building.

Of all the medical celebrities at the meeting, none was as acclaimed as Great Britain's Joseph Lister. He was thin and of average height, distinguished only by the side-whiskers that flared wildly off his ruddy cheeks. Lister was professor of clinical surgery at the University of Edinburgh and renowned for discovering antisepsis, which explains that germs are the source of infection and can be controlled through certain precautionary behavior—Listerine would later be named for him in recognition of his work. He eventually received a baronetcy and later became the first medical man raised to the peerage.

At forty-nine years of age he was a poised and confident speaker who was attending the Congress as part of his ongoing travels to promote his ideas. He had recently completed a successful lecture tour on antisepsis through Austro-Hungary and Germany; the king of Saxony, intrigued by Lister's bold claims, had even requested that an antiseptic-based operation be performed in his presence. Lister was worth a listen.

None of the American physicians anticipated Lister's scheduled remarks on antisepsis more than Frank Hastings Hamilton, dean of the old-guard American clinicians. The sixty-three-year-old, battle-hardened Civil War hero was a nationally recognized expert on the legal aspects of medicine, public hygiene, and surgery. He had graduated from Union College, whose trustees later awarded him an honorary doctor of laws, and from the University of Pennsylvania Medical School. Hamilton was not only a prolific author but was long active in the politics of organized medicine. He cofounded both Manhattan's Bellevue Hospital Medical College and Brooklyn's Long Island College Hospital, and served as president of the New York State Medical Society and the New York Medico-Legal Society. "There are few men of modern times, in this country," wrote one of his contemporaries, "who have advanced so steadily or obtained so rapidly the justly merited reputation of a well qualified surgeon as Dr. Hamilton."[4]

Hamilton relished the opportunity to confront the Englishman publicly over what he considered radical scientific theories and revolutionary surgical techniques. "A large proportion of American surgeons seem not to have adopted your practice [of antisepsis]," Hamilton told Lister. "Whether from a lack of confidence or for other reasons, I cannot say."[5] It was a one-sided exchange, for the impatient Hamilton spoke out during an open discussion a day prior to Lister's scheduled presentation. As a result of the timing miscue, the unassuming British surgeon never had the opportunity to respond directly to the New Yorker's observations. Hamilton's preemptive strike, however, set a confrontational tone for the gathering, one that shaped American attitudes toward Lister's antiseptic methods for years to come.

On the day following Hamilton's comments, Lister flattered his hosts by telling them that "American physicians are renowned throughout the world for their inventive genius, and boldness and skill in execution." He reminded them that it was to their credit that civilization enjoyed the blessings of anesthesia, "the greatest boon ever conferred upon suffering humanity by human means." And he made certain that the Americans knew he was on a proselytization effort regarding the principles of antisepsis. This was important to Lister because physicians in the United States, unlike most of their European colleagues, had been slow to embrace his views. "I should be pleased, indeed, if the discussion which is about to take place should have the effect of strengthening the belief of the profession in the truth, the value, and the practical application of the principles of Antiseptic Surgery."[6]

Lister gave a three-and-a-half-hour discourse explaining the nuances of his antiseptic system, concentrating on the intertwined relationships among bacteria, dirt, pus, and wound infections. He based his ideas on the earlier work of Louis Pasteur, who showed that the presence of living microorganisms in a nutrient broth was attributable to the dust that settled on the substance rather than to the previously believed spontaneous generation. Expanding on Pasteur's notions, Lister deduced that these airborne microorganisms, or germs, caused putrefaction in a wound in the same way they produced mold on living matter. The Englishman's conclusions were brilliant in their simplicity: destroy germs on the wound during an operation, prevent their access to the incision during the healing process, and no pus will form. "The germ theory of putrefaction is the foundation of the whole system of antisepsis," Lister told the Americans, "and, if this theory is a fact, it is a fact of facts that the antiseptic system means the exclusion of all putrefactive organisms."[7]

Lister explained to his audience that wounds should never be manipulated with unclean instruments, especially not to root about aimlessly in search of an elusive bullet or other foreign object, and that unwashed fingers must never enter an injury or touch a fracture with exposed bone. "The skin being thoroughly cleansed, the instruments soaked, the hands washed, fingernails brushed," explained Lister, "it is the close attention to these minute details that renders this system so absolutely certain and safe."[8] The matter-of-fact Lister even demonstrated antiseptic techniques on an actual patient and later displayed an atomizer used to spray an antiseptic solution on a wound and throughout the air of an operating room.

For many, Lister's talk was an unqualified triumph. "Modesty is stamped upon his every act and word," wrote an eyewitness to Lister's performance, "and he does believe in antiseptic surgery."[9] The reporter for the prominent *Boston Medical and Surgical Journal* declared that "the great event of the day was the discourse by Professor Lister."[10]

Lister's doubters, however, dotted his audience as well, and many were upset with the length of his talk. As strange as it sounds today, physicians in the pre-Listerian era regarded the presence of pus as desirable. They believed wounds to be lined with dead tissue that needed to be expelled in the form of purulent matter. When an injury healed without an abundant flow of what was termed "healthy" or "laudable" pus, doctors considered it a medical aberration. Hamilton pointed out that there were other popular methods for treating wounds as well, "for which their advocates have made special claims, all of which may be considered as contending with the method advocated by Prof. Lister, for respectful consideration, if not for preference."[11]

At the Congress's Friday-night closing banquet, Lister sat next to Samuel Gross, the esteemed American surgeon, who was president of the Congress and the subject of the Eakins painting that hung in the main hall. Gross had recently penned a celebratory essay praising the contributions of American physicians to the art of surgery. As a finishing aside in his article, he quipped, "Little, if any, faith is placed by any enlightened or experienced surgeon on this side of the Atlantic, in the so-called treatment of Professor Lister."[12] It was a study in contrasts at the banquet as the self-important Gross toasted the self-effacing Lister with platitudes. Gross's insincerity was evident to many at the table.

Lister followed his appearance at the Congress with a transcontinental train journey to persuade the nation's surgeons of the supremacy of antisepsis. The Englishman and his wife were also going to experience the wilds of North America—just three months earlier Lakota and Northern Cheyenne warriors, under Crazy Horse and Sitting Bull, had annihilated George Custer and his 264 soldiers at the battle of the Little Bighorn River in the eastern Montana Territory. Lister dutifully traveled over the Rockies to San Francisco and back via Salt Lake City and Chicago. Leaving the Midwest, Lister passed through Boston and finished up in New York City, where he performed an operation using antiseptic techniques before a crowded audience of students and surgeons at Charity Hospital, located on Blackwell's Island (now Roosevelt Island). "His minute attention to all such details made this lecture of unusual interest and importance,"[13] related an eyewitness. Despite the widespread publicity surrounding Lister's appearance, Hamilton, a Manhattanite, was noticeably absent from the gallery.

Two days later the Listers left for London, uncertain of Joseph's success in convincing American doctors of the significance of antisepsis. This doubt was well founded. Although some journal articles attested to the growing use of Listerian antisepsis in America, others were less complimentary. "It should be remembered," cautioned one cynic, "[Lister's ideas] are the words of a theorist, who, as the Italians wittily say of such, has a grasshopper in his head."[14]

The Slow Embrace of Listerism

European physicians had broadly embraced scientific medicine in the early 1870s, but Listerism, and the scientifically based principles it embodied, divided the older generation of American physicians from their younger colleagues. Most elder and clinically conservative doctors listened politely, but refused to accept the new thinking, especially the underlying notion that microscopic organisms, so-called germs, were the main culprits behind infection, pus, and disease. They considered Lister's system of fingernail scrubbing, hand washing, instrument cleaning, and skin spraying burdensome. Doctors like Hamilton belittled Listerism as the needless rinsing of a wound with a cleansing liquid while the up-and-comers argued that the technique involved more than just the flushing of a wound; bandages, fingers, instruments, and even a physician's operating clothes needed to be antiseptically clean.

The country's older physicians had meager backgrounds in scientific medicine and no exposure to clinical research. Consequently, they had little comprehension of the new discipline of bacteriology and its fundamental bulwark, the germ theory, on which Listerism depended. "Do not be biased too quickly or strongly in favor of new or unsettled theories based on physiological, microscopical or chemical experiments," cautioned one well-known physician. "If you abandon the practical branches of medicine for histology, post-mortem researches, refined diagnostics, and abstract reasoning, your usefulness as a physician will almost surely diminish."[15] Such thinking stymied acceptance of both the basis of Lister's theories and their practical applications. These poorly educated physicians (even, as in the case of Hamilton, when they were among the country's medical elite) simply distrusted scientific medicine and found it incomprehensible that recently discovered microbes could cause so many terrifying problems.

Many of the older doctors also failed to grasp the sophistication and scope of true Listerism, not to mention the amount of diligence it required. They pointed to repeated antisepsis failures, even when surgeons supposedly followed the rules, without understanding the difference between sloppy antisepsis in practice and refined antisepsis in theory. Each surgeon had his own opinion as to what Listerism was and was not. Many practiced a bastardized form, in which some aspects of antisepsis were utilized while certain hard-to-break habits remained. Physicians worked with carefully cleansed operative sites and used instruments dipped in antiseptic solution, but refused to wash their fingers or clean their bloodstained operating coats. Some sneezed into their hands and proceeded to manipulate wounds or held the scalpel between their teeth as they completed tying a knot, all the while claiming to practice Listerism because they showered the operating room air with his antiseptic solution. "A showy thing like the spray attracted attention at once," acknowledged one practitioner while reminiscing about the ignorance of germs. "Physicians understood the spray (really the least important part of the whole business) and they understood rinsing their hands in carbolic solution and laying their instruments in it; but beyond that they could not go."[16] Then there were those American doctors who relied on a unique form of regional medical chauvinism as the justification to back off from Lister's thinking. "The pure country air in Virginia," claimed a southern healer, "being in itself antiseptic . . . our country physicians will very rarely have to lament a case of pyemia [severe blood poisoning]."[17]

Despite this entrenched resistance, a vanguard of American physicians imported true Listerism from their studies abroad and fought for its acceptance back home. Younger doctors had been traveling to Scotland since 1868 to learn Lister's techniques as part of their postgraduate European medical tour. They returned to the United States filled with an unabashed enthusiasm for the antiseptic method. For example, John Collins Warren, the twenty-six-year-old namesake grandson of ether's "codiscoverer," wrote of his experience in Scotland, "This visit to Lister left a deep impression upon me." When the younger Warren proposed using antisepsis at Massachusetts General Hospital, a committee of old-line physicians bluntly informed him that the "treatment had already been tried and discarded."[18] Warren disregarded their admonition and performed a mastectomy using Listerian antisepsis. Despite the patient's successful (and pus free) recovery, Harvard officially banned antisepsis. Still, Warren and other American medical novitiates continued to experiment with antisepsis, wrote articles describing their clinical successes, and attempted to interest their older mentors. It was to no avail. The older generation would never fully accept Listerism.

Whatever trepidations the American medical profession had about Bernard's, Pasteur's, and Lister's work, the lay community had few. "The germs whose existence is to be decided are confessedly invisible," wrote an editor in the *Atlantic Monthly*. "We shall have to look about therefore for as extensive a mass of facts as possible, and see which theory, that of germs or that of spontaneous molecular reconstruction, is, on the whole, the simplest and easiest 'fit.' "[19] Nonmedical journals trumpeted news of bacteriological research activities and increasingly presented scientific medicine in a more favorable light than medical journals.

Those physicians who failed to embrace bacteriology, as well as pathology and physiology, continued to treat the symptoms of disease instead of the underlying causes. Rush's heroic therapy, with its reliance on bloodletting, emetics, and purgatives, was no longer de rigueur, but America's doctors still depended on heroiclike therapies intended to demonstrate their control of the clinical situation.

Stimulants or tonics, particularly beverage alcohol, became new wonder drugs. Similar to heroiclike therapies, they could alter appetite, breathing, heart rate, mentation, and skin color. By the mid-1870s, tonics and analgesics, specifically opium and its derivative morphine (given through hypodermic injection), were the profession's prime medicinal agents. With whiskey or brandy and occasionally champagne leading the way, patients found the large doses of the new therapies to their liking. Alcohol was affordable and ubiquitous, an ideal antidote to the enervating nature of illnesses and a first-rate therapy to overcome the physical collapse that accompanied gunshot wounds or other injuries. "When the heart is suddenly enfeebled by hemorrhage," wrote one doctor, "alcoholic stimulants may be cautiously given, care being had not to bring about violent reaction."[20]

Physicians clashed with members of the Woman's Christian Temperance Union, which promoted abstinence in the consumption of intoxicating liquors, denying them even as a clinical therapeutic. One doctor cautioned, "The cause of temperance cannot be promoted by ignoring or denying the often proved and constantly recurring benefits obtained from the use of alcoholic liquors as a therapeutic agent."[21] This physician, like many of his peers, confused cause and effect, disease and symptom, panacea and poison, and pushed his profession into untenable, and often ridiculous, clinical positions. Most of the nation's physicians were still no better therapists than their "bleed, blister, puke, and purge" predecessors.

"Doctor, I am a dead man"

When President James A. Garfield prepared to leave Washington for a vacation in July 1881, he never could have imagined that his fate was linked to Lister's lecture in Philadelphia and Hamilton's offhand but powerful comments at the medical congress.

Garfield was born in a log cabin and grew to become a college president, Union army general, and congressman—all by the age of thirty-two. During an eighteen-year congressional career he had signed out more books and spent a greater amount of time at the Library of Congress than any other politician. His erudition was complemented by political pragmatism. Garfield worked diligently to become a successful Republican strategist.

His nomination for the presidency was unexpected, the result of a political deadlock at the Republican convention. Though he had gained the presidency, he had landed in the middle of a bitter row between warring factions of his party over political patronage. The four months after his inauguration were particularly demanding as both factions of the Republican party continued to assert their claims to federal power.

On Saturday morning, July 2, the stressed president was looking forward to a relaxing train ride and an extended retreat through New England. Garfield had barely entered the Baltimore and Potomac Railroad depot when a destitute-looking man approached him, pulled a snub-nosed revolver from his coat pocket, and fired twice. Wounded in his midback and grazed on his upper arm, the president slumped to the wooden floor as police arrested the shooter, Charles Guiteau, a schizophrenic religious fanatic who had long pestered White House officials regarding patronage positions.

Confusion reigned as stunned onlookers gathered around the semiconscious Garfield. Even though Abraham Lincoln had been assassinated fifteen years before, the American president still traveled without medical attendants. When Garfield fainted, someone held him upright instead of keeping him flat and raising his legs. Individuals rubbed his extremities to stimulate his senses, but to no avail. One bystander placed a wet cloth on the president's forehead, but Garfield remained lethargic. Despite the panic of the situation, an onlooker had the sense to dispatch messengers to locate any available physician.

In ten minutes, a health officer from the District of Columbia arrived. He had no particular expertise in gunshot injuries, but he assisted the minimally alert Garfield to sniff and swallow a stimulant mixture of brandy and smelling salts. The president perked up. He was turned on his side and his coat lifted to reveal the tiny back wound with its slight but steady stream of blood. The physician then became the first of over a dozen individuals to place their unwashed fingers and unclean instruments directly into the bullet hole in Garfield's back. "I did nothing further than to remove with my finger a small clot of blood from its mouth,"[22] the doctor innocently recalled several months later. Garfield inquired about the injury and when the physician told him it was not serious—the doctor lied, for he thought the damage was fatal—the president shook his head sideways, demonstrating his disagreement with the assessment. "Doctor," said Garfield, "I am a dead man."[23]

Onlookers transferred Garfield to a more private area in a second-floor lounge as the enlarging crowd grew unruly. Another doctor arrived and ordered bottles of hot water placed around the president's legs to counteract his feeble pulse and shallow breathing. This physician gave Garfield a further shot of plain brandy to stimulate his bodily functions. Then, thirty minutes after the shooting, a fifty-five-year-old doctor, Doctor Willard Bliss—his first name was actually Doctor—arrived.

Bliss assumed control. He was considered an expert on gunshot wounds from his days of Civil War surgery, and as Bliss attempted to determine the direction that the bullet traveled, he took the little finger of his unwashed left hand and, in his words, "passed it to its full extent into the wound."[24] Not satisfied with the results of his examination, Bliss grabbed a dirty metal probe and inserted it directly into the bullet track. He twisted and turned the slender rod, whose bulbous head became entangled in bullet-fractured rib fragments. Bliss then pressed on Garfield's breastbone in an attempt to relieve the mass of splintered bones. He finally removed the instrument and announced that the slug had entered Garfield's liver and that the president would shortly bleed to death. By this time ten physicians surrounded Garfield as Bliss asked several of them to place their unwashed and manure-tainted fingers—some of the doctors had arrived on horseback—into the wound and confirm his findings. The doctors, who agreed that Garfield had a mortal injury, opted to have the president transported to the White House, where he could die in peace.

Once home, Garfield took morphine to treat the onset of severe leg pains. The only medical treatment the president received during the first day were these injections, along with alcoholic stimulants and an occasional sip of lime water mixed with milk to control vomiting (among the unpleasant side-effects of morphine are constipation and nausea). The use of antibiotics, blood transfusions, intravenous fluids, and X-rays, let alone the simple task of monitoring blood pressure, did not exist. In light of the unsophisticated state of clinical medicine, Garfield's recovery—assuming that his physicians were incorrect and the bullet had not injured any vital organs—was going to depend on much good fortune and the problematical process of self-healing.

Over a dozen physicians were congregating in the hallways of the White House when Bliss decided that four of them should reexamine the president. At least one of the doctors, the surgeon general of the U.S. Navy, stuck his unwashed fingers into Garfield's wound. The others probed and prodded and, after an hour of deliberation, determined that Bliss was correct in his original assessment concerning a life-threatening liver wound. In a last-ditch medical effort consisting again of tonic therapy, they handed Garfield a flute glass filled with champagne and told him to drink up and go to sleep. Several hours later, and much to the physicians' amazement, the president's physical condition and mental state had improved. "The patient is decidedly more cheerful," reported the doctors in the first of what became a steady stream of medical bulletins, "and has amused himself and watchers by telling a laughable incident of his early career."[25] The optimism did not last long. By late Sunday evening, thirty-six hours after the attempted assassination, Garfield's pulse rate was a rapid one hundred twenty beats per minute, he was taking twenty breaths every sixty seconds, and his temperature had spiked to 102 degrees.

News of Garfield's shooting and his critical condition shocked the nation. The public was swept up in the drama as medical communiqués flashed through newly strung telegraph wires to every frontier town and country hamlet from the Atlantic Ocean to the Gulf Coast and out to the Pacific shores. Reports told not only of Garfield's fight for life but of incipient verbal clashes, even fisticuffs in a White House hallway between Bliss and other doctors over the president's treatment. The physicians argued with Bliss about his authoritarian and unscientific ways. This chorus of doctors accused Bliss of egomania and lambasted his professional credentials. They did not consider a private practitioner, bereft of scholarly achievement, worthy of caring for an American president. One doctor pointed the finger directly at Bliss's lack of understanding of Listerism. "I am afraid Bliss will probe the wound," said the detractor, "and if he does, inflammation will set in and the president will die."[26] Bliss's comeback was direct and God-like: "If I can't save him, no one can."[27]

"His case is very hopeful"

Bliss needed to defuse the bickering and spread the medical blame should Garfield die. He turned to Hamilton, Lister's old foil, and entreated him to leave New York at once for Washington to evaluate the president. Bliss knew Hamilton from their Civil War stint as military physicians. Bliss had been surgeon in chief to the U.S. Army's Armory Square Hospital in Washington, while Hamilton, who placed second in the nation on his military entrance examination, had held the prestigious title of inspector, U.S. Army, with a rank of lieutenant-colonel. Bliss also knew that Hamilton's medical opinions would be politically circumspect because of his past association with the Washington establishment—his brother-in-law, the recently deceased Henry Wilson, had been vice president under Ulysses

Grant. Hamilton welcomed the opportunity to be involved in such a historically important medical case and booked passage on a Sunday-evening train. He arrived at the White House at 6:30 the following morning.

One hour later, Hamilton, as well as another consulting physician, were ushered into Garfield's room. The president's condition had improved during the night. A reassured Bliss briefed the two men on the situation. Garfield was upbeat but had little to say when Hamilton asked him to turn over. For twenty minutes, the New Yorker examined the surface of the wound with his unwashed hands while using unclean bougies and probes to determine the depth of the bullet's damage. Hamilton concurred with Bliss's treatment plans, and a public bulletin was issued stating that he approved of all that had been done. "When I left Washington at 3 o'clock this afternoon," Hamilton later told a reporter for the *New York Times,* "President Garfield was no worse than he was at 6:30 o'clock this morning, when I arrived there. There was no evidence that he was sinking—nothing to lead to a suspicion that he was."[28] Hamilton effectively quelled initial doubts about Bliss's clinical judgments. Back in Manhattan, Hamilton received lengthy daily telegrams on Garfield's progress.

For a moment, these old-guard doctors believed that their clinical judgment had staved off disaster. What Bliss and Hamilton did not realize was that as soon as they and the other physicians placed their unwashed fingers and sullied instruments into Garfield's wound, they compromised the president's life. These supposed authorities had taken a relatively clean bullet track and converted it into a highly contaminated one; forceful and blind manipulations had spread bacteria ever deeper. Most wound infections do not become clinically evident for three to five days. It requires that amount of time for the bacteria to increase in number to produce symptoms, especially fever spikes. The unfortunate Garfield was sicker than anyone imagined. Within two days of the shooting, his fever was over 102 degrees and was soon spiking every evening to as high as 104 degrees.

A modern physician knows that when a patient has daily temperature increases, this implies the presence of a brewing infection or, worse, an undiscovered abscess. If an abscess is incised, allowing free drainage of its foul contents, then natural immunologic defense mechanisms should overwhelm the bacteria and bring about healing. If, however, an abscess goes untreated or is inadequately opened, it festers and grows, and, in the worst of cases, the bacteria spread throughout the body, leading to irreversible sepsis, shock, and death. With Bliss and Hamilton ignorant of these facts, Garfield was a clinical time bomb.

Six days after the assassination attempt, Garfield's wound began to discharge pus. The president was listless but restless as his heart and breathing rate ran up, all consistent with a sizable infection. The outpouring of pus would come to serve as a day-to-day gauge of Garfield's fluctuating health. For several weeks Bliss reassured Hamilton that all was copasetic. "July 19th, [the president] has had a better day today than on any day since he was injured," Bliss telegrammed Hamilton. "The wound looks well, and is discharging healthy pus freely."[29]

It was reported on numerous occasions, to both Hamilton and the public, that Garfield's "wound was dressed antiseptically."[30] To the president's physicians this meant that the opening of the bullet's entry site was swabbed with an antibacterial solution after which the same fluid was injected into the orifice to bathe the underlying tissues. Disregarding Lister's caution that all aspects of the antiseptic system must be adhered to, the president's doctors continued to probe his injury with dirty instruments and placed unclean rubber tubes inside the bullet's track to facilitate the drainage of pus. "Here again was the fatal mistake," noted one reporter. "Day after day the burrowing pus was aided on its way downward among the tissues by the disturbing tubes of the surgeons."[31]

As Garfield's case dragged on, debates concerning Listerism and the president's treatment filled the pages of medical journals and lay newspapers. "The difference principally lies between the extreme advocates of 'Listerism' and those who continue the methods in use before the introduction of antiseptic precautions," explained one editor. "The former condemn all probing of the wound."[32] Citizens wrote to the White House expressing their viewpoint. "Do not allow probing the wound," pleaded a Kansan. "Saturate everything with [Lister's] carbolic acid, one part to 20 parts water about. Use quite freely of this about the wound. Probing generally does more harm than the ball."[33]

Despite the hullabaloo Hamilton continued to profess little concern about Lister's precepts and the relationship between germs and pus. When a local reporter asked the doctor whether the increasing amount of pus held any clinical relevance, the New Yorker had an almost boastful reply: "Oh no, it is a favorable sign, and indicates that the wound is doing well. The discharge is nothing more than what was expected. It is safe to say that the President is getting along admirably, and his case is very hopeful."[34]

"Ignorance is bliss"

In late July, Garfield's wound discharged an extraordinary amount of purulent material. The president began to have "rigors," an antiquated medical term for intense shaking chills accompanied by a high fever (104 degrees) and a rapid heart rate (over one hundred twenty beats per minute). The onset of rigors usually signified the occurrence of septicemia, or "blood poisoning"—an idiomatic expression with which physicians in 1881 were well acquainted. Garfield, who could no longer eat (he vomited all that was given to him), became delirious and a large pocket of pus appeared on his back. One of his physician attendants anonymously informed reporters that the president was dying and proposed the reasons for it: "Pus had through carelessness and neglect been allowed to be in the wound till it rotted and pyemia had done its perfect work."[35] Septicemia, the doctor believed, had advanced into pyemia with its deadly consequence of metastatic abscesses. Bliss had run out of medical options and was forced to summon Hamilton back to Washington.

As the microbes multiplied and the abscesses expanded, Hamilton (along with another consultant physician, this one from Philadelphia) decided that the bullet hole itself did not provide a wide enough opening for the pus to drain adequately; another point of egress was needed. With dirty scalpels in their unwashed hands and without anesthesia, the two doctors made a two-and-a-half-inch incision into the pus pocket. Unfortunately, Hamilton had misjudged the clinical situation. The incision was too narrow, and two days later, again without anesthesia or adequate antisepsis, he further enlarged the opening. Hamilton removed fragments of rib and fastened two bacteria-laden rubber drainage tubes in place. As the pus poured out, Garfield temporarily rallied. Hamilton assured an anxious public that there was no evidence of pyemia nor any need for absolute Listerism as called for by younger American physicians. "Science died with each generation, and the next had to begin anew," Hamilton said. "There were those who had not even seen the case who assumed to know more of it than the group of physicians who were in daily attendance at the bedside."[36]

Over the next six weeks Bliss and his team incised multiple abscesses. One was so extensive that it necessitated general anesthesia. Garfield's condition never improved. So poisonous was the president's mix of bacteria that when Bliss cut his own finger while opening up an abscess, he developed a secondary infection. Despite Bliss's injury with its presence of pus, he still prevented other doctors from treating the president, and these physicians soon criticized him for ignoring Lister's antiseptic principles in his own wound while continuing to treat Garfield. "There is reason to suppose that he would, by so doing," wrote a detractor, "not only place his patient's life in additional danger from blood poisoning, but that he would also be acting in violation of the most ordinary precautions of modern surgery."[37]

Garfield was starving to death, a consequence of the overwhelming bacterial infection. In less than two months, his weight had fallen from 230 pounds to 130. His ribs stuck out, his arms and legs resembled matchsticks, and his face appeared skeletal.

With Garfield hallucinating and clearly incompetent, most observers realized that his life was at an end. Not so with Hamilton. Four days before Garfield died, this most renowned of American physicians insisted that all was still well. "The president is gradually getting rid of his septicemia, and, in my opinion, will successfully do so altogether," a straight-faced Hamilton told a newspaper reporter. "It will probably take at least five weeks. Thereafter his recovery will be very rapid."[38]

Garfield died on September 19 with Hamilton at his side. The following morning, eighty days after the shooting, an autopsy showed that the bullet was lodged deep in the tissues of the president's back. Not one vital organ was damaged in the initial injury. However, the examining doctors found multiple pus-filled cavities, all caused by the incessant probing with unwashed fingers, dirty instruments, and bacteria-laden tubes that spread microbes wherever they were poked.

Bliss and Hamilton vehemently denied that their actions caused any of Garfield's problems. In fact, the doctors consigned Garfield's demise to the bullet's passing through the president's vertebral column and the consequences of a deeply situated shattered bone with its supposed predilection to produce a sinister strain of pus. Afterward, when questioned about the importance of Lister's techniques and the validity of the germ theory relative to the autopsy findings, Hamilton assured the nation, "Throughout the whole course of the treatment, contrary to what has been publicly said repeatedly, so far as it was possible to apply the system of antiseptic surgery advocated by Mr. Lister to a wound of this character, it was rigorously employed."[39] Hamilton still regarded the partial use of Lister's system as more than adequate.

But younger doctors knew that the old-guard surgeons had mishandled the Garfield case through their intransigence on the topic of Listerism. They understood that it was an all-or-nothing proposition—everything from bandages to equipment to hands must be antiseptically fresh, every time. "It is indeed humiliating to the historian," wrote one physician, "to record such a mass of irretrievable [clinical] blunders."[40] The younger Warren, in reaction to Garfield's death, wrote (with some degree of sarcasm), "From an antiseptic view, we might criticize the introduction of the finger of several surgeons into the wound ... [T]hese examinations were not in accord with the prevailing present theories."[41] One young doctor noted in his private memoirs that his cohort of physicians considered the Garfield case a situation "where ignorance is Bliss."[42]

Even Garfield's assassin argued that the doctors had killed Garfield through their recalcitrance. At his trial Guiteau vehemently opposed the prosecution's attempt to pin the president's death on him, shouting: "Nothing can be more absurd, because General Garfield died from malpractice."[43] He might have been a lunatic, but his courtroom utterances rang true. And while Guiteau was merely attempting to save his life, his opinion was in line with those of many laymen throughout the country who were outraged over the medical aspects of Garfield's case, specifically the lack of Listerism. The jury ultimately found Guiteau guilty of murdering Garfield and he was hanged in June 1882.

The case for medical malpractice, however, was never pursued against Bliss or Hamilton, in no small part due to the personalities involved. Hamilton publicly had long opposed the practice of suing for medical malfeasance. In courtrooms throughout the country, he would flaunt his honorary doctor of laws degree and testify on behalf of physicians who were prosecuted. "Reputable lawyers never publicly criticize the practice of a professional brother during the progress of a trial," wrote Hamilton, "and I cannot but regard the public criticism of medical men under such circumstances as disreputable."[44]

Despite Bliss's and Hamilton's genuine attentiveness toward Garfield, their sincere desire to see him get well, and their faith in the probity of their clinical habits, their actions, stemming from the generational split over the merits of bacteriology and Listerism, resulted in the death of an American president. The two doctors through their last days refused to accept the validity of Listerism. "Mr. Lister and his disciples deceive both themselves and their audiences," wrote an unrepentant Hamilton. "Antisepsis has in no degree abated any dangers and difficulties."[45] Several decades later one of Hamilton's trusted assistants placed everything in a more practical perspective: "Dr. Hamilton was an old man, and not likely to be a pioneer in a new field of surgery."[46] Hamilton died in 1886 from repeated bouts of bleeding in his lungs brought on by several decades of tuberculosis.

The Garfield tragedy made the public more aware of bacteriology, germ theory, and antisepsis. "Now every intelligent citizen is enabled, as the result of a pardonable interest in Garfield's diagnosis and treatment," noted an editor, "to appreciate, in a great measure, the relative value of the many important questions involved."[47] From literary journals to popular culture science magazines, this new knowledge and its promise to revolutionize healing enthralled writers and readers. Observers credited much of this fervor to the awareness of medical facts and terms that the public acquired in following Garfield's case. They finally began to believe that medical science could take on disease in earnest—one of the best illustrations of this was the quick reception given to the discovery in 1882 that a bacterium was the direct cause of tuberculosis.

The Physician Himself

In the waning decades of the nineteenth century, the younger doctors who embraced scientific medicine could suddenly, almost unbelievably, cure the ill. Heroic therapy had ruled only a generation earlier, but the era of bleeding, blistering, puking, and purging was nearly forgotten, and these new men of science stood at the forefront of a half-century advance that had taken clinical medicine from uncertainty to modernity. Admittedly, the science of healing came to mean different things to different people, but the all-encompassing influence of microbiology, pathology, and physiology soon extended beyond clinical therapeutics to include education and training, hospitals, licensing, schools, and societies. The result was that American medicine was slowly escaping the divisiveness of proprietary medical schools, of anti-Listerian curmudgeons, and of irregular healers disparaging bedrock principles of science.

But against this backdrop most practitioners still lacked direction in establishing and managing a modern-style practice, something they would need to assure an increasingly finicky public. In addition, many doctors were simply careless of the social graces. For all the medical advances since the Civil War, physicians continued to wrestle with the fundamental question of how does one become a good doctor in America? The answer appeared in the form of a short manual called *The Physician Himself*, a road map for professional success that became the bestselling medical book of its age.

The man who penned this seminal primer was unknown outside of his native Baltimore, as anonymous as his book would be popular. Daniel Webster Cathell studied briefly with Hamilton, one among thousands for the great physician-teacher, and received his medical degree in 1865 as salutatorian from the Long Island College Hospital. He spent his entire professional life in private practice in Maryland and served a few years as professor of pathology in Baltimore's poorly managed and underfunded proprietary College of Physicians and Surgeons. There were no great breakthroughs or discoveries, no famous patients or feuds, no eponyms or honorary titles to his name. Cathell was medicine's everyman, a steadfast and unassuming member of Baltimore's numerous civic and professional societies.

Cathell was forty-three when he completed *The Physician Himself* in 1882. He intended the 194-page manual to be a practical vade mecum on how a physician could succeed in medical practice. The book was distinguished by its absence of convention and freedom from abstruse medical claims. Cathell simply packaged prevailing wisdom of his day and a fair deal of common sense. "What shall you add to the strictly scientific, to make your success in practice more certain, more rapid, and more complete?" he asked. "You will find that intellect, genius, temperance, correct personal habits, and other excellent qualities, will all fail unless you add ambition, self-reliance and aggressiveness to them."[48]

Physicians welcomed his wisdom in all its banality. *The Physician Himself* went through three editions of six thousand copies within six months, and its popularity would not wane for several generations. Cathell expanded his thoughts with each revision—the book had doubled in size after ten years—and addressed the leading medical questions of his day. The 1892 edition advised doctors to "shun politics and electioneering tactics,"[49] the 1902 recommended that "the telephone is both a luxury and a necessity,"[50] and the 1922 counseled that "in these days of rapid-transit, the automobile has great advantage over horse and carriage."[51] The book, which remained in publication through 1931, is now a rare antiquarian treasure, extant copies bearing evidence of frequent rereadings through torn pages and shaken bindings.

Cathell explained to his colleagues how to appear as affable but learned community leaders, as men of professional behavior and public decorum. He took doctors to task for any and every offense: the unseemly office with shabby furniture, the inappropriate clothes, the bedraggled personal appearance, dalliances with prostitutes, or the poorly-cared-for horse pulling the poorly-cared-for carriage. If Cathell could have knotted the tie, combed the hair, and stood by the side of each physician, he very well might have tried. "What is a more disgusting spectacle than a drunken, swearing, reckless sot-of-a physician with whiskey-soaked breath, staggering around the bed of a sick or dying person, profaning the occasion by the thoughts he excites, and by his grossness?"[52] No detail that could ruin economic success was too inconsequential or unpleasant to escape the Baltimorean's pen. As a book reviewer noted, "The advice given by Cathell to guide the physician in his conduct towards his patient and the public is sufficiently sound and sensible, and may be read with profit by all."[53]

Cathell believed that the guise of expertise was even more important than true scientific competency. "You will find that your placeboes not only amuse and satisfy people," claimed Cathell, "but you will be surprised to hear that some full-of-faith persons are chanting your praise and are actually willing to swear that they are cured of one or another awful thing by them."[54] The message was that good medicine was more than just good science, it was an art as well. "If a physician be especially refined in manner and moderately well versed in medicine, his politeness will make him a troop of friends," suggested Cathell, "and will be professionally more effective with them than the most profound acquaintance with histology, microscopic pathology, and other scientific acquirements."[55]

While some of Cathell's book focused on artifice, in the end he had a clear picture of what a doctor was and was not. Consequently, he was ruthless in his dismissal of nonmainstream practitioners. Such people were a bane on the profession and undercut the accomplishments of American medicine. Until scientific medicine unified the profession, the medical world remained a treacherous and unsympathetic place where too many unsophisticated healers competed for too few paying patients. This situation persisted until early-twentieth-century scientific advances brought about more objective evaluations of medical school curricula and facilities and of the competency and therapies of physicians. "Let your love of these twin virtues, *truth* and *honor,* prevent you from ever entertaining a thought of consulting with Eclectics, Homeopathists, Hydropathists, or other irregular practitioners, under the specious plea of duty to humanity," counseled Cathell. "Let their retirement be the prime consideration under which you assume charge."[56]

While Cathell's ideas advanced American medicine toward professionalism, in one respect he remained heavily rooted in the late nineteenth century. He had an unwavering devotion to the concept of the general physician. The entire premise of his book was that every true American physician should be of a similar mold. In defending this viewpoint he opposed not only threats from without the mainstream profession but also threats from within, most notably specialization. The emergence of specialists worsened the overcrowding in the medical marketplace created by lax standards and nonmainstream healers. Cathell saw the congestion issue as so severe that he wrote, "Do not induce young men to study medicine, as there are already three doctors where one is required."[57] General practitioners skirmished against the rise of specialists and their claimed technological superiority. "Never turn your cases over to specialists," warned Cathell in 1882. "You will lessen your own scope, and degenerate into a mere distributor of cases, a medical adviser instead of a medical attendant."[58]

Cathell the teacher. Cathell the schoolmaster. Cathell the autocratic principal. Cathell, a man most contemporaries would not have known if they ended up on his examining table, authored the one book that told the late-nineteenth-century physician how he should view himself. But not all social progress comes with one man, or one pen. New science and new manners meant doctors could cure the sick and regard themselves as professionals in the late nineteenth century more than any time before. But clinical improvements in the late nineteenth century only came one person at a time, and in the nation's cities, overrun by floods of immigrants, health problems mounted by the tens of thousands.

Saving Lives, Millions at a Time

Doctors needed to establish in the citizenry's mind an unshakable faith in the power of scientific medicine. A belief emerged that public health, if properly promoted, was the one medical discipline that would allow physicians to achieve this goal. This consensus grew as bacteriologists discovered that microorganisms were the cause of epidemic diseases, especially cholera, diphtheria, and typhoid. Such knowledge changed the manner in which contagious illnesses could be managed. Quarantine was no longer the sole solution.

Physicians, especially those who served in the Civil War and understood hygienic principles, laid claim to the nascent field of public health with its increasingly respected, bacteriologically based sanitary codes. The clinical authority and social standing of the profession would be elevated as physicians began to save lives, millions at a time. By the closing years of the nineteenth century, public health had evolved into a discipline based on medical and scientific expertise in which physicians guided sanitary engineers, scientists, nurses, and public-spirited citizens as they worked in relative accord. Of all the physicians who commanded prestige in America's burgeoning public health circles, few were as respected as Stephen Smith.

Smith was born in 1823 and his life spanned some of the most important milestones in American medical history, from the discovery of anesthesia in 1846 to the acceptance of microbiology and antisepsis in the 1890s to the global ascendance of American medicine following World War I. Of Smith's many mentors, few were as influential as Hamilton. Smith started as Hamilton's office assistant in 1849, and his professional interests closely paralleled those of his preceptor through medical school, internship, and beyond. Whether it was studying the legitimacy of medical malpractice suits or perfecting surgical operations, Smith was always considered one of Hamilton's outstanding students. Smith's clinical acumen and technical skills were so remarkable that within four years of receiving his degree he was appointed to the surgical staff of New York City's Bellevue Hospital. Smith joined Hamilton and several other prominent physicians in organizing the Bellevue Hospital Medical College in 1861. The two men remained friends and collaborators on its faculty for over two decades.

Unlike Hamilton, Smith was not only a distinguished clinician but also the ablest of authors. "We have no right to ridicule the man who frequently communicates his views to the profession," argued Smith.[59] He believed in the power of the written word in a time when physicians were often less than literate. His *Hand-book of Surgical Operations* became one of the most widely read clinical texts during the Civil War, while his *Manual of the Principles and Practice of Operative Surgery,* published in 1879, was a surgical classic for almost three decades. But more than just a prolific author of clinical tomes, Smith was one of American medicine's first men of letters. He wrote a weekly column for the widely read *American Medical Times,* penned several lengthy essays on the history of surgery in the United States, and authored numerous pieces on the role of the profession in society. Smith's literary endeavors continued well into his later life, when he composed the critically acclaimed *The City That Was,* describing the history of sanitary reform in New York City, and *Who Is Insane?* with its call for improved treatment of the mentally ill.

Though he accomplished much in clinical medicine and writing, his most lasting achievements came in public health, a field of study that hardly existed at the outset of Smith's career. In 1859, Hamilton commented that the profession of medicine had failed to promote and teach civic hygiene and sanitary reform. "There is everywhere, among the people a most fatal ignorance upon this subject," he told a group of graduating medical students, "and if physicians are not responsible for it, I do not know who is."[60] Smith agreed with his mentor's concerns and began to address these problems. He supervised a survey of Manhattan sanitary conditions that produced the Metropolitan Health Bill (1866); served five years (1870–75) as commissioner of the Board of Health of New York City; organized the American Public Health Association in 1872; presided over the section on sanitary science at the 1876 International Medical Congress (the same conference where his mentor, Hamilton, confronted Lister); assisted in creating in 1879 (at the request of President Rutherford B. Hayes) the short-lived National Board of Health; and, in 1894, traveled on behalf of President Grover Cleveland as a delegate to the ninth International Sanitary Conference in Paris.

Smith's mission to improve the nation's public health would not be easy given this starting point. Piles of horse manure fouled urban streets where flies swarmed over any living creature. Livestock roamed the alleys and the animals' odors permeated all. City dwellers abandoned their dead and dying horses without concern, much like junked automobiles would shortly litter the nation's landscape. Through the 1890s, offal contractors hauled away an average of eight thousand dead horses a year from New York City's thoroughfares. Smith spoke of "fat-boiling, entrails-cleansing, and tripe-curing establishments,"[61] which polluted the air and yards of neighboring buildings. In the most loathsome of slaughterhouse tales, a two-block stream of blood and liquefied animal parts snaked from an abattoir on West Thirty-ninth Street to the Hudson River. With droves of cattle, hogs, and sheep arriving daily at New York's two hundred slaughter pens, many located in the most densely populated neighborhoods, the city desperately needed new sanitary codes based on principles of bacteriology and hygiene.

As bad as life and death were for these animals, their masters may have had it worse. New York City's buildings towered upward, but beneath their sheen clustered people in poverty. Street after street of tenement houses bore names conveying their inhabitants' dreadful standard of living. From "Rotten Row" to "Bummer's Retreat," the medical evil of packed housing was frightening. Smith termed it "tenant-house cachexy." "The eye becomes bleared, the senses blunted, the limbs shrunken and tremulous, the secretions exceedingly offensive," he explained. "There is a state of premature decay."[62] Raw sewage flooded tenement basements.

Dark and damp air, with no chance for circulation, suffocated all in its stink. Infectious diseases rampaged and the sickening odor of cholera or typhus was unavoidable. Whether Boston, Chicago, New York, or Philadelphia, the public health problems were the same and growing as the immigrant poor crowded into the nation's cities.

Much of Smith's public health acclaim stemmed from his efforts to clean New York's streets. In dramatic testimony before an investigatory hearing of the New York State Legislature, he referenced statistics, supplied graphs, exhibited pictures, and dramatized and personalized the problems associated with inadequate sanitation and substandard housing. Smith brought the medical reality of filth as a cause of cholera and slovenliness as a cause of typhoid to the legislator. "Intestinal diseases, as cholera infantum, diarrhea, dysentery, typhoid fever, etc., which arise from, or are intensely aggravated by the emanations from putrescible material in streets, courts, and alleys, or from cesspools, privies, drain pipes, sewers," he warned, "were prevalent in the tenant-house districts, creating a vast amount of sickness, and a large infant mortality."[63]

Smith's endeavors turned into a cause célèbre. The city's dailies covered the hearings with front-page news. "The only persons who are doing anything for the public health are the agents of [Smith's] Citizens' Association," wrote a *New York Times* editor. "The subject of cleaning streets, the plan and ventilation of tenement-houses, the removal of offal, the number of persons lodged in a given space, the existence and removing of nuisances, the cellar population, and similar topics, ought to be put in the hands of a competent board or commission."[64]

After months of deliberation and facing increasing public pressure, the politicians agreed with Smith's assessments, and the Metropolitan Health Bill, which in large part he had drafted, became law. The new legislation was a major triumph in the history of public health and American medicine. It afforded the country's greatest urban metropolis the beginnings of effective sanitation codes and civic hygiene regulations that trained physicians would enforce. Smith, in an uncharacteristic burst of egotism, boasted that the law was "declared, officially and judicially, to be the most complete piece of health legislation ever placed on the statute books."[65] He was correct in his evaluation. Passage of the Metropolitan Health Bill led to the creation of the first effective urban health department in a major city. Supporters hailed the law as a victory for American democracy and a signal that medicine was undergoing profound changes.

Smith's success fostered the merger of medical and civic responsibilities. More important, his labors brought order to the disordered state of public health, introduced science into backward sanitary codes, and improved the authority and status of physicians by uniting doctors and laymen in a common cause. The city organized a corps of vaccinators as well as a bureau of vital statistics. Physician inspectors studied outbreaks of communicable diseases and inspected tenement houses for defective plumbing and inadequate ventilation. Leaflets explained the ravages of diphtheria, including details about how the disease spread and safeguards to be taken.

These efforts brought about the beginnings of organized public health education in the United States. Other cities and states followed New York's example in quick succession. As additional health departments opened, Smith's followers suggested a national organization for the promotion of public health. Some physicians promoted the AMA's newly formed section on state medicine and public hygiene as a starting point. The Association, however, remained hamstrung in its capacity to act as the overall representative of the medical profession, and its initiatives on the topic generated little attention. "I must confess," wrote one public health enthusiast, "judging from the small number of members attending the Section on Hygiene, that subject seems to afford less interest than any other."[66]

In 1872, Smith called together some of the more prominent men involved in public health to discuss the national situation. All agreed that any such organization needed to be less concerned with establishing sanitary standards or defining the limits of preventive practice and more focused on increasing managerial support for existing municipal and state health agencies. Smith suggested that an organization mixing professionals with scientific expertise and citizens with an interest in sanitation "would greatly facilitate the enlightenment of the public and promote the appointment of more competent health authorities."[67]

The lay press embraced Smith's endeavors. Journalists welcomed the new organization and extensively covered its meetings. "The business before this association is so urgent, so vital in its importance, so new to the general public, and so inexorably practical, that the physicians should not waste a moment in sentimentalism," wrote an editor for the *New York Daily Tribune*. "It is for this Association to tell us what we need and that in as plain and direct words as possible."[68] Articles in popular magazines reinforced the surging interest in sanitary reform and the new wonders of the germ theory and bacteriology.

While public health reforms changed the way citizens viewed doctors, the growing acceptance of scientific medicine changed the way doctors dealt with sickness. "Once the priests were physicians," wrote an observer at the time, "but now the physicians are becoming, in their way, priests, and giving laws not only to their own patients, but to society, and revising the rubrics and shaping the Epos and the Ethos of the race."[69] A series of startling discoveries by America's bacteriologists reinforced this new-found cultural authority of physicians. During the 1890s the first treatment with diphtheria antitoxin was administered to a child; the filtration of water to decrease bacterial pollutants was instituted; the commercial production of pasteurized milk became available; fly-control as a means of preventing typhoid fever was formulated; and the nation's earliest specialized hospital for tuberculosis patients opened. The astonishing rapidity and impact of these scientific accomplishments provided a clear backdrop to the growing professional esteem and influence of physicians.

The medical profession, like the nation, was urbanizing, specializing, and uniting. While traditional medicine, with its dogmas, had divided physicians, the acceptance of scientific medicine and bacteriology brought healers together. By removing uncertainty science gave rise to a new professional consensus that immeasurably strengthened the social position of physicians and allowed them to assert their cultural authority. Emergent financial and professional incentives to conform and adapt offset any desire to differentiate oneself in the daily practice of medicine. This consolidation of power could only be complete when sectarian practitioners, particularly the prickly but powerful homeopaths, joined the regular profession in their embrace of the bacteriological revolution and the fundamentals of medical science.

✤ Four ✤

CONSOLIDATION OF POWER

An Ignorant Fanatic

B Y THE LATE NINETEENTH CENTURY America's homeopaths, with their gentle therapeutics and hands-on style of health care, were at the acme of their clinical successes. Homeopathic medical schools could be found in most major cities, including facilities associated with Boston University and the Universities of Iowa, Michigan, and Minnesota. Homeopathic medical societies, clinics, dispensaries, and hospitals were present in over thirty states. Homeopathic medical books and journals covered every conceivable clinical subject. Almost ten thousand healers practiced homeopathic medicine, approximately 10 percent of all doctors nationwide. "It is accurately safe to say," claimed a homeopathic enthusiast, "that in the aggregate at the lowest calculation fully one-third of the taxable property [in the nation's major cities] is held by people who employ homeopathic treatment."[1] The assertion might have been an idle boast, but homeopathy's popularity was difficult to deny, especially among the country's influential and wealthy.

Samuel Hahnemann, a German physician, had formulated the original theories of homeopathy out of a series of studies on the pharmacologic characteristics of herbal medicines. He had become disillusioned with traditional medicine and its inability to cure patients of their ills. Based on his research, Hahnemann concluded that a weakening of the vital spirit, an indefinable force within the human body, produced disease. He also postulated that there was an intense interrelationship between the spiritual and material aspects of life. Healing, according to Hahnemann's abstruse philosophies, could not follow rational physical principles because it required reanimating the intangible vital spirit.

Some labeled Hahnemann an "ignorant fanatic"[2] because he flouted medical conventions, but when these conventions included ineffective heroic therapies, such contrarianism showed more common sense than ignorance. And Hahnemann was in fact well educated, even scholarly. He earned a medical degree with honors from the University of Erlangen in 1779 and claimed to speak proficient Arabic, Chaldaic, English, French, Greek, Hebrew, Italian, Latin, Spanish, and Syriac. Hahnemann relied on these many tongues when he traveled through Europe lambasting his fellow doctors, denouncing their barbaric and harmful medical therapies. He became one of his era's most strident critics of traditional medicine, with a vigor and irascibility that betrayed his elfinlike features and small frame. The viciousness of his opinions impeded any financial or social success as a doctor, and after years of frustration, he renounced day-to-day practice and turned to translating the era's great medical treatises and studying pharmacology.

In 1790, Hahnemann was working on a book concerning the properties and preparations of herbal-based drugs. He was intrigued by the author's claim that malaria could be cured by the astringent qualities of cinchona, a medicinal found in the bark of a South American tree. Hahnemann knew that other astringent-like medicines were ineffective against the disease. His inquisitiveness led him to conduct a series of self-experiments regarding the actions of this so-called Jesuit's bark. After two weeks, Hahnemann found that cinchona evoked malaria-like symptoms in himself: "My feet, finger tips, etc. at first became cold; I grew languid and drowsy; then my heart began to palpitate, and my pulse grew hard and small; intolerable anxiety, trembling, prostration throughout all my limbs; then pulsation in my head, redness of my cheeks, thirst, and—in short—all those symptoms which are ordinarily characteristic of malarial fever."[3] When he discontinued the drug, the symptoms abated and he was again well. This led Hahnemann to consider that a substance could inexplicably create symptoms that it can also relieve.

Hahnemann began systematically testing herbal medicines for their pharmacologic effects on healthy individuals. He attempted to deduce from these studies, or "provings," as they became known, the diseases that herbal drugs would cure. After six years and thousands of experiments, Hahnemann formulated the basic principles of homeopathy. First, he identified the key homeopathic law of *similia similibus curantur* (like cures like). Sicknesses could be alleviated and the vital spirit rejuvenated by herbal medicines that produced in a healthy person the symptoms found in those who were ill (akin to fighting fire with fire). Hahnemann then determined that administering these herbal-based drugs in minute quantities increased their effect (the law of infinitesimals or potentiation); smaller doses were more successful in supporting the vital spirit of the body. Hahnemann carried this concept to an extreme, believing that dilutions as small as one one-millionth of a presumed normal dose were effective. He claimed such decreased strengths worked because the body in illness was more sensitive to drug therapy than it was in health. However, the concept of dilutions was insufficient by itself—further action was necessary. Hahnemann called for the flask holding the watered-down curative to be struck against a special leather pad to release the liquid's healing powers. Once the solution was ingested and the homeopathic medicine displaced a patient's natural disease, the new weaker artificial disease could be easily treated.

To his defenders, Hahnemann epitomized the solitary genius shaking off the shackles of traditional knowledge through the sheer power of his intellect. To his detractors, Hahnemann's words were medical gobbledygook. However, with homeopathy billed as both an experimental and philosophical method of healing, many lay individuals considered it more "scientific" and "logical" than time-honored conventional medicine and embraced its tenets. Homeopathy's favorable reception also likely arose because its practitioners prescribed commonsense activities, like eating well and exercising vigorously or walking in the fresh air and sunshine, while mainstream physicians shunned such advice and instead readied the bleeding lancet and prepared the calomel.

Hahnemann termed his physician critics "allopaths" (derived from the Greek *allos,* other, and *pathos,* suffering), explaining that their patients endured unnecessarily from the popular medical treatments they gave. He taught that his detractors' therapies were antiquated and based on the ancient Latin medical maxim, *contraria contrariis curantur* (contrary cures contrary). Hahnemann's followers colloquialized "allopath" to represent any physician who prescribed drugs with actions opposite to the symptoms of an illness. Over the course of the next century, the words "allopathy" and "allopathic" became pejoratives and were highly provocative for any doctor who was not a homeopathic enthusiast.

Lifeless Delusions

Hahnemann died in 1843 an acclaimed and wealthy individual. A decade earlier his homeopathic theories had spread across the Atlantic Ocean to the new world, where German-speaking immigrants and their physicians embraced his principles. These new homeopaths (also known as irregular, unorthodox, or sectarian healers) recruited converts from the ranks of America's mainstream doctors (so-called regular, orthodox, or traditional practitioners). In 1848, a state-chartered, proprietary homeopathic medical school was established in Philadelphia and, one year later, a proprietary homeopathic college was founded in Cleveland. By 1860 the nation's twenty-four hundred homeopaths appeared more prosperous and united than their orthodox colleagues. It helped that homeopaths were supported by a national medical society (the American Institute of Homeopathy), six medical colleges, and five monthly journals. America's emboldened homeopaths called themselves the New School and ridiculed the practitioners of traditional medicine. "We are the regular physicians," argued one professor of homeopathy, "for the practice of the old school is very irregular, and in consequence its practitioners are irregular also."[4]

Despite the occasional haughtiness of the irregulars, orthodox physicians generally welcomed homeopathic theories as an appealing and alternative style of medical practice. This was understandable given the public's harsh criticism of heroic therapy. Orthodox societies opened their membership rolls to homeopaths, many of whom had graduated from traditional medical schools. Hahnemann, who never set foot on American soil, received honorary membership in the Medical Society of the County of New York in 1832. Even the editors of the staid *Boston Medical and Surgical Journal* recognized homeopathic activities. "We are open to conviction," wrote an editor, "and to show that we entertain no hostility to homeopathia or the scientific followers of Hahnemann, everything found in homeopathic magazines, which can be of interest or utility to the profession at large, will be transferred to the pages of our Journal."[5]

But all was not well. Since homeopaths assumed the designation of "doctor," unschooled laypersons were usually unaware of the doctrinal differences. The sick simply wanted to be cured and homeopaths were masterful at gaining their confidence. It did not take long for orthodox doctors to realize the financial and professional threats inherent in homeopathy's rapid growth.

Traditional physicians began to ridicule the experimental and supposed scientific basis of homeopathy. In 1842, Oliver Wendell Holmes—physician, poet, and father of Supreme Court justice Oliver Wendell Holmes Jr.—stood before members of the Boston Society for the Diffusion of Useful Knowledge and scoffed at Hahnemann's theories as just another in a long line of "lifeless delusions" that mainstream medicine met. "Homeopathy," he told the crowd, "is a mingled mass of perverse ingenuity, of tinsel erudition, of imbecile credulity, and of artful misrepresentation. The new doctrine is not truth, it is a dangerous and deadly error."[6] Shortly thereafter, a member of the Rhode Island Medical Society explained that the profession's attitude toward homeopaths would have been different if "they had not excluded themselves by their bad conduct, and by their association with illiterate and dishonorable men, and especially with irresponsible foreigners."[7] The *Boston Medical and Surgical Journal* ran an editorial about-face: "We regard as ridiculous and farcical the whole subject of Hahnemannism."[8] The newly organized AMA passed a code of ethics in 1847 that forbade its orthodox constituency from dealing with their unorthodox detractors or treating any patient under their care.

These hostilities compelled the homeopaths to leave the company of the regulars. It was more of a sacking than a secession. The orthodox doctors may have been hurling criticisms that were justified, but the underpinnings of traditional medicine were themselves unscientific, and in several decades orthodox medicine would renounce its own confused ways. For now, homeopaths and allopaths, like blind men arguing over the colors of the rainbow, were fueled by their own ignorance. And the groups prepared for further battle as the nation itself plunged headlong into civil war.

When President Abraham Lincoln called for doctors to serve as army volunteers, the orthodox physicians who dominated the army medical corps systematically denied entry to any suspected homeopath. Most Americans agreed with the decision. "The fact is, what the country and the army now want is hard fighting with the enemy, and speedy and decisive victories over him; and they will be very glad to leave the questions between the allopathic and homeopathic schools for decision in the coming halcyon days of peace," wrote an editor for the *New York Times*. "Till then, let Congress postpone homeopathy and everything else but the main question in hand."[9] It would be sheer insanity, declared one senator who supported traditional medicine "to introduce clairvoyancers, spiritual rappers, homeopathists, and practicers of all other systems of medicine that are known at the present day, in order to gratify the caprice of every soldier."[10]

Homeopaths followed their principal of *similia similibus curantur* and fought right back, enlisting as army physicians—albeit under the guise of orthodox converts—and bringing their own politics and politicians into the fracas. "The devotees of that old institution [allopathy] are every whit as desperate towards homeopathy as the rebels of the cotton states are towards the government," proclaimed a homeopathic supporter, "and, if they come out of this contest in much the same way as the rebels will, they have themselves to thank for it."[11] In Congress, pro-homeopathic senators fought with their pro-orthodox colleagues.

As ridicule and invective poured forth, angry editorials filled the pages of orthodox and homeopathic journals. Homeopaths championed personal freedoms and a soldier's right to choose a doctor. They carried on an aggressive campaign questioning the constitutionality of the government's right to support one system of medical care. The arguments did little to further tolerance for military medical pluralism. "Allopaths feared medical anarchy," wrote one historian, "and used it to justify their continued exclusion of homeopaths from the army."[12]

Uncertainties concerning therapeutic distinctions between regulars and homeopaths muddied the debate. "I believe the difference between the two systems is the size of the dose, the homeopathists give less," remarked one senator. His opponent disagreed: "They have different medicines entirely."[13] No one in Washington seemed certain of the answers, least of all the congressmen doing the talking. Congress ultimately refused to act and the army remained an institution without sanctioned homeopathic practitioners.

After the war, homeopaths were further incensed when the regulars sought to extend their exclusionary tactics into the civic arena. Orthodox physicians in Chicago refused to treat patients in the new city hospital if homeopaths were granted admitting privileges. Similar boycotts broke out in Boston and New York.

The gentler ways of homeopathy were catching on with patients despite the regulars' prohibitions, and the press and the public soon called for more professional tolerance and less medical partisanship. "The two schools, which originally were diametrically hostile in theory and practice, now differ in name rather than in fact," wrote a newspaper editor, "and in most important respects there is little real difference between the practice of an accomplished regular physician, and that of the intelligent homeopathist."[14]

Orthodox physicians initially succeeded in preventing sectarians from working in municipal institutions, but a number of wealthy patients of homeopathic practitioners established private homeopathic clinics, dispensaries, and schools. When the well-heeled trustees of Boston University decided to organize a medical college in the mid-1870s, they solicited only homeopathic practitioners to form the faculty. "For the first time in the history of homeopathy," gushed a homeopathic leader, "have we secured a medical school in connection with a university or other educational institution."[15] Of the institution's original two dozen educators, eight were Harvard medical school graduates who had converted to homeopathy, three were women, and half of the staff had trained in Europe. The well-educated teaching staff gained approbation from the city's medical community.

The experience at Boston University was not unique. From its beginnings homeopathy appealed primarily to the nation's influential and well-to-do as they sought an alternative to the dreadfulness of traditional healing. This attraction came about for several reasons. Americans copied old-world customs, and homeopathy was fashionable among Europe's nobility and upper classes. In turn, the social standing of homeopathy's patrons influenced the type of physician who turned to homeopathy.

Early American homeopaths were generally better educated and more worldly than their peers. These practitioners were fluent in French and German and able to read the original versions of the homeopathic literature. Homeopaths also encouraged patients to treat themselves, an idea abhorrent to the practitioners of heroic therapy.

Such intellectualism, libertarianism, and sophistication, bolstered by homeopathy's faith in one's vital spirit, also attracted America's influential clergymen and the Transcendentalists. Intellectual giants such as Amos Bronson Alcott, his daughter Louisa May Alcott, Henry Ward Beecher, Ralph Waldo Emerson, Nathaniel Hawthorne, and Henry David Thoreau touted homeopathic-inspired medical reforms as one way to foster new religious and social norms. By the mid-1800s, Transcendentalism was among the most fashionable of the nation's pop-culture movements, and its leaders filled their speeches and writings with references to the salubrity of homeopathy. "How is your throat?" one of Louisa May Alcott's characters asked in *Jo's Boys*. "Throat? Oh, ah! yes, I remember. It is well. The effect of that prescription was wonderful. I'll never call homeopathy a humbug again."[16]

Homeopathy's success, along with the country's lax attitudes toward physician licensure, enabled the movement to broaden and diversify. Starting in the 1880s, clinical specialization by homeopaths closely paralleled and occasionally preceded similar developments in the regular profession. The members of the elite American Institute of Homeopathy established specialty sections in gynecology, laryngology, pediatrics, psychological medicine, public health, ophthalmology, otology, and surgery. Nonclinical issues were addressed by other organizations, like the American Homeopathic Health Resort Association, the American Institute of Homeopathic Pharmacies, the Homeopathic Intercollegiate Congress of the United States, and the National Association of Superintendents and Managers of Homeopathic Hospitals for the Insane. Among the various homeopathic associations, one group stood out for its rapid evolution, the bizarreness of its clinical claims, and the fanaticism of its followers: the American Association of Orificial Surgeons.

"The rectum is the focus of existence"

Edwin Hartley Pratt was the quintessential medical charlatan. Ambitious, authoritative, self-promoting, and smart, he turned the fringe homeopathic practice of orificial surgery into one of America's more intriguing and popular late-nineteenth-century medical disciplines. He stood greater than six feet, weighed over two hundred fifty pounds, and carried the most ample of abdominal girths. Pratt preached that diseases could be treated through a variety of operations on bodily openings, and when this giant man with the thinning hair and Vandyke beard went to work, no mouth, penis, rectum, or vagina was safe from a manipulation or scraping. "Bring me an individual with clean lips; a palate of proper length and unobtruding tonsils; a rectum that presents neither piles, prolapsus, fissure, ulcers, pockets nor pappillae—an individual whose sexual orifices are smooth and free from all irritation," Pratt assured the faithful, "and I will show you a human being whose digestion is good, whose sleep is sweet and restful, whose capillary circulation is superb, whose very existence is a constant source of uninterrupted delights."[17]

Pratt was initially regarded as an up-and-coming general practitioner, praised for his clinical skills and noted for an uncanny ability to sell himself and his ideas. He received his diploma from the Hahnemann Medical College of Chicago in 1873. Less than three years later Pratt helped organize the Chicago Homeopathic Medical College, a crosstown rival that provided him a receptive audience for his theories. He and the other founders pledged to elevate the academic requirements for admission and introduce broader studies in basic medical education. In reality, the new institution was just another in the long line of proprietary medical schools that did little more than enrich faculty members and produce mediocre physicians. Within its halls, Pratt lectured each year's class of seventy-five students on the virtues of homeopathic therapeutics. He also solidified his thoughts about orificial surgery.

In an era characterized by the audacity and mendacity of its medical con men, Pratt's theories stand out. Nonhomeopathic practitioners chafed at his specious claims, especially the abilities to snip off a hemorrhoid or two and thus cure illnesses like arthritis, constipation, eczema, insomnia, menstrual cramps, syphilis, tuberculosis, and even insanity. "The logical conclusion to be formed from the teachings of orificial specialists," dead-panned a detractor, "is that the rectum is the focus of existence, contains the essence of life, and performs the functions ordinarily ascribed to the heart and brain."[18]

Despite his critics' taunts and opposition, Pratt proved an outstanding self-promoter, spreading his doctrines through private classes and writing a textbook. He established the American Association of Orificial Surgeons in 1888. Four years later the monthly *Journal of Orificial Surgery* began with Pratt serving as editor in chief. He even performed orificial surgeries on his own students at the Chicago Homeopathic Medical College.

Pratt's orificial philosophy began with the noncontroversial assumption that good health depended on the normal circulation of blood. The logic of orificial surgery then went as follows: the sympathetic nervous system was the sole determinant of blood flow; fatigue of this system caused blood to stagnate, which led to disease; vast numbers of sympathetic nerves controlled muscles at the openings of the sexual organs and rectum (a fact discovered by nineteenth-century anatomists); any problems in these sensitive areas—inflamed hemorrhoids, redundant skin over the clitoris, a tight foreskin—created muscle spasms that exhausted the sympathetic nervous system and produced poor circulation and disease. "The weakness and the power of the sympathetic nerve lies at the orifices of the body," Pratt told his disciples. "Surgery must keep these orifices properly smoothed and dilated."[19] Pratt further argued that local problems involving sympathetic nerves instigated illness in distant parts of the body. For example, lacerations of the cervix were responsible for brain seizures and excess folds of rectal tissue caused asthma. Modern physicians understand that the circulatory system, like all complex physiological networks, is influenced by a myriad of factors, only one of which are the sympathetic nerves, whose main function is to control a person's fight-or-flight reaction.

Just as Hahnemann's words were scientific gobbledygook, Pratt's ideas were medical gibberish. Yet as senseless as orificial surgery seemed to orthodox physicians, Pratt's fame and influence continued to expand. His prolific writings and nonstop lecturing brought him much attention. Pratt seemed to have it all, from membership in the chic Chicago Automobile Club and the expensive Evanston Century Club to the presidency of the Illinois Homeopathic Association. As testament to his financial and professional success, Pratt constructed a private hospital known as the Lincoln Park Sanitarium, for which he published a fifty-page public relations selling piece with a collection of glossy pictures. He established the Lincoln Park Training School for Nurses as a department within his hospital at a time when the formal training of nurses was in its infancy. "The nurses are selected with great care," wrote an observer, "and are exceptionally competent in every way."[20] Thus, Pratt greatly expanded his clinical activities with the help of his ready supply of knowledgeable assistants. Meanwhile, Pratt trumpeted his new position as orificial surgeon to Chicago's Cook County Hospital as evidence of the legitimacy of his clinical theories and medical credentials. City officials had granted him and other homeopaths municipal admitting privileges on the belief that there were no substantive differences between orthodox and homeopathic medical school graduates.

With continued success, Pratt's confidence in his theories increased and he began to see himself as a prophet. Pratt made this evident at the International Homeopathic Congress at the 1893 Columbia World's Fair. "Almost all the patients have been under treatment elsewhere for a series of years," he told the assembled, "and have lost faith not only in doctors but in humanity, and they are not in the frame of mind to brook delay." Pratt predicted, "In good time the sympathetic nerve and its uses will receive the consideration to which they have long since been entitled and yet denied."[21]

By the early 1890s, Pratt's sympathetic nerve theories were in ascendance. Orificial surgery was an established homeopathic discipline and homeopathic physicians had performed tens of thousands of orificial surgical operations—Pratt himself had done well over one thousand. The American Association of Orificial Surgeons had almost three hundred dues-paying members and held its annual meeting in Chicago's priciest hotels. Orificial surgeons from as far away as California, Oregon, and the territories of Arizona and Utah told of their clinical experiences while lauding Pratt's accomplishments. "The philosophy he evolved was not an invention, but rather the development of principles so great as to affect life in all its complexities," wrote an admiring homeopath from Columbus, Ohio, "an awakening, as it were, of principles and policies which had remained unrecognized until his genius and foresight revealed their power and force to the waiting world."[22]

Science, the Final Arbiter

Pratt's medical theories were suspect, but his surgical technique was sound by the standards of his day. Even when the rationale for a particular procedure depended on unsound theories of sympathetic nerves, little about his operations fundamentally differed from surgery as practiced by the traditionalists. Pratt had formulated a clinical plan that incorporated old-time homeopathic therapeutics with up-to-date orthodox surgical techniques and claimed the best that both had to offer—anatomic and physiologic theories unique to homeopathy with surgical operations patterned after those devised by renowned orthodox surgeons. This melding was not surprising since a decades-old common ground existed between regular and homeopathic physicians regarding the technical practice of surgery. "So far as the manual operations are concerned," wrote one sectarian surgeon as far back as 1851, "the homeopath most cheerfully records his approval and admiration of the perfection to which they have been brought by the scientific investigation, ingenuity, and untiring industry of the allopathic profession."[23] It was only in the pre- and postoperative use of homeopathic preparations that the two sides disagreed.

The long-standing consensus on surgical technique opened the door for agreement on related scientific and medical advances. Anesthesia and antisepsis had turned surgery from a crude and dangerous art into the most influential and prestigious of all late-nineteenth-century medical specialties. The American Institute of Homeopathy's Bureau of Surgery issued a generally favorable commentary on Listerism and antiseptic surgery in 1883. Seven years later the Bureau's physicians reported to its membership: "The year's experience has seemed only to strengthen the general faith in antiseptic surgery. Indeed, its practice may be said to have had almost no opposition, at least so far as open demonstration against it is concerned."[24] Homeopaths accepted these findings and educators like Pratt taught students to use Lister's carbolic acid or even "Listerine" as antiseptic agents.

Homeopaths began to acknowledge (or resist) the significance of medical science exactly as members of the regular profession did, and as clinical therapeutics incorporated scientific know-how, past differences between regulars and homeopaths diminished ipso facto. Growing financial, professional, and scientific inducements to accommodate and adapt offset any reason to separate oneself based on dogma and empiricism. Old-style medicine, with its guesswork and ineffectual results, had caused rifts between doctors, but scientific medicine unified them through logic and results, setting the basis for a new collective professional consensus.

Many of the era's orthodox physicians argued that they had defeated homeopathic medicine through science. In turn, some modern medical historians contend that today's medical doctors descended directly from orthodox practitioners and deny homeopaths any lineage. Both claims are incorrect. Revolutionary changes in the natural sciences transformed the whole of medical theory, medical education and training, and medical practice. As much as orthodox physicians deemed homeopathy a medical sect based on nonsensical theories, their own clinical activities were haphazard and unscientific. The regular profession was little more than orthodox sectarianism with its own exclusive dogma of bloodletting boondoggles and irrational druggings. The truly meaningful difference between the two groups was that regulars enjoyed mainstream support because they outnumbered homeopaths. "Today our profession is regarded by the State," explained a thoughtful orthodox physician, "as only a numerically strong medical sect."[25]

Thus, neither group can be regarded as the true ancestor of the modern medical doctor. Developments in scientific medicine snuffed out illogical and unscientific thinking for the whole of healing. In contrast to the clinical disagreements and personal feuds that plagued nineteenth-century medicine, therapeutic convergence and professional compromise between regulars and sectarians characterized the beginnings of twentieth-century American medicine. "Modern medicine has little sympathy for allopathy or for homeopathy," wrote one perceptive observer. "It simply denies outright the relevancy or value of either doctrine. It wants not dogma, but facts. It countenances no presupposition that is not common to it with all the natural sciences, with all logical thinking."[26]

The overpowering authority of scientific medicine dramatically changed the makeup of the profession. Patients no longer asked physicians from whose name they derived their medical authority—whether it be Hahnemann, Rush, or some other empiricist. A growing number of regulars came to understand that many sectarians were as well trained as they were and that the AMA's long-standing code of ethics, with its decree against dealings with homeopaths, was an anachronism. "Surely, if the object of this code were the suppression of quackery," wrote one critic, "its success can hardly be described as brilliant."[27] The emerging group of medical and surgical specialists opposed the code's restriction on consulting because without referrals from homeopaths they would lose a significant source of revenue. "Professional men of acknowledged ability and great reputation," reported one physician, "have said that they could not tell how many thousands of dollars they have lost by adhering to the old code, in declining consultations with irregulars."[28]

By the time of the Spanish-American War in 1898, there had been enough of a political rapprochement between medicine's factions that President William McKinley commented: "I have reviewed the subject and could find no law to prevent homeopaths from becoming surgeons and assistant surgeons in the army and navy."[29] Even the surgeon-general of the navy said that he was pleased to have homeopaths in the service because "it would be a great saving to the government by doing away with a large drug bill."[30]

The leadership of the AMA ultimately conceded that maintaining the half-century-old code of ethics was antithetical to medicine's future growth. "The time has come when we can not absolve ourselves from the responsibility of doing away with the inconsistencies for which we may now be properly criticized," wrote the president of the Association in 1902.[31] The organization replaced the rule the following year with a statement of principles that omitted any references to a physician's style of practice. "The new code frees us from the old charge of bigotry and it will kill the old cry of persecution," wrote Daniel Cathell, the previously homeopath-hating author of the bestselling *The Physician Himself*. "It will have a great and far-reaching effect on our material interest; it will everywhere promote and foster professional unity; and, far above all else, by putting an end to partisan agitations it will increase the good repute of every worthy medical man in America."[32] Cathell even reversed his earlier stance on specialization: "Be friendly and fair and show hearty good-will toward your brethren, 'The Specialists.' "[33]

Science, the final arbiter between valid and invalid clinical therapies, soon toppled Pratt's orificial surgical theories as well. Doubters long believed that orificial surgery's benefits included the power of suggestion and that Pratt's claims were little more than clinical exaggerations. "I have never from my own personal experience in a single instance seen any beneficial results from anal dilatation," wrote a prominent homeopathic cynic. "I express my own convictions from personal experience. In doing so, I claim the same right to think for myself and express my conclusions as I grant to others."[34] The death knell of orificial surgery was rung to the rhythm of homeopathic physicians fleeing to join the more broad-minded AMA.

With fewer referrals and a dwindling patient base, Pratt eventually closed his private hospital. He flirted with bankruptcy as his practice situation worsened, and he suffered a personal tragedy when his wife and only child died. In 1901 the *Journal of Orificial Surgery* abruptly ceased publication and the Chicago Homeopathic Medical College soon closed its doors. Pratt was no longer a professor of surgery and there was talk of disbanding the American Association of Orificial Surgeons. Damned by its illogical theories and its association with a weakened homeopathy movement, orificial surgery died a swift and silent death. It was but a vague memory in the minds of the nation's doctors by the end of World War I.

Much like orificial surgery, the rest of homeopathy also faded away. As science took hold and political squabbles lessened, younger men shied away from strict adherence to Hahnemann's theories and disavowed the relationship between healing and a vital spirit. Several homeopathic medical societies passed resolutions denying the validity of Hahnemann's drug laws. "The theory of dynamization of drugs promulgated by Hahnemann," wrote a committee of the Albany County (New York) Homeopathic Medical Society, "is false in theory, and should be discarded by the homeopathic profession."[35] In 1881 American homeopathy formally split into two opposing factions, the "purists," who organized the International Hahnemannian Association and denounced anybody attacking Hahnemann's ideas, and the "eclectics," who remained members of the American Institute of Homeopathy and prescribed both traditional and homeopathic remedies. Four decades later there were only two homeopathic medical schools in existence and fewer than one thousand avowed homeopathic physicians.

Despite its decline, homeopathy never completely retreated from the public's fascination. Remnants of the country's nineteenth-century homeopathic heritage remain in Hahnemann University Hospital in Philadelphia and with a massive bronze statue of Hahnemann dedicated in 1910 at Massachusetts Avenue and Sixteenth Street in Washington, D.C. In the 1970s, homeopathy's popularity began to revive and it has once again become an alternative system of therapeutics.

Irreconcilable Differences

The rise of scientific medicine not only led to clinical cooperation between regulars and homeopaths but also produced support for the restoration of medical licensing standards. Licensure laws had been swept away during the era of Andrew Jackson's self-help style of democracy and for over fifty years there were few limitations on the practice of medicine. As medical degrees had become easier to obtain, anyone who wanted to call himself a doctor could. New medical schools had opened at an alarming rate and the number of practicing physicians had skyrocketed in proportion to the population explosion following the Civil War: 64,000 in 1870; 85,000 a decade later; and, by century's end, 120,000 doctors cared for 76,000,000 Americans.

Since a medical degree was the only qualification needed to open a practice, a lucrative black market for bogus diplomas developed. Unscrupulous profiteers operated diploma mills. Parents bought degrees for their children or purchased them for themselves with the expectation that possession alone would improve their financial lot. The scandal reached international levels when immigrants, portraying themselves as fully trained American physicians, returned to their European homelands with a fake degree in hand. In Birmingham, England, the government prosecuted an individual for passing himself off as "M.D., Indianapolis." The investigator at the trial disparagingly noted that "such a title could only be one of those American degrees which could be got for a dollar or two."[36]

As the diploma mill scandal continued unabated, reputable practitioners concluded that state and federal governments needed to reestablish licensing legislation to close the medical degree loophole. "We need uniform state laws exacting of every one aspiring to practice medicine," declared a delegate to the AMA's annual convention. He further added that "proof of personal fitness and professional competency would prove the most potent agency in improving the standards of medical education and in enhancing the dignity and usefulness of the medical profession."[37]

Licensing improved the quality of physicians and science the quality of medical care, but specialization changed the character of American medicine at the turn of the century. It was one thing to apply an expertise, like obstetrics and gynecology, in the general practice of medicine but it was another to limit clinical cases to such expertise, forgoing unrelated work and assuming financial risk. John Morgan tried in the 1760s and ended up penniless. Specialization could not be monetarily rewarding until scientific medical knowledge expanded enough that generalists were no longer capable of handling the volume of the newly treatable ailments and the sophistication of newly discovered techniques. By the beginning of the twentieth century, these requirements had been met. "Doctors began to realize that by devoting themselves to one branch instead of working up a general practice," declared the president of the AMA, "they could often do more good, earn more money, and have less arduous work to perform."[38]

Generalists feared the competition from specialists, who threatened to cut into their profits and slowly whittle away their responsibilities. "The only question which can arise relates to the manner in which the specialist shall proceed," cautioned a prominent general practitioner. "Whether any or no attention shall be paid to the feelings and wishes of the profession; whether an individual shall pursue that course which is generally considered gentlemanly and honorable, or assume an ideal superiority over his brethren, and thus temporarily obtain a meretricious reputation and an undeserved reward."[39] Generalists regarded themselves as compassionate bedside clinicians and viewed specialists as aloof technicians, more interested in the wizardry of science than the art of healing. For two decades, the members of the AMA debated whether a specialist should be required to serve several years as a general practitioner before having the right to advertise his specialty. While the Association's doctors dillydallied, specialism flourished, propelled by the meteoric rise of scientific medicine, and the political strength of specialists grew.

These physicians, with their extra education, sophisticated gadgetry, and entrepreneurial ways, became powerbrokers within the profession. The specialists, who used hospital outpatient clinics and dispensaries more extensively than general practitioners, began to receive recognition from the institutions. Several big-city hospitals, spurred by increasing patient revenues in the 1870s, opened departments of dermatology, laryngology, neurology, and ophthalmology. Specialists established their own organizations with interests distinct from those of general practitioners. The American Ophthalmological Society and the American Otological Society, formed in the 1860s, presaged the mania for national specialty societies in the 1880s and 1890s, when the profession would expand to recognize gastroenterologists, gynecologists, laryngologists, neurologists, orthopedists, pediatricians, psychiatrists, urologists, and even proctologists.

Generalists were irate. They argued that specialty societies fragmented medicine and reduced the effectiveness of the AMA. "We have lost in some measure the unity of our professional organization," declared a two-time president of the Association, "and in the same proportion we have come to perceive clearly the existence of diverse, if not directly antagonistic interests. So much so, indeed, that it has become quite common to hear the interests of the general practitioner and the wants of the specialist spoken of as essentially distinct."[40] Specialists cared little about the criticisms. "If it be said that we are striking a blow at the AMA, we deny the soft impeachment," asserted the founder of the American Surgical Association. "On the contrary, we shall strengthen that body by rousing it from its Rip Van Winkle slumbers, and infusing new life into it."[41]

Railroads and Doctors

Initially confined to eastern cities, specialists spread across the land as their influence grew. "Every cross-road village has its ophthalmologist, aurist or gynecologist," observed a bemused medical writer at Fort Scott, Kansas, "not mentioning the gentlemen who in a minor way make the rectum, urethra, throat, nose, pharynx, etc., their particular field of onslaught."[42] Much of this was due to the explosive growth of railroads, whose steam-powered carriages bridged the physical gap between rural and urban America. Not only did railroads facilitate the spread of specialization, but the field of railway medicine was itself among the most prominent of early specialties.

Americans reveled in their expanding nineteenth-century railroad network and travelers used the railways as often as they could. The glamour and excitement of moving at breakneck speeds enchanted them. But railroads, that nineteenth-century metaphor for progress, had a sinister side. The Interstate Commerce Commission reported that at the turn of the century one of every 28 railroad employees was injured and one in 399 died on the job. "That much danger to life and limb is incurred by those who are thus engaged in this special vocation is self-evident," wrote one contemporary expert. "Even in localities where the strictest supervision and management are employed to avoid danger, the number of accidents is painfully large."[43]

Each year railway accidents also injured thousands of passengers. There was the widely reported 1876 Ashtabula River disaster in Ohio that resulted in ninety-two fatalities when a bridge collapse caused eleven passenger cars to plunge one hundred fifty feet into a frozen creek. Even more spectacular was the 1882 crash in Spuyten Duyvil, on the northern border of New York City, where a rear-end collision triggered a massive conflagration killing eight prominent politicians and dozens more— local farmers rolled giant snowballs down a hillside in an attempt to extinguish the blaze. Railway medicine arose out of necessity, and a new breed of physician, the railway doctor, emerged to care for these patients and advise railroad officials on public health, workplace safety, and sanitation issues.

Railway medicine quickly developed into a de facto medical specialty with its own textbooks, journals, and national, state, and local associations. Railway physicians were usually small-town general practitioners who learned their trade on the job. They offered a full spectrum of medical and surgical care for railroad employees and passengers, from completing routine physical examinations to delivering babies to repairing hernias. In 1888 the National Association of Railway Surgeons was established and several years later it had over fifteen hundred dues-paying members. "The associations of railway doctors are wholly scientific, in their objects, and you might say philanthropic," asserted one railway specialist, "and only seek to improve themselves by coming together and discussing the various methods of taking care of the maimed and injured victims of accidents."[44] The Association's annual meetings were among the best attended medical conventions in the country (hardly surprising as the far-flung members all had direct connections to the nation's transportation network). Whether it was in Galveston, Omaha, or St. Louis, hundreds of doctors gathered to learn the latest research in railroad medicine. Manufacturing and pharmaceutical companies also came to promote their products. At the tenth annual convention in Chicago in 1897, representatives from Eli Lilly, Johnson & Johnson, McKessin & Robbins, Parke-Davis, the Pasteur Vaccine Company, and Searle & Hereth attended.

Thousands claimed expertise in railway medicine, but few influenced the specialty like Christian Stemen. He was a well-traveled and experienced doctor, who served as chief physician to the Pennsylvania Railroad Company and as a medical consultant to the Pittsburgh, Fort Wayne and Chicago Railway and the Wabash Railroad. Stemen was a religious evangelical and president of the National Association of Local Preachers. His medical education, which included regular and sectarian schools, was typical of that of many midwestern practitioners. Stemen initially had an itinerant practice based wherever Ohio's railway lines transported new settlers. This wearisome routine changed in the mid-1870s when he moved to Indiana and organized the proprietary Fort Wayne College of Medicine. As the school's business-minded professor of medicine, Stemen influenced much of the delivery of health care in that region, and his prior work experience convinced him that alliances with railroad companies were critical to medicine's future prosperity.

"Railway medicine is rapidly becoming the leading specialty of medical and surgical practice in the United States," Stemen told his students and other physicians, "and requires special study and preparation."[45] Private railroad carriers needed to develop some manner of medical organization to better care for their employees and passengers. Stemen foresaw that such efforts would turn into large-scale bureaucracies with sizable budgets and become a windfall for thousands of doctors. Acting on his entrepreneurial hunches, Stemen founded an organization, the awkward-sounding Surgical Society of the Wabash, St. Louis and Pacific Railway East of the

Mississippi River, to act as a liaison between physicians and railroads. He organized a second group, the Surgical Society of the Pittsburgh, Fort Wayne and Chicago Railway, several months later in late 1882.

Stemen also traveled throughout Europe investigating the methods railways used to care for their workers. He admired the vigor of the foreign railway medicine movement and agreed that scientific medicine, especially bacteriology and Listerism, should be the catalyst for shaping the American movement into a more cohesive and influential force. "Having been a strong believer in antiseptic dressing before going abroad," proclaimed Stemen, "I have returned with a stronger belief than ever in this mode of dressing wounds."[46]

He wrote the country's first textbook on railway medicine and promoted a new journal, *The Railway Surgeon,* as the official organ of the National Association of Railway Surgeons. The magazine proved an effective lobbying tool for thousands of railway physicians, with advice columns, editorials, national news reports, and scientific articles.

The National Association pushed for railroads to maintain medical departments and build private hospitals under the authority of a chief surgeon. Company executives agreed, and by 1896 thirteen railroads managed twenty-five hospitals that treated over 165,000 patients annually. Several of the larger hospitals were state-of-the-art facilities and became celebrated as first-class training centers for interns and residents. In these financially flush hospitals, managers could be forward-thinking in their philosophies regarding inpatient care. "In all ways the policy of the management is broad-gauge and liberal. No effort is made to economize in any matter wherein the welfare of a patient is concerned,"[47] wrote a reporter describing the availability of surgical specialists, horse-drawn ambulances, and a twenty-eight-hundred-volume library at the Missouri Pacific Hospital in St. Louis. Administrators also provided novel outpatient services through specially equipped "emergency department" railroad cars. These relief cars reached the far-flung outposts of any railway system and foreshadowed the U.S. Army's famed Mobile Army Surgical Hospital—MASH—units. They had full-service operating and recovery rooms and hot water from the locomotive's boiler to sterilize bandages and instruments. "The patient has more chances of recovery," wrote a railway physician describing the emergency car, "and he himself, as well as the surgeons and officials of the road, rests content with the knowledge that every effort has been made for the best possible results."[48]

The railroad industry led the development of employee medical programs at the turn of the twentieth century, with hundreds of thousands of workers, tens of thousands of physicians, and hundreds of hospitals, clinics, and outpatient dispensaries. These services, ranging from prepaid medical and hospital plans to long-term-care benefits, were rudimentary precursors to modern-day managed care. Railroads used mandatory payroll deductions to fund the programs, leaving the employees little choice but to use company-assigned doctors. Many workers disliked the system because they could not choose their own physician. In cases of work-related injuries, where a medical evaluation determined compensation awards, the injured employee naturally distrusted any physician paid by the company.

Many physicians also opposed the program, which challenged the conventional view of the doctor as an independent decision maker with unquestioned authority. Stemen and other leaders attempted to counter such hostility. They stressed the financial security of working for a railroad and how a physician's presence decreased fraudulent injury claims; by protecting railway companies from lawsuits, doctors maintained the financial well-being of an industry vital to the country's growth. "Railway physicians are serving the best interests of the company," suggested one doctor in a speech before the New York Medico-Legal Society, "and on the principle that 'a dollar saved is as good as a dollar earned' we hold that we are constantly protecting the company."[49]

Critics rejected these explanations and rarely concealed their contempt for and suspicion of company doctors. Medical societies denied memberships to railway physicians and passed resolutions declaring contract medicine an ethical abomination. Some saw contract practice as exploitive, especially when companies had physicians bidding their fees down against each other. "Too much of the spirit of trade has already found its way into the profession, and its further encroachment should be resisted, not encouraged," cautioned a report from the AMA's Committee on Railroad Practice. "Let us continue to maintain, so far as that is yet possible, the old relations of perfect freedom between physicians and patients, with separate compensation for each separate service."[50]

Most of the men who became railway physicians did so to supplement their meager incomes as general practitioners, not due to their political or professional embrace of corporate medicine. In rural and poorer areas companies paid higher salaries for doctors willing to relocate. The vast majority of railway physicians were general practitioners who performed surgical operations, provided obstetrical care, and proffered advice on personal and family matters. They had neither the financial wherewithal nor the clinical willingness to limit their practice to specialties like operative surgery or obstetrics and gynecology. Indeed, their use of the term "surgeon," as evidenced in their journal, *The Railway Surgeon,* or their national organization, the National Association of Railway Surgeons, was a professional misnomer and a public-relations disaster. Perhaps railway doctors were trying to capitalize on the rising medical status, compensation, and social recognition of specialty surgeons. To suggest that railway doctors during this era were more surgeon than physician is inaccurate.

Despite the rapid ascent of the railway doctor, the specialty failed to gain traction within the medical profession and suffered a swift decline. Although railway care made up a considerable portion of the country's total medical practice, no railway physician ever assumed an important leadership position within mainstream medicine. Other specialty societies rarely recognized railway doctors. The nation's physicians opposed the contract practice of railway doctors and feared that corporate capitalism could dominate medicine. The National Association was moribund by 1920, and the journal, *The Railway Surgeon,* dropped the word "railway."

Stemen's fate typified the lost legacy of railway physicians. Leaders of mainstream medicine snubbed him and the standard biographical listings and various medical bibliographies of the period omitted his name. Medical historians forgot Stemen despite a string of accomplishments that included his being the successor to ex-president Benjamin Harrison on the board of trustees of Purdue University; one of the few American physicians to be a member of the British Medical Association; father of one of the first female doctors in Kansas; founder of Taylor University; and railway medicine's most seminal thinker.

Despite the demise of the specialty, ex-railway doctors continued to practice their brand of general medicine, which included dabbling in surgery. General practitioners, however, could no longer be conversant with the growing intricacies of medicine. As specialization advanced, they were less capable of treating complex illnesses, less skilled at managing difficult emergencies, and less adept at performing technically complex operations. The generalists seemed displaced by a more sophisticated profession. "Specialism is a necessary phenomenon of progress, and cannot be ignored," claimed one individual. "Nay, I would go farther and would say that it should be fostered and encouraged, for in this direction, only is healthy growth to be obtained."[51]

Discussions during the first years of the new century about how to restrict the activities of generalists led to a political stalemate. With new licensing legislation already curbing the public's selection of physicians, specialists battled generalists over the right to provide any manner of specialty-style care, especially surgical operations. Doctors would long be perplexed by how to draw a professional line between the self-professed specialist, who remained a general practitioner, and the growing class of highly skilled, clinically focused specialists.

American medicine had become a shifting patchwork of overlapping factions: generalists and specialists; regulars and irregulars; national, state, and local medical societies; licensing boards and medical school administrators; public hospitals and private practitioners. The nation's physicians nonetheless had a measure of the organizational unity and clinical competency that eluded them throughout the nineteenth century.

Part Two

COMING OF AGE

❧ Five ❧

SCIENTIFIC ADVANCEMENT

Lehrfreiheit and *Lernfreiheit*

I N THE DECADES that followed American independence, medical education in the new nation improved, but it still lagged behind that of Europe, despite the fact that most of the country's great physicians—John Morgan, Benjamin Rush, and Franklin Hamilton among them—had studied abroad. By the middle of the nineteenth century the center of academic medical study on the Continent had once again shifted. This time from France to Germany and Austro-Hungary, where men like Engels, Nietzsche, and Schopenhauer forged the modern intellectual canon. Great Britain's medical reputation, unparalleled in Morgan and Rush's day, had long ago given way to French clinical innovations, which now yielded to Germanic authority in the sciences.

American doctors educated and trained after the Civil War looked increasingly to German-speaking universities, known for sophisticated teaching methods and specialized medical knowledge. "The French had something to teach, namely, the importance of opening the hospital wards freely to medical students," wrote a contemporary observer, "but we had more to learn from the German method of building up medical education in an orderly fashion to the end that the student first acquired the tools and the technique with which gradually to win his independence."[1]

The trickle of American physicians traveling to German-speaking countries soon became a flood. Over fifteen thousand American healers—students, recent graduates, middle-aged practitioners, even retir-

117

ees—took courses, completed research, or received a medical degree at German-speaking universities between 1870 and 1915. It almost seemed a requirement to have studied in Austro-Hungary or Germany to have any influence in American medicine during this time.

The exodus of American medical students spawned a cottage industry of Baedekers, advice columns, and travel narratives, each promising to help navigate the process of foreign study. Some suggested acclimation at a smaller university like Freiburg, Halle, Göttingen, Rostock, or Würzburg before moving to a larger urban campus: "In these [smaller] places there are not so many novel things to distract, and also the professors and their assistants will devote more time to a single person. They are all more or less fond of Americans, especially if they find them to be diligent."[2] Others offered more pragmatic advice: "If a young medical man is to go abroad, let him do so after his moral habits have become so fixed that they are not easily upset by such deceitful vanities as wine and profligate women."[3] Henry Hun's 1883 *A Guide to American Medical Students in Europe* left little to chance—it listed Atlantic Ocean steamship lines, gave baggage-handling tips, and even inserted a last-minute appendix showing changes to university faculties since the initial manuscript had been submitted.

American doctors marveled at the well-financed, ever-growing state-sponsored universities in Austro-Hungary and Germany. They featured fully equipped laboratories, intense rivalries between professors, and bustling hospitals with bedside teaching. Universities expected their junior and senior faculty to conduct scientific and clinical research, the sine qua non of an academic medical career, and students benefited from exposure to such work. "The German and Austrian hospitals were practically a part of the universities," wrote an American physician, "and M.D.'s pursuing graduate courses of study had much freer access to patients than was allowed to undergraduate students in this country."[4] Students performed hands-on examinations ("touch classes")[5] of pregnant women, operated on cadavers, studied patients using cystoscopes, laryngoscopes, ophthalmoscopes, otoscopes, proctoscopes, and stethoscopes. "The object of these courses is not to discuss the theory of the disease," wrote Hun, "but to train the students in the use of their eyes, hands, ears, and medical instruments in the examination of patients."[6]

Germanic schools offered Americans unprecedented educational freedom. *Lehrfreiheit* (free teaching) and *Lernfreiheit* (free learning) meant that bureaucracy was removed from the educational environment and that both teachers and students were encouraged to study whatever topics interested them. "There is such freedom in the laboratory [in Germany]," said one American, "that one has the opportunity of seeing everybody else's work, so that if I did nothing myself, I could not fail to learn a great deal."[7] The system allowed easy transfer from one academic center to another, and each city's university had its particular strength. In Breslau, Leipzig, and Strasbourg, schools boasted the basic sciences, those of Dresden and Prague offered obstetrics, while Heidelberg was famous for nervous diseases.

No city had greater appeal than Vienna, with its rich history and varied medical opportunities, and its professional establishment both embraced and exploited foreign doctors. Schools offered classes in English and used high tuitions to boost revenues. Exchange students and expatriates formed an American Medical Association of Vienna to organize information and provide a meeting place. It recalled the Virginia Club of Edinburgh that American students had established over a century earlier in Scotland. Membership was prestigious and the University of Vienna acknowledged this with certificates and other documentation. Returning American physicians papered their office walls with these records that attested to their newly acquired knowledge and technical skills.

"Popsy"

William Henry Welch, like many in his generation, had traveled to Germany to complete his medical education. He had graduated from Yale University and earned his medical degree from Columbia University's College of Physicians and Surgeons before heading to Europe. His experience with German medical education would shape him and, in turn, all of medical education in America. Balding, bearded, and portly, Welch would eventually become the dean of the Johns Hopkins School of Medicine—the "dean of American medicine," according to many—and in that role he would mold the character of early- to mid-twentieth-century American health care.

Welch was a medical visionary, insightful and imaginative. Drawing on his exposure to German universities, he realized that important medical breakthroughs would occur if American doctors related laboratory research to their clinical practice. These advances in patient care would in turn lead to increased professional and social prestige for doctors. Welch also felt that physicians could better secure a cultural authority to complement their rising professional status by demonstrating their humanism, and he advocated a medical education that encompassed the humanities: "The study of the languages, history and philosophy, which give a culture not to be derived solely from the study of the natural sciences should add greatly to the intellectual pleasure, satisfaction, breadth of vision and even efficiency of the man of science."[8]

He was no mere medical theoretician, however, and his research and laboratory work alone made up a successful medical career. He made one of his era's most significant contributions in 1891 when he isolated the bacterium that causes gas gangrene, which kills living tissue and produces dreadful, often lethal, outcomes. While serving during World War I, Welch helped develop an antitoxin for this gas gangrene bacteria that minimized the impact of thousands of combat-related injuries. Welch's passion for research also facilitated the rapid expansion and acceptance of the field of bacteriology: "He immediately began spreading the new heretical doctrine that disease was caused by microscopic bodies," wrote a magazine reporter. "He found a fertile field for his missionary work and set up a laboratory, studied, taught, and practiced what he preached."[9]

Many characters in American medical history—Morgan is the classic example—outlived their contributions and died in anonymity, but Welch remained influential all his years. On his eightieth birthday in mid-April 1930, Welch appeared on *Time* magazine's cover. That same week he was honored at a celebrity-filled event in Washington that was carried live by the nation's major radio networks (shortwave transmissions broadcast the proceedings overseas). President Herbert Hoover, accompanied by his military and naval attachés, sat next to the famous physician and described him as the country's "greatest statesman in the field of public health." "He has happily combined in his character and intellect," remarked Hoover, "the love of truth and the patient experimental habit of the pure scientist, with the ingenuity of the inventor and the organizing vision and energy of the promoter of sound enterprise—and combines all these things with a worldly vision and gracious charm that have made him a leader amongst men."[10]

While the world at large celebrated Welch's medical achievements, he was known to his Baltimore community as much for his personality as his professional prowess. His enthusiastic and paternalistic nature led friends and students alike to nickname him "Popsy." He had a hearty laugh, was an engaging conversationalist, enjoyed the pleasures of eating and drinking, and delighted in being a memorable dinner companion. He lived life as a bachelor and fed the gossip mills of Baltimore (reputedly, at his death, an enormous collection of pornography was found in his house). Welch was a beloved oddball who habitually walked the city's streets during the late hours of the night, left for the weekend without revealing his destination, took nonstop roller-coaster rides at Coney Island, and refused to employ secretaries. His infamous behavior spawned the Johns Hopkins ditty "Nobody knows where Popsy eats, nobody knows where Popsy sleeps, nobody knows whom Popsy keeps, but Popsy."[11]

"If we only had such laboratories in America"

The roots of much of Welch's success and his irrepressible devotion to scientific medical research can be traced back to when he first studied in Europe in 1876 and 1877. His letters from this period contrast the cohesiveness and vitality of German medical schools with the underfunding, poor equipment, and chaotic organization of American facilities. "The laboratories are richly endowed by the government and are intended to give every encouragement to research," Welch wrote to his father. "If we only had such laboratories in America I am sure that we should be as productive in scientific discoveries as the Germans, for with such opportunities there would be no lack of patient, conscientious workers."[12]

For American medicine to advance properly, Welch came to believe that he and like-minded enthusiasts needed to press for significant new roles for scientific research in medicine. He would work to demonstrate that, as with the German-university model, a physician could make a living solely by teaching medicine and performing scientific research, a vision many American doctors found foolish and impractical. "How is it that no scientific work in medicine is done in [the United States], how is it that many good men who do well in Germany and show evident talent there are never heard of and never do any good work when they come back here," he wrote to his sister. "The answer is that there is no opportunity for, no appreciation of, no demand for that kind of work here. In Germany on the other hand every encouragement is held out to young men with taste for science."[13]

While Welch admired the research and rigor he found in German universities and laboratories, he readily dismissed certain aspects of German medical education that struck him as commercial or exploitive. He had little regard for Vienna, the center of medical culture for Americans abroad, where savvy, cash-hungry institutions offered every variety of clinical coursework in English. The city was overrun with American doctors seeking such clinical experience. "Vienna is in almost all respects much as I had pictured it in my mind to be and I do not regret that I have not spent more time here," he wrote. "Everything is given up to practical subjects, and the courses are conducted chiefly by young men who have no reputation and whose only aim is to make money."[14] Welch felt that his profession would be doomed if doctors simply maintained a sophisticated, profitable clinical practice without improving medical treatment through scientific research.

Following his return to New York in 1878, Welch struggled for several years to advance his cause. He taught the country's first laboratory course in pathology at Bellevue Hospital Medical College. This initial effort brought too little money and required much time. Moreover, Welch could not focus on scientific research in a city (and a nation) where laboratory facilities were virtually nonexistent. "I sometimes feel rather blue when I look ahead and see that I am not going to be able to realize my aspirations in life," he wrote his sister. "I can teach microscopy and pathology, perhaps get some practice and make a living after a while, but that is all patchwork and the drudgery of life and what hundreds do."[15]

In early 1884 a visitor appeared at Welch's pathology workroom door with a proposal that would change his days. John Shaw Billings, a tall, handsome figure with a mane of silver hair and walrus-style mustache, had been scouring the world for the medical staff of a new hospital, and Welch was to be his prized catch. Billings, a well-respected physician, was chief medical adviser to the president of Johns Hopkins University. It was his latest role in a distinguished medical career that also included founding the Library of the Office of the Surgeon General of the United States (now the world-renowned National Library of Medicine). In his position at Johns Hopkins, he oversaw the planning of the new university-affiliated hospital and was even the actual designer—he eventually achieved greater fame designing the iconic Beaux Arts building of the New York Public Library on Fifth Avenue.

Like Welch, Billings was intrigued by German medicine and its close links with science. Billings had traveled to Europe to familiarize himself with the German-speaking universities while researching design ideas for the Johns Hopkins complex. "The German universities are great corporations, with special powers of jurisdiction over their inmates," Billings told an audience upon his return, "and it is considered a special honor and privilege to come under this peculiar jurisdiction."[16] He determined to recruit a hospital staff and medical school faculty only from Americans who had studied abroad, which largely meant German-speaking countries.

Billings summed up his thoughts of his first encounter with Welch in a letter to the president of Johns Hopkins University: "I saw Dr. Welch, had a long talk with him—heard him lecture—and saw him directing work in his laboratory.... I think he will develop well."[17] Welch, who later said that "of all the men I have ever known, [Billings] was about the wisest,"[18] took little time to accept the offer to join the new hospital.

The trustees of Johns Hopkins University pronounced Welch the inaugural professor of pathology in April 1884. His responsibilities included staff planning for the hospital, which would not admit patients until 1889, and curriculum development for the medical school, which would not officially open until 1893. The New York medical profession was shocked. Never before had there been an instance of so ambitious and able a young man exchanging a brilliant future in practice for an academic professorship. Welch's atypical decision changed the course of medicine in America by raising academic research to the level of clinical practice.

The professorship freed Welch of financial worries and a liberated Welch devoted the next year to doing everything in his power to prepare for his new responsibility. At the urging of the Johns Hopkins's trustees, he returned to Europe to keep abreast of the most recent scientific developments. For twelve months, Welch worked with Austro-Hungary's and Germany's leading bacteriologists and interviewed the region's hospital administrators and medical educators. Welch finally arrived in Baltimore in the fall of 1885, prepared with rigorous scientific training and knowledge of the world's up-and-coming medical scientists. He was full of get-up-and-go, spending days and nights outfitting his pathology laboratory and preparing a series of lectures on bacteriology for the city's physicians. In the midst of this, Welch also traveled about the nation to visit its hospitals and medical schools. He found himself, according to an acquaintance, "in a place in the world that was perfect to his needs and desires."[19]

When the Johns Hopkins Hospital opened in 1889, it quickly became a center of medical research and a financial success. A jubilant Welch reported to its board that patient beds were filled to capacity. Since his laboratory was the hospital's academic center, it set the tone for the whole institution. The sophisticated level and extraordinary amount of scientific research carried out under Welch's supervision astounded visitors. Enthusiastic clinicians and laboratory men lived and worked together. "Each one was interested in all that was going on," remarked an eyewitness.[20] Increasing numbers of recently graduated medical students from throughout the country arrived to perform scientific research in Welch's laboratory. They even included the son of the most outspoken critic of Welch's departure from New York for Johns Hopkins as well as one future surgeon general of the U.S. Army, George Sternberg and his brilliant protégé Walter Reed.

"We are lucky to get in as professors"

The Johns Hopkins Medical School opened in the fall of 1893 and departed dramatically from its forebears in American medical education. Welch organized the new medical school according to the medical education paradigm developed in the universities of Austro-Hungary and Germany. For the first time in the history of American medicine, a medical college was fully integrated into the academic workings of a larger university. "There is no saving grace in merely calling a medical school a department of a university," explained Welch. "The medical school must be a vital, integral part of the university."[21]

Johns Hopkins quickly attracted the country's best talent as students and as professors. The large number of premedical applicants and the small class size had created a spirited competition for admission. The initial class comprised fourteen men and three women (Hopkins guaranteed the acceptance of women, a major advance for medical education). "We are lucky to get in as professors," quipped a faculty member to Welch, "for I am sure that neither you nor I could ever get in as students."[22] The faculty was first-rate. They were also young, most in their thirties. As time passed, the reputation of the medical staff became extraordinary, and a list of their names read like a who's who of America's healing great.

Welch and his colleagues, for the first time in American medical education, required all students to familiarize themselves with the progress of disease in patients. During the first two years, students studied the pathological and physiological workings of diseases in the laboratory, took case histories, and began to examine the sick on the hospital's wards. Third- and fourth-year students, spurred to work day and night, followed the progress of their patients until discharge or death. These doctors-to-be discussed their cases with attending physicians, performed clinical laboratory tests, assisted at surgical operations, and aided with autopsies if their patients died.

In essence, a Johns Hopkins medical education meant learning by doing. The intensive laboratory work of the first two years mitigated the tedium of basic scientific instruction. The around-the-clock bedside care of the last two years ensured that the academic medical knowledge developed into professional and practical competency. The gradual increase in clinical responsibility given to the students made this educational experience unique and rewarding. No American medical school had ever provided a system that afforded appropriate education at all levels. It was a revolution in medical schooling of the first order.

Verdeutsched

To implement his vision of reform in medical education, Welch needed men with scientific know-how, medical savoir faire, and a gusto for teaching. These qualities did not frequently intersect in late-nineteenth-century medicine—recall the Garfield disaster earlier in the decade—but Welch chose wisely and recruited a faculty that would go on to found many of the various branches of modern medicine. One of them, William Stewart Halsted, stood out with his passion for scientific research and his zeal for the German approach to medical education and training.

Welch chose Halsted to be the professor of surgery—a title that conveyed professional esteem and job security—and the young doctor would become the preeminent surgeon of his generation and one of the greatest of all time. Most agreed that Halsted was a technical genius in the operating room, a brilliant innovator in the laboratory, and a guiding taskmaster in the classroom. Welch admiringly called him a "genuinely scientific surgeon," who was "animated in high degree by the spirit of scientific inquiry." He also called Halsted "notable" for his "work as teacher and leader of a school of surgery."[23] While Halsted stood out for his professional success and technical abilities, his appointment stemmed from his long-standing personal relationship with Welch. It was Welch's devotion to Halsted that resurrected the surgeon's career, and probably saved his life, when this greatest of all operating room technicians fell victim to his own medical curiosity and became addicted to cocaine.

Halsted grew up in Manhattan, where his father was a well-to-do wholesaler of European dry goods. The wiry youth took advantage of all the opportunities that mid-nineteenth-century America offered its Anglo-Saxon upper class, from the family's stately mansion on Fifth Avenue and Fourteenth Street to its country estate in Irvington-on-the-Hudson. The family fortune supported his various pursuits, which included stints at Yale, Columbia, and Bellevue, the same educational path as Welch.

Halsted also lived for two years in Europe, where he came under the sway of Germanic university education. Arriving in Vienna in November 1878, he studied anatomy and embryology for six months and devoted the remaining eighteen months to observing physicians and surgeons at university hospitals. "I sat upon the benches, often seven hours a day, listening to medical lectures," wrote Halsted. "I was so impressed with the characters and lives of some of my teachers that I believed they represented all that was most advanced in medicine."[24] A Johns Hopkins colleague once said Halsted was "very much *verdeutsched*."[25]

He returned to New York in September 1880 with an enthusiasm and a depth of knowledge that marked him as one of the city's up-and-coming physicians. Halsted was a whirlwind of activity over the next four years during which he joined numerous hospital staffs and began counting some of the most eminent names in New York medicine among his close friends. "Halsted was the most talked-of of the younger surgeons of that period in New York and many of the older ones shook their heads over his innovations," recalled Welch.[26]

Halsted's gumption especially impressed Welch when, in 1883, the thirty-one-year-old surgeon snubbed Bellevue's physicians over their antipathy to Listerian principles of antisepsis. Halsted had come to favor Listerism while studying abroad, where his Germanic professor-surgeons had been among the first to employ Lister's spray. Upon his return, he generally refused to perform surgical operations without proper sterile conditions. Bellevue's older operating rooms did not fit his needs, so he raised $10,000 and erected his own operating room in a tent on the hospital's grounds. Halsted's new surgical tent had piped-in gas, hot and cold running water, apertures for light and ventilation, a central drainage gutter, and a maple floor as "fine as a bowling alley."[27] Only in such a controlled environment could Halsted apply his methods of antisepsis. "He ranks among the first," wrote an astounded Welch, "if not the first, to develop in this country on the basis of these principles a consistent and thorough antiseptic technique."[28]

Halsted approached his social life with the same dedication and care he gave to surgery. He was an integral part of Manhattan's Gilded Age party scene, with a luxuriously furnished bachelor pad at Madison Avenue and Twenty-fifth Street and membership in the nearby University Club. There were endless dinner parties, musical soirées, and open houses, all attended by a revolving group of prominent young professionals and businessmen. Welch, among the more frequent guests, recalled Halsted the host as a "model of muscular strength and vigor, full of enthusiasm and of the joy of life."[29] These were pleasant times for Halsted, who was becoming one of New York's more successful physicians.

Then, in mid-1884, a series of scientific events forever altered his life. In Vienna, Sigmund Freud authored a comprehensive review of the physiological effects of cocaine and its potential use in treating certain neurological diseases. In the report, he noted the anesthetizing effect that cocaine had when it encountered the skin. One of Freud's colleagues then discovered that applying a few drops of liquid cocaine could numb not only the skin but the eye. When these startling findings were discussed at a medical meeting in Heidelberg, a visiting American physician reported it to a New York–based medical journal, introducing the profound discovery to an American audience that included Halsted.

The Professor and Cocaine

Although less dramatic than the 1846 announcement of ether anesthesia, the news of the discovery of cocaine's anesthetic qualities sparked widespread reaction in America. Physicians began to experiment with it in a haphazard fashion—the drug's use was not yet regarded as a social problem. People wrote books about cocaine's application in ear, nose, and throat surgery, articles flooded the medical journals, and scientific magazines carried full-page pharmaceutical company advertisements about the wonders of the drug. General stores freely offered derivatives of cocaine to treat health-related complaints, from the gastrointestinal consequences of infected food and polluted water sources to nasal congestion from allergies and colds. The drug was a key ingredient in a variety of all-purpose health tonics, including a recently developed carbonated, nonalcoholic refresher named Coca-Cola. Demand for the drug exploded and the lay public believed it could relieve anything. As physician investigators soon realized, cocaine cured little.

Halsted, an indefatigable medical innovator, also began evaluating the usefulness of cocaine for surgery. Through experiments on himself and others, he determined how to inject the drug to block nerves and obtain local anesthesia in differing areas. It was an impressive scientific achievement made all the more spectacular since he served as his own guinea pig.

But Halsted began to enjoy the pleasant side effects of cocaine. He found that the stimulating results of the drug's use gave him increased stamina in the lab and made even mundane social encounters feel exhilarating. Halsted snuffed it at the theater and even injected his friends. Unaware of cocaine's addictive qualities, Halsted used it freely and indiscriminately. He was drug dependent within six months, acting irrational and facing professional ruin.

Halsted's personal crisis unfolded during Welch's yearlong sabbatical to Europe in 1885. Welch sensed the seriousness of his friend's problem upon his return. After settling in Baltimore, Welch determined to help Halsted. Physicians in this era barely understood drug addiction and effective medical treatments were unavailable—seclusion combined with fresh air and exercise was the routine therapy. Welch convinced Halsted to join him for a therapeutic sailing trip to the Caribbean's Windward Islands (now the southern islands of the Lesser Antilles). The voyage, in February and March of 1886, was an unmitigated disaster as Halsted filched cocaine and alcohol from the ship's supply room.

Welch despaired over his friend's behavior and urged Halsted to admit himself to a mental hospital. Seven months of treatment transformed Halsted from a straight cocaine addict to a mixed cocaine and morphine user. At the same time, his father pleaded guilty to embezzlement, leaving the family's finances in ruin.

Realizing there was neither a professional nor a social future for Halsted in New York, Welch insisted that he move to Baltimore. There, under his friend's watchful supervision, Halsted would work in the new pathology laboratory, undertaking what one medical historian called "a form of occupational therapy."[30] Welch promised Halsted little besides a chance to regain his footing. There was no pledge, implicit or otherwise, of an academic appointment to the inchoate Johns Hopkins faculty. Halsted's attempt at recuperation failed nonetheless, and he returned to the mental hospital, spending most of 1887 as an inpatient.

The romantic tale of Halsted, an upstart surgeon wending his way through the chaotic world of 1880s American health care, seemed to have reached its end. Drug dependent, socially disgraced, and financially weakened, he found little pleasure in science or medicine. But the unexpected happened during Halsted's latest confinement. He managed to lessen his unrestrained abuse of cocaine and morphine and replaced it with a controlled addiction solely to morphine. Halsted's use of morphine was no less a habit and would remain his lifelong nemesis, but he regained control over his day-to-day existence.

Halsted's Resurrection

Halsted moved back to Baltimore in January 1888 and resumed his research in Welch's laboratory. During this time he devised some of his landmark studies on wound healing, the proper handling of tissues during an operation, and elements of the modern mastectomy and groin hernia repair. Halsted gradually began seeing patients and performing operations at hospitals around the city. Undoubtedly, he hoped to obtain a staff position at the Johns Hopkins Hospital when it opened the following year. Just three months after the hospital's start, Welch wrote a faculty member, "Halsted (popularly known in hospital circles as Jack the Ripper) does nothing but operate the whole forenoon and it must be admitted with brilliant results."[31]

Halsted the clinician, educator, and scientist had returned, but these reincarnations vastly differed from what they had been. His changed personality and demeanor were obvious to those who had known him earlier in his career. Drug addiction had taken its toll. The bold and enterprising surgeon was gone, as was his joie de vivre. Instead, there was an aloof, overly deliberate physician, who wielded his scalpel in a cautious, laborious, and perfectionist manner. Some younger medical students sarcastically referred to his sophisticated clinical discussions as "shifting dullness,"[32] an allusion to Halsted's ability to make things boring. The outspoken scientific researcher had turned into an obsessive and reclusive investigator who relished the privacy of the laboratory. When Halsted walked through the corridors of Johns Hopkins Hospital he characteristically bowed his head low, so as to avoid personal interactions. It was this incarnation of Halsted, whom faculty members and students solemnly referred to as "the Professor,"[33] that the nation's doctors would come to recognize as the quintessential researcher, surgeon, and teacher, an unapproachable medical genius.

Halsted's progress pleased Welch and, in February 1889, he convinced Johns Hopkins's doubting trustees (how much they knew of Halsted's drug difficulties remains an open question) to appoint Halsted to an interim staff position. Others, including the recently named professor of medicine William Osler, supported the appointment as well: "Halsted is doing remarkable work in Surgery. I feel that his appointment to the University and the Hospital would be quite safe."[34]

Despite his ongoing addiction, Halsted never experienced any further mental deterioration and his academic career took off. Three years later, the trustees made Halsted's appointment permanent, testament to Welch's instincts and devotion. "No greater good fortune could have befallen The Johns Hopkins Hospital and later the Medical School," recalled Welch, "than to find Halsted here on the ground."[35] Halsted was now surgeon in chief to the hospital and would shortly be named the school's first professor of surgery. For the next three decades, his legend would grow, as both the courtly, punctilious professor and the absentminded laboratory loner.

Halsted's scientific successes attracted worldwide attention and, over the years, thousands of physicians traveled to Baltimore to witness Halsted with scalpel in hand. They came to observe the latest operating techniques practiced at the epicenter of American medical education. Some marveled at the precision and control Halsted displayed: "He never seemed nervous, he was never in a hurry, neither blood nor unusual difficulties disturbed his equilibrium."[36] Others were less impressed. "Four hours to do a breast. Think of it," said a doubter. "Four solid hours for an operation that ought to take but an hour and a half at the most. Whew!"[37] While these contrasting attitudes were both objectively correct, the former eventually pushed out the latter.

Halsted conducted surgery as a form of scientific inquiry, a manifestation of Welch's maxim that good medicine meant good research. Gone were the centuries-old speed counts way of doing things. He introduced rubber gloves and scrubs into the operating room. Halsted banned rapidity and roughness as the surgeon's way of doing things, replacing them with accuracy, carefulness, and thoroughness in the handling of tissues. His methods went beyond simple safety in surgery. Halsted pioneered a series of innovative surgical procedures that supplanted the old-fashioned, helter-skelter slicing away of disease. His operations of the bile ducts, blood vessels, intestines, and thyroid were meant to restore form and function to as near to normal as possible. Halsted's acolytes labeled these practices and principles "Halstedian technique."

The Halstedian technique symbolized an American revolution in surgery that soon spread far beyond the American operating theater. The Halsted school of painstakingly slow but safe surgery, with its outstanding results, transformed surgery the world over. Modern surgery started here. Halsted's influence became so great that more than a century later surgeons can still attribute many of their methods to those of the Baltimore master.

Surgeons of the Highest Type

Welch said that Halsted, despite his acclaim as a technical innovator, "found the greatest satisfaction of his life in the training of surgeons."[38] Halsted began devoting his energy to figuring out how best to institutionalize surgical training. "We need a system," he told a group of Yale doctors, "which will produce not only surgeons but surgeons of the highest type, men who will stimulate the first youths of our country to study surgery and to devote their energies and their lives to raising the standard of surgical science."[39] Halsted's system would soon set the standard for how postgraduate medical training and its end result, specialization, would evolve.

Welch, Halsted, and the other Johns Hopkins faculty members agreed that the current single-year internship (the term "intern" implied that the doctor lived in the hospital) left the medical graduate too inexperienced. "He acquires a confidence in himself and a self-complacency which may be useful in time of emergency," warned Halsted, "but which tend to blind him to his inadequacy and to warp his career."[40] Internships had been part of the country's medical education in some form since midcentury. They allowed a small number of recent graduates an opportunity to become skilled at examining patients in a controlled hospital environment in an era when medical schools did not provide such clinical settings. The majority of doctors simply learned practical medicine at the bedsides of their private patients.

The country's internship infrastructure could not keep pace with the late-nineteenth-century explosion in medical knowledge. Traditional internships, which provided a modicum of experience without formalized continuing medical education, trained the old-fashioned general practitioner, not the modern, science-oriented specialist. With the growth in medical knowledge, internships eventually had to divide into medical and surgical types. They also became entries into specialization, but one or two years was not enough time to produce capable specialists. Aspiring specialists, particularly surgeons, sought some type of hospital appointment to gain sufficient technical skills. Candidates were competing vigorously for such training opportunities in the last decade of the nineteenth century.

The Johns Hopkins Medical School sought to fill this need with a more rigorous and sophisticated post-medical-school training program. "Medical education is not completed at the medical school, it is only begun,"[41] Welch told a group of Harvard doctors. He, Halsted, and other faculty members wanted to imitate in Baltimore the German-speaking university system of "assistantships" for postgraduate medical education and training. In that system, "assistants," the brightest medical school graduates, competed for hospital positions and the eventual opportunity, after many years and advancing levels of responsibility, to serve as chief associate to a professor. German universities structured the assistantship program like a pyramid—every year, less competitive assistants dropped out until only one remained.

Halsted designed his surgical residency program at Johns Hopkins after these Germanic assistantships. The surgeons-to-be (all of them had completed an obligatory internship) supervised those junior to them, allowing one professor to maximize his teaching presence. The program demanded residents to spend years—upward of a decade at times—surviving physical rigors, constant competition, and financial hardship. The residency did not guarantee that participants would retain their status year over year. Their motivation, besides a desire to acquire knowledge and skills, was the opportunity to have Halsted designate them as his house surgeon (in today's parlance, chief resident), the pinnacle of surgical success. "These positions are not for those who so soon weary of the study of their profession," warned Halsted, "and it is a fact that the zeal and industry of these young assistants seem to increase as they advance in years and as their knowledge and responsibilities become greater."[42] The hospital's departments of medicine and gynecology instituted similar residency systems. "I think that this new and different [residency] system," wrote an admiring observer, "was the biggest single all-embracing contribution the Hopkins has made to American medicine."[43]

Halsted resolutely believed that great surgeons should breed great surgeons, and he achieved exactly this at the hospital. Of Halsted's seventeen house surgeons, eleven later implemented Halstedian residencies at other hospitals, from which another 166 house surgeons graduated. Even Halsted's 55 residents who did not become house surgeons profoundly influenced American medicine. Men in this group established the country's first residency programs in otorhinolaryngology, orthopedics, and urology. Halsted was American surgery's Adam, and most surgeons still trace their professional pedigree to him and his early followers.

Instruments of Precision

The era of ineffective postgraduate medical education, with its "undergraduate repair shops" that ignored science and attempted to "mend a machine that was predestined to break down,"[44] was ending. Johns Hopkins–style residencies transformed the average medical graduate into a thoroughly trained, science-and-technology-oriented, modern doctor. "After all," explained Halsted, "the hospital, the operating room and the wards should be the laboratories, laboratories of the highest order, and we know from experience that where this conception prevails not only is the cause of higher education and of medical science best served, but also the welfare of the patient is best promoted."[45]

Specialists with university education and Halstedian-style training were replacing the half-trained, ersatz expert. Physicians refused to accept, professionally or socially, the men who declared themselves specialists following makeshift, month-and-a-half-long classes in electronic gadgetry, medical instrumentation, and operative techniques. The success of residencies confirmed that specialists were exclusively the product of intensive, hospital-based training, and postgraduate medical and surgical training developed even greater sophistication in the first half of the twentieth century.

The makeover of postgraduate medical training and of the nature of science and specialists also changed the relationship between physician and patient. Case histories and physical examinations ceased being the sole sources of diagnostic information. Healers stopped relying on vague clinical answers and untested remedies, and when physicians refused to abandon such traditions, the new generation of hospital-trained doctors dismissed them as ineffective charlatans. "The provision of laboratory equipment has become a necessity," asserted Welch. "Modern methods of diagnosis require in ever-increasing measure trained experts and the necessary rooms and equipment for biological, physical and chemical diagnostic procedures."[46] The sick increasingly expected doctors to diagnose problems with objective facts and figures.

Patients believed that doctors who used newly available medical equipment and technologies would discover more effective treatments. The public viewed the medical technology itself as invaluable for optimizing care—a phenomenon that continues into the twenty-first century. Popular magazines told of astonishing medical technologies delivering accurate clinical information. The public read about X-ray machines and how they produced miraculous pictures of the insides of the body and about powerful microscopes that could see the smallest of cancer cells. Hospital administrators located clinical laboratories with the new equipment near wards to ensure that patients and their families saw the science and technology of the new medicine.

Medical students and residents working in well-equipped hospitals thus shaped their practice patterns around medical apparatuses and technologies. Hospitals offered blood tests and urinalyses around the clock. Clinical information increasingly derived more from technology than from a physician's diagnostic abilities. Doctors grew dependent on these results, as patients clamored for technology-based examinations.

These new technologies strengthened the professionalism of medical treatment both by further segregating medical knowledge from lay understanding and by bringing greater uniformity to certain clinical practices. The precise information these pieces of equipment produced gave doctors a new and convincing vocabulary, full of exotic words and concepts. As has often been observed, a profession is defined by its vocabulary, and this burgeoning lexicon added to medicine's scientific and social power. In addition, this new data, largely incomprehensible to the general public, were easily shared among physicians, meaning that several could simultaneously evaluate a case. Clinical decision making was no longer solely in the hands of a solitary practitioner, and this collegiality strengthened the assertion that the new style of medicine was based on more objective judgments. Clearly, a paradigm shift had occurred: panels of experts could now provide a clinical conclusiveness previously impossible.

While the most conservative physicians resisted these new technologies, mainstream American medical leadership embraced their potential. This generation of American doctors favored experimentation, research, and science, a dramatic departure from the previous generation that had derided the discoveries of Lister. William Williams Keen, the all-powerful president of the AMA and American Surgical Association, spoke of "instruments of precision"[47] and how, within just a few months, their presence had revolutionized medical care. He told audiences that 75 percent of a physician's knowledge of internal diseases came from information derived from technology. "Without these ingenious instruments," warned Keen, "physiologists, physicians, and the surgeons and specialists would be as utterly helpless as if in our community life our railroads and steamships, our telegraphs and telephones were suddenly abolished."[48]

Few in the medical community could challenge the views of a man of Keen's stature. He was at the height of a career that included time as a Union army physician during the Civil War, travels through the medical outposts of Europe, a teaching appointment for artistic anatomy at the Philadelphia Academy of Fine Arts, and a long-standing professorship of surgery at Jefferson Medical College. Keen's medical career was distinguished not only for its long duration—he lived ninety-six years—but also by the patients who sought his advice. His well-known compassion and clinical competence drew the rich and famous, from President Grover Cleveland (Keen helped to remove his cancerous left upper jaw in 1893) to Franklin Roosevelt (in 1921 Keen misdiagnosed the budding politician's incipient polio, then a three-day-old case of paralysis, as "a clot of blood from a sudden congestion that settled in the lower spinal cord").[49]

Keen, like Halsted, recognized that the increasing dependence on science and technology added to the professionalism and authority of medicine. He authored the earliest American surgical book based on Listerian principles, and his eight-volume *System of Surgery,* with its vivid descriptions of thermometers, electrocardiograms, and other gadgets, was a preeminent text for the nation's physicians during the first decades of the twentieth century. In his later years, Keen spoke effectively for various scientific causes, including the theory of evolution and animal experimentation in biomedical research. He often discussed his causes célèbres and how to best lobby for them with his close friend Halsted (Keen referred to the Baltimore surgeon as a "treasury of knowledge"),[50] who urged him to emphasize the need for even greater use of medical technologies. "Research, Research, Research," extolled an eighty-year-old Keen, "that is the method by which we shall enter into the Paradise of Health."[51] Having begun his career in the pre-Listerian era, Keen helped convince Americans, including many within the medical establishment, that the art of healing had become a science.

"Hidden Solids Revealed"

Few technologies fascinated the public and the medical profession more than the X-ray machine, the magical device that turned man inside out and revealed what nature had secreted away. William Roentgen, a German physicist, formally discovered X-rays in late 1895. His early X-ray machine was relatively simple—it passed an electrical current through a partially evacuated cathode-ray tube and sent the invisible rays this generated against a photographic plate. The medical uses were obvious immediately, and when the *New York Times* broke the news in January 1896 ("Hidden Solids Revealed"), the article concluded that it would transform "modern surgery by enabling the surgeon to detect the presence of foreign bodies."[52]

The X-ray created a "delirium of enthusiasm, experimentation, and expectation,"[53] according to *Popular Science Monthly,* as people queued up to glimpse their bones or see the inner recesses of inanimate objects. Individuals rushed to obtain shadowgraphs, skiagraphs, or radiographs of any and everything—these interchangeable terms avoided the idea that they were real-light photographs. Friends held hands and had pictures taken of their entwined fingers; lovers exchanged notes of affection on X-ray images of different portions of their bodies; pet owners hung X-rays of their favorite animals on parlor walls. Private investigators marketed their X-ray skills as an ability to see through doors for use in divorce proceedings. The X-ray was the nation's newest toy, but it also exposed the human body's inner workings to physician scrutiny as never before. Doctors hurried to determine what body parts could be meaningfully X-rayed and how to apply the information to treat disease and injury.

In March 1896, Keen authored the first detailed American contribution regarding the use of roentgenography. In this report, he described the X-ray as a useful aid for identifying foreign bodies, including bullets under the skin, and detecting abnormal conditions of bones, especially fractures. Keen also showed that certain tumors of the bone and other types of cancers could be seen on X-ray images. "It seems not improbable that in consequence of this discovery," he wrote, "our views of light, heat, electricity, and vibratory manifestations in general may have to undergo revision and possibly serious alteration."[54]

Despite these contributions, Keen could not foresee nearly all the future medical functions of X-rays. His early experiments, for example, had convinced him that X-rays did not impede bacteria growth: "In fact, if there was any change, the [bacterial] cultures made afterward seemed to be more luxuriant than usual."[55] Other researchers were more optimistic and believed that in the future increasingly powerful X-rays would possess "a germicidal action."[56] History favored the sanguine scientists, and formidable X-ray machines, with high-energy beams capable of destroying dangerous bacteria, now irradiate commercial foodstuffs and sterilize biologically hazardous material on medical equipment.

Doctors in Keen's era responded quickly to the early possibilities the X-ray created. In May 1896, less than half a year since Roentgen's discovery became public, X-ray images were demonstrated for the first time at a scientific program, the tenth annual session of the American Orthopedic Association. By the end of that year, local medical societies commonly exhibited X-rays at their meetings. Physicians boasted about being the first in their town to employ the device. Pundits went even further and claimed that no doctor could deliver adequate care without one of the new machines. "No consulting room is fully equipped without an apparatus for X-ray investigation," wrote a Harvard professor. "Unless the physician has the apparatus at his elbow, information can be obtained only by sending the patient to a hospital or to an expert . . . reasons which themselves justify the assertion that every physician should do his own skiagraphy."[57]

By the turn of the century, doctors were using X-rays for more than displaying skeletal fractures and detecting metal objects in the body, and with scientists and inventors constantly discovering new applications, the X-ray quickly infiltrated American medicine. At the 1897 meeting of the Association of American Physicians, one physician reported that X-rays could detect, earlier than other methods, the era's most feared disease, tuberculosis of the lungs. A researcher, several years later, developed a method for X-ray visualization of the intestinal tract, permitting doctors to locate colon cancers. Then, Thomas Edison informed the medical community that he was developing a practical and powerful type of X-ray that would contain "a fluorescent lamp, photographic plates, and the best form of electric oscillation to energize the lamp."[58] Within a few months, he had perfected the fluoroscope, a machine that showed bones in motion. Edison, who had been patenting electric devices at an amazing rate of frequency, chose to leave the apparatus in the public domain for the benefit of medicine, a tribute to the rising respect and professionalism that would have been unfathomable a generation earlier.

With X-ray technology gaining prestige and value, physicians began specializing in electricity and radiography. These men became known as radiologists, and like other nascent specialists of this era, they pushed for greater reliance on science, research, and technology. By 1900, radiologists had organized the American Roentgen Ray Society and were publishing their own journal. These experts lobbied for much greater use of X-rays. The president of the American Roentgen Ray Society, speaking at Johns Hopkins Hospital, claimed that a physician's failure to employ X-rays "either shows his ignorance of a valuable modern method or his willful neglect of his patient's interests."[59] The American public, already benefiting from technological advances in agriculture, manufacturing, transportation, and even housework, took their cue from the radiologists and began to ask that an X-ray be taken routinely as part of a physician's workup. Patients expected to be photographed, categorized, and quantified by a machine that did away with clinical uncertainties.

As the public's and profession's reliance on X-rays increased, lawyers started to use them to settle medical disputes, and doctors found themselves suddenly accountable to the supposedly unerring testimony of technology. Expert witnesses in skiagraphy populated the country's courtrooms to explain to juries the whys and wherefores of X-ray technology. "I have no doubt that advantage will be taken of this to the disadvantage of the physician,"[60] warned Keen. Other doctors were less hesitant: "An X-ray picture is very convincing and would be sure to have great weight with a jury."[61] Some, in turn, voiced concern that X-rays were sometimes taken out of fear of legal repercussions: "It is coming to this, a surgeon is not safe unless he has a shadowgraph taken before and after each operation. It is surprising to see the number of damage suits now pending against corporations, individuals, and especially surgeons, depending entirely on the shadowgraph as evidence."[62] Numerous committees investigated the medicolegal aspects of X-rays, but few of their conclusions slowed the move toward defensive medicine and the ordering of costly but unnecessary tests. Technological medicine did not arrive without its costs.

Medicine's newfound tools and wisdom had transformed the physician's role in providing health care from one of ineffectual luxury to beneficial necessity. The scientific and technological discoveries of this era continued to mount: in 1905 alone, doctors described the normal chemical composition of urine, discovered the causative agent of syphilis, resuscitated the heart with injections of epinephrine, completed a successful blood transfusion, and froze thinly sliced sections of tissue to rapidly analyze them under a microscope for an intraoperative surgical diagnosis. The result was that medicine could no longer be the closed, self-centered avocation that it had once been.

As patients became more dependent on the expanded healing powers of their physicians, doctors would need to focus on the coordination of efforts to deliver, finance, and organize the nation's medical services if their professional status was to continue rising unabated. In an era increasingly concerned with reform and accountability, this would not occur without some struggle.

"We do not sell Humbug"

The rise of technology and scientific medicine shifted care away from people's homes and toward hospitals, institutions earlier considered little more than a final stop on the way to the cemetery. A boom in hospital building—the number of new institutions far outpaced the percentage rise in population—facilitated this change, providing centers for physicians' services and for expensive medical technologies. Nineteenth-century hospitals had been medically primitive and ramshackle, but architects and urban planners designed the modern facilities as architecturally original, organizationally sophisticated, scientific institutions for all of a community's citizens. New hospitals offered advanced patient care and assisted in educating medical students and residents.

Leaders within American medicine called for the profession to assume managerial control of hospitals and their staffs. They argued that the ultimate power of accreditation, licensing, policy, and standardization needed to be in the hands of the medical professional. They believed that only doctors could rightfully determine the content of medicine as well as the character of the profession's future, especially how its new home base, the hospital, was to be governed. At the same time, the rising costs of new technologies and scientific medical treatments in this period forced a hospital's lay trustees and administrators to turn increasingly to patients as an additional source of income. Since doctors referred patients to hospitals, boards expanded the number of positions for doctors, especially those with high-volume practices. As their ranks swelled, physicians became the dominant voice in hospital administration, which increased the public's perception of their clinical authority and social privilege.

Hospitals became an indispensable element in the American health care scene, offering a sophisticated clinical setting in which physicians clustered and availed themselves of expensive equipment. In these physically impressive buildings, the results of costly bacteriological and chemical tests, as well as the findings of elaborate microscopic and X-ray studies, were readily available. As medicine became unalterably institutional, any doctor who desired to be viewed as scientifically responsible and socially respectable needed to join the staff of a hospital. The transformation was so complete that, by the early 1930s, five out of every six doctors had some form of hospital admitting privileges.

Clinical medicine was more easily evaluated in hospitals than in the far-flung offices of individual practitioners. The more doctors congregated and isolated themselves in these medical institutions, the simpler it was to study and regulate their practice routines. Reform-minded doctors, nurses, and administrators in the early twentieth century—this was the height of Progressivism, when reformers in every major U.S. city worked to improve public institutions—began asking fundamental questions. How long did it take for the hospitalized individual to be diagnosed? Did the patient recover? If not, were the physicians or the hospital to blame?

They demanded answers that correlated hospital outcomes with physician performance, especially the use of scientific and technological advances. Much as doctors used science to improve the outcomes of clinical care, these activists hoped to transform hospital care through new scientific approaches to management and industrial production.

"Efficiency" became a key word, a simple metric for interest groups to determine if doctors and hospitals were providing optimal care. The era's most renowned efficiency expert, Frank Gilbreth (an early advocate of scientific management who is best remembered as the father and central figure of *Cheaper by the Dozen* fame), had used time and motion studies to show how an operating room nurse could be more efficient in passing instruments to a surgeon. Efficiency experts touted the conviction that a well-organized hospital and staff would offer excellence in therapeutics. Progressive hospitals needed to impose order and discipline on their staffs, especially with regard to the scrutiny of patient outcomes, and they established regulations and routines over an increasingly specialized workforce. Audits, statistics, and success-or-failure data also came into use for the first time.

Among the medical reformers, Ernest Amory Codman, a Boston Brahmin surgeon, became the most militant of all when it came to efficiency. Codman's early career was conventional and, as an associate recalled, marked by "squareness."[63] He attended Harvard for his undergraduate and medical education, completed an internship at Massachusetts General Hospital, studied at Europe's German-speaking universities, and taught at Harvard Medical School. And, much like Halsted, Keen, and Welch, Codman believed in the potential for science and technology to cure mankind's medical ills.

As Codman's career progressed, he implacably advocated accountability and competition to reduce the costs of health care and improve its quality. The quixotic healer initiated a crusade with a bold message: medicine faced a moral failure because it had not capitalized on the promise of science and technology to improve patient care. He wanted to gather private clinical data, analyze them, and publicize the information so that patients would better understand a doctor's work. Codman believed medical science, in its clinical applications, could progress only if it were utilized and evaluated appropriately. "Has the time come when we can face the facts in a truly scientific manner?" he asked. "Can we let others look at the results of our experiments?"[64] He antagonized his peers with his assiduity. "A few centuries ago [Codman] would have been burned at the stake, would have gloried in it and have sought the opportunity to make the sacrifice,"[65] wrote one of his backers.

In 1910 the forty-one-year-old surgeon developed a method he called the "End Result System." The proposal was a practical method to standardize hospital records and allow for a comprehensive audit of medical and surgical outcomes. He argued that just as industrial processes were judged by the quality of manufactured goods, the health care system (he concentrated on patient care, nursing conditions, and ancillary services, particularly the presence and sophistication of X-ray equipment) should be similarly evaluated for how well it achieved "end results." At participating hospitals Codman's researchers would place in the chart of every hospital patient an end result card that summarized their stay, including symptoms, diagnosis, treatment, and complications. These investigators would then record the results of yearly follow-up visits.

Codman's plan disregarded a physician's clinical reputation or social standing as well as bedside manner or technical skills. All that counted were the clinical consequences of a doctor's effort. The redoubtable Codman further alienated physicians when he urged that hospitals use his audits to determine promotions and that they be made public so patients could better select where to obtain care. "The end-result system is something like a thunderstorm," wrote Codman. "It is an unwished for hospital guest. It is blown on us by the winds of progress and is inevitable. Let us accept it, since we have to, with the best grace we can."[66] To his supporters, Codman's system boldly and sensibly solved the problem of medicine's unregulated growth. To his detractors, it was an outlandish attempt to undermine the privacy of the physician/patient relationship.

Medical staffs, somewhat expectedly, resisted Codman's entreaties and the idea was not easily realized. It demanded hospitals to employ a costly end result clerk or, in modern terminology, a quality assurance specialist. It also required committees on efficiency to assure that audit results were standardized and published in a comprehensible format. And physicians would have had to relinquish a measure of their patient control, something that had strengthened immeasurably thanks to scientific medicine, hospital-centered care, and the power of their newfound professionalism. "The factors which have militated against the general adoption and continuance of such an obviously good system," wrote one of Codman's friends, "are the frailty of human endeavor, often called staying power, and the lack of anything individual and effulgent in the results."[67] Despite weighty opposition, Codman labored undeterred to implement the end result system. He lobbied members of medical societies, organized open discussion sessions, handed out sample end result cards, and made his views known whenever possible.

Codman became one of medicine's most persistent gadflies. He insisted that the trustees at Massachusetts General Hospital, where he practiced, use the end result system and link errors to outcomes. Codman protested against promotion by seniority rather than merit and demanded that he be the hospital's surgeon in chief. The managers of the hospital repudiated his ultimatum and, in a counterattack, stripped him of his admitting privileges. Emboldened by this denunciation, Codman opened his own ten-bed facility, which he called the End Result Hospital, and set prices lower than those at Massachusetts General. "We do not sell Humbug," he told Bostonians, "the question is whether there is a demand for Honest Medicine and Surgery."[68] For years, Codman paid for and published an annual account of his patients' outcomes. He highlighted complications as well as mortalities and even sent copies of his reports to rival area hospital administrators, challenging them to prepare similar documents. In his words, the idea was "to apply a little ridicule to Harvard and its affiliated institutions [which included Massachusetts General]."[69]

Codman's campaign against the Boston hospital climaxed in 1915 when he chaired a local medical society meeting on hospital efficiency. There, Codman unfurled an eight-foot cartoon for the incredulous audience, which included the city's mayor. The sketch depicted an ostrich, intended to represent the public, with its head buried in a pile of humbug. The bird is laying golden eggs that it kicks into the waiting hands of Massachusetts General's staff. Physicians hold on to these temptations, meant to be a snub against medical science. Hospital bureaucrats in the background (some drawn with faces true to life) question one another: "If we let her [the ostrich] know the truth about our patients, do you suppose she would still be willing to LAY?" Across the way, Harvard's president inquires, "I wonder if clinical truth is incompatible with medical science? Could my clinical professors make a living without humbug?"[70]

Pandemonium broke out as accusations flew back and forth. The medical society terminated Codman's membership and Harvard relieved him of teaching responsibilities. Acquaintances said Codman's action was "too impulsive" and that he would "pay in loss of dignity, prestige and professional income."[71] "For weeks some of my friends did not speak to me," admitted Codman, "and if I entered a room where other doctors gathered, the party broke up from embarrassment or changed their subject."[72]

He had been indiscreet and hardheaded, but any negative aspects were a small price because the hue and cry over Codman's cartoon created a nationwide buzz. Medical efficiency and the end result system were suddenly the hot topics of the day. As the profession and the public learned about Codman's ideas, a growing number of hospitals across the country implemented his scheme. Codman became a sought-after speaker and when the fledgling American College of Surgeons formed a commission on hospital standardization, he was appointed its first chairman. In the national movement for hospital standardization that followed, physicians, led by Codman, focused hospitals on the business and science of curing through a set of criteria concerning case records and operative notes, educational benchmarks for staffing, equipping clinical laboratories and wards, teaching principles for students, residents, and nurses, and prohibitions against fee-splitting. Doctors who specialized in surgery particularly favored these standards to ensure well-managed and efficient facilities for their increasingly complex and risky operations.

The revolution in science and technology had produced a sustained confidence in the diagnostic talents and therapeutic competence of America's physicians. In turn, doctors converted this professional self-assurance into higher incomes, improved social status, and expanded economic and legal clout. In the most dramatic of changes, medicine became a highly desirable career choice. In the nineteenth century, rejections to medical school were unheard of, but by the late 1920s, almost twice as many individuals were applying as there were available openings. Well-equipped and expensive laboratories along with expansive libraries and clinical buildings were now essential to medical education and students wanted in. These changing educational realities were underscored when a detailed report concerning the status of medical education in the United States brought about the closing of all the country's commercial medical schools and forever altered the face of American medicine.

❦ Six ❧

PROFESSIONAL AUTHORITY

A Layman's Job

I T WAS EARLY April 1909 and Abraham Flexner stood at a railroad depot in Des Moines, Iowa, waiting for his host, the dean of the city's medical school, to disappear from sight. Flexner was three months into a yearlong mission that industrialist and philanthropist Andrew Carnegie had sponsored to evaluate the teaching methods and facilities of each of the nation's one hundred forty-eight medical schools. To an administrator, the name Carnegie initially brought visions of endowment windfalls. After all, the financier had recently funded the construction of three thousand public libraries across the United States. Shortly before Flexner's arrival, however, the dean had discovered that Carnegie's agent was no philanthropic emissary, but an ironfisted investigator.

The dean had rushed through his appointment with Flexner, his answers defensive and evasive. Flexner saw the words "anatomy," "chemistry," "physiology," and "pathology" stenciled on doors, but was never permitted inside the rooms. Every department was locked and keys could not be located. Faculty were unavailable for interviews, financial ledgers could not be accessed, and students were nowhere in sight. Flexner had faced similar situations, but never this confrontational or concealing. Having expressed his satisfaction with the visit, Flexner asked the dean to drop him off at the depot so he could board the next train to Iowa City.

Once the physician drove away, an exasperated Flexner hired a horse and carriage and returned to the school. He searched for a janitor and, after he slipped him five dollars, the janitor unlocked the doors. "The equipment in every one of the rooms was identical," noted Flexner. "It consisted of a desk, a small blackboard, and chairs; there were no charts, no apparatus—nothing!"[1] There were no laboratories, no clinical facilities, and no patients either. Nor were there course guidelines, graded examinations, or graduation requirements. Yet one hundred fifteen students would soon call themselves physicians, treat people, and prescribe medicines. Their tuition went directly to a consortium of greedy local physicians who owned the school and recruited students and patients with false and tacky newspaper advertisements. The school was among the worst of America's medical diploma mills. "Everything about the school indicates that it is a commercial business,"[2] wrote Flexner. In his subsequent white paper to Carnegie, Flexner described this proprietary medical college as a disgrace to Iowa and simply recommended, "The school should be summarily suppressed."[3]

Flexner's investigation and subsequent report would catalyze an evolving process of medical education reform. Academic physicians had realized that new, stricter educational standards would create more full-time teaching positions. Office practitioners knew that educational reforms would decrease competition from poorly educated doctors. The result was that by the time of Flexner's investigation medical powerbrokers largely agreed how to teach medicine properly.

Johns Hopkins was the model and they wanted it applied throughout the United States. Schools had to teach the basic sciences of microbiology, pathology, and physiology, and such essential instruction required fully equipped laboratories in well-funded schools. Just as essential was the educational concept of learning by doing. Young doctors needed to examine patients, and patients needed hospitals with a full array of technological advances.

This winning strategy initially had found its strongest backing from the Council on Medical Education, a committee of the recently reorganized and revived AMA. No longer preoccupied with fighting the homeopaths, the Association prioritized medical school reform. In 1906 they decided to conduct a survey of the nation's schools. The council, however, never made the results of the investigation public—half of the institutions were found lacking—because members of the governing board deemed it ethically irresponsible for the Association to criticize its member schools. Many critics complained about the secrecy and holier-than-thou attitude of the council and its survey.

Under growing pressure, the leadership of the council decided that an independent party should redo the survey, this time for public consumption. The council members found a natural partner in Carnegie's Foundation for the Advancement of Teaching. Carnegie and members of his foundation's board had long felt that America's medical schools, much like the country's undergraduate colleges and graduate universities, should provide not only superior teaching but more full-time research positions, so that doctors could view academic medicine as a secure career choice. The foundation's board expressed further concern that commercial interests dominated medical education, which meant that greed compromised health care. The council and the foundation agreed at a joint meeting in December 1908 to pool their efforts and conduct another, more detailed evaluation of America's medical schools. Carnegie and his foundation would fund the survey and provide staffing, while the council would direct from behind the scenes.

The task of carrying out this enormous assignment fell to a relatively obscure, forty-three-year-old educator, who was ignorant of medical schools, postgraduate training, and hospitals. Abraham Flexner's detractors said those were not his only shortcomings. They described him as erratic, quarrelsome, and stubborn, and he was all of these. But he was also one of the most knowledgeable critics of the nation's educational systems and able to understand medical educators when they discussed teaching philosophies or the differences among classroom, laboratory, and clinical settings.

Flexner was born in Louisville, Kentucky, to impoverished Jewish immigrants from Bohemia. He overcame this humble beginning and, when he was only nineteen years old, received a bachelor's degree from Johns Hopkins University. He then returned to Kentucky to organize a private college preparatory school where, for two decades, this serious young man advocated a philosophy of secondary education marked by hands-on teaching, one-on-one attention, and small classes. Flexner's school attracted attention—the president of Harvard once sent a note congratulating him on the success of his students in coming to the famed university younger and graduating in a shorter period of time than matriculants from any other high school. Despite his success, in 1904, Flexner decided that "in a remote town like Louisville and under the limiting conditions of a school preoccupied with admission to college, I had done all that I could hope to accomplish."[4] He and his wife moved to Boston where he pursued graduate work at Harvard. Flexner studied philosophy and psychology and also completed master's degree research in Europe, paying particular attention to the Austro-Hungarian and Germanic educational systems.

While living in Heidelberg, he wrote a monograph critiquing America's scheme of higher education. Flexner argued against the disorganized nature of the nation's colleges and universities, emphasizing his distrust of both large unwieldy lectures and freedom of choice in coursework. In what became typical of his no-nonsense style, Flexner demonstrated little concern about who might be offended. His language was pugnacious, his thoughts confrontational. "The college has come down from the mountain," he warned. "It dwells among men."[5] Despite the book's commercial failure, it gained the attention of the board of the newly organized Carnegie Foundation for the Advancement of Teaching.

Flexner writes in his autobiography that he believed the foundation administrators confused him with his brother Simon, who was the director of the Rockefeller Institute for Medical Research in Manhattan and a protégé of William Welch, the professor of pathology at Johns Hopkins. Abraham assured the foundation's staff that he knew little about medicine or medical schools. "That is precisely what I want," the board's president wrote back. "I think these professional schools should be studied not from the point of view of the practitioner but from the standpoint of the educator. I know your brother, so that I am not laboring under any confusion. This is a layman's job, not a job for a medical man."[6]

Time was of the essence and Flexner gave himself slightly more than a month to master the history and current status of medical education. He read voraciously, including a detailed treatise on the teaching of the medical sciences in German universities, and spent several days with his brother. He traveled to Chicago to confer with the staff of the council and later to Baltimore to interview Welch and Halsted. The influence of the Johns Hopkins educational model, with its German-like standards and ideals, on Flexner's thinking cannot be overemphasized. "I became intimately acquainted with a small but ideal medical school, embodying in a novel way, adapted to American conditions, the best features of medical education in Germany," recalled Flexner. "Without this pattern in the back of my mind, I could have accomplished little."[7] Hopkins would be the standard-bearer, the exception to the rule of American medical education.

Flexner began a hectic year of travel in January 1909 following his preliminary readings and interviews. During an age of railroads and horse-drawn carriages (augmented by the recently developed automobile), he managed to crisscross America dozens of times, traveling to ninety-eight cities and conducting one hundred seventy-four separate investigations of medical schools (some more than once). In April 1909 alone, the same month that he toured schools in Iowa, Flexner inspected thirty medical colleges in a dozen cities.

Bulletin Number Four

In 1910, Flexner's report, *Bulletin Number Four* of the Carnegie Foundation for the Advancement of Teaching, was published. It was a landmark policy statement and one of the most important documents in the history of American medicine. It incorporated thirty years of educational reform, reflecting social and economic changes in America itself. A product of the Progressive Era and its push for general equality, public safety, and social justice, the *Bulletin* argued that the move toward professional education must also include medical educators.

While the *Bulletin* embodies Progressive Era ideals, it also ranks among the best works of the muckraking era, a classic piece of investigative journalism masked as a technical study. Like his contemporaries Samuel Hopkins Adams, famous for his exposés of the patent medicine industry, and Upton Sinclair, whose book *The Jungle* spurred federal legislation regulating food and drug practices, Flexner used words as weapons, rarely shying away from the pithy insult. The schools he reviewed were often "poorly equipped," sometimes "wholly inadequate," and occasionally he encountered a facility that simply "defied description." It was not only the style of the writing. Flexner named names and uncovered skeletons in medicine's long-closed closet. In his judgment, "such a rattling of dead bones has never been heard in this country before or since."[8] The book became a widely read tour de force, one that shocked the nation.

The country could no longer tolerate inferior medical educational institutions, including all proprietary facilities, according to the *Bulletin*. Flexner portrayed commercial school owners as contemptible figures deserving popular derision for placing their financial interests above the public's health. "They know more about modern advertising than about modern medical teaching,"[9] warned Flexner. He lumped these men with other betrayers of public confidence, acquisitive industrialists and corrupt politicians among them. "The medical profession is a social organ," wrote Flexner, "created not for the purpose of gratifying the inclinations or preferences of certain individuals, but as a means of promoting health, physical vigor, happiness—and the economic independence and efficiency immediately connected with these factors."[10] He demanded that Americans, using law and public opinion, destroy what he termed "mercenary concerns that trade on ignorance and disease."[11]

Flexner quickly became a celebrity and a target. Owners of the proprietary schools threatened him with lawsuits and, in one case, actually sued for libel for $150,000. Several people threatened his life anonymously—one letter writer warned that Flexner would be shot if he ever showed up again in Chicago. Members of various state boards of medical examiners, dumbfounded by the ruthless exposure they received, attempted to scapegoat Flexner for their own failures. It was all to no avail.

Americans listened and supported Flexner, especially when he suggested that the number of medical schools be severely reduced. "The improvement of medical education cannot be resisted on the ground that it will destroy schools and restrict output," he explained. "That is precisely what is needed."[12] Although some considered Flexner's viewpoints too Draconian (he would have left almost one-half of the states without any medical schools), newspaper editors recognized both the sensational and commonsense aspects of the *Bulletin* and repeated its findings in graphic headlines. "Factories for the Making of Ignorant Doctors; Carnegie Foundation's Startling Report that Incompetent Physicians Are Manufactured by Wholesale in This Country"[13] was the title of the lead story in a Sunday

New York Times Magazine section. Few knowledgeable physicians argued with its major conclusions. At a time when Congress passed the Federal Food and Drugs Act, the medical profession had to also reform or face the growing threat of federal and state regulatory efforts.

With its logical approach to medical education, Flexner's work swiftly accomplished its purposes. The number of the country's medical schools fell to under a hundred within five years of the report's publication, and the number of graduates decreased from 5,440 to 3,535. Only eighty-five schools remained by 1920 and, ten years later, the number was down to sixty-six. State medical licensing boards' increasing unwillingness to recognize graduates of the remaining low-grade schools hastened the downsizing. Since the AMA's Council on Medical Education had the only rating system for medical schools, the profession rapidly monopolized control over educational regulations and the development of strong schools.

The principal cost of these positive developments was that the practice of medicine suddenly became limited to those who could afford both college and four years of medical school. Flexner countered that higher standards, although initially denying opportunity to some, would engender better health status for the many. In turn, improved health care would raise living conditions, increasing the opportunities to partake in better education and enter the medical profession. Flexner, like so many others of his generation, believed in a trickle-down theory of medical education. The enriching and democratizing effects of first-class public education would eventually bring superior schooling to all.

Flexner, however, was incorrect in his belief that medicine would become democratized. It became the exclusive preserve of upper-middle-class white men for the half century following the *Bulletin*. The profession would welcome neither ethnic and religious minorities nor females until the last decades of the twentieth century.

Despite such criticism, most contemporary educators and physicians agreed that Flexner analyzed a chaotic situation properly and proposed a remarkably straightforward solution. The *Bulletin* also made it clear that successfully reconfiguring medical education and training would require considerable financial assistance from outside the profession. Private individuals, foundations, and philanthropic organizations needed to support improvements in modern medical education. Flexner's catchphrase for the monetary answer was "abundant benefaction."[14] The *Bulletin*'s recommendations might have faded away like so many good ideas had Flexner not left the Carnegie Foundation and become an administrator at the General Education Board, financed by John D. Rockefeller Sr.

"Flexnerian" Philanthropy

One of the great ironies of Flexner's investigation was that Carnegie, who had established his foundation to advance American education, decided to no longer fund any medical education projects. The industrialist, always a pragmatic businessman, told Flexner that he saw little point in helping institutions that had allowed themselves to get into such financial difficulties. "You have proved that medical education is a business," a forthright Carnegie explained to Flexner. "I will not endow any other man's business."[15]

The major power in medical philanthropy from the 1910s through the 1930s instead was Rockefeller's General Education Board. Flexner might not have been able to convince Carnegie to fund medical education, but his appeals to Rockefeller resulted in a $50 million bequest, a staggering sum that would forever change the face of American medicine. The endowment also ensured what many individuals had long believed: only Flexner could direct a bold initiative to transform America's medical schools. Flexner proved a decisive personality within the board's administration and would negotiate scores of agreements with medical schools. "The road was clear," wrote Flexner. "The country at large knew that the Board was prepared to go forward and for some years thereafter my attention was devoted almost entirely to medical education."[16] The *New Yorker* termed Flexner the nation's educational "Robin Hood," noting that he was "a fierce partisan and a passionate antagonist."[17]

Flexner administered all of the board's medical philanthropic activities for a decade and a half, creating a vast financial and educational empire. His policies determined which schools would endure, which teaching hospitals would be built, and how universities would administer their medical complexes. Flexner became academic medicine's closest friend, but his influence extended far beyond the profession. He lectured and wrote articles in popular magazines like the *Atlantic Monthly*. Flexner became known as a "knight errant" who, noted an editor at the *New York Times,* "had the temerity to raise the question whether we Americans really value education in spite of the amount we spend for it."[18]

Flexner's efforts shaped the modern medical school and his educational paradigms and attitudes about social responsibility continue to affect American medicine. His name even became an adjective, "Flexnerian," meaning a firm conviction about the importance of basic science in medical school curricula. Indeed, every medical doctor educated and trained in this country owes the essence of their professional identity and thinking to the century-old work of Flexner. On his retirement from the board, Flexner remained active in higher education. He organized the Institute for Advanced Study at Princeton, served as its first director, and facilitated Albert Einstein's immigrating to the United States.

As forward-thinking as Flexner was, his wide-ranging investigations and his seminal *Bulletin* did not deal with one significant component of American medical education and training: specialization. Specialism, exemplified by railway physicians as well as doctors interested in eye, ear, nose, and throat illnesses, had been on the rise since the 1880s. Backed by journals and societies, specialization was turning into a prominent element of American health care. Despite its growth and the vociferousness of the debates about specialism's future, the organizational politics surrounding specialization were haphazard. There were no defining details as to who was a specialist or even what constituted a specialist's clinical work. Part of the problem was that the nation's medical schools had done little to characterize specialties or specialists. The result was that physicians at first saw Flexnerian-style medical education, which emphasized broad-based scholarly learning, as protective of the modern general practitioner. However, the increasing research orientation of medical schools as well as scientific and technological advances in clinical practice heightened demands for all manner of specialists by the mid-1910s.

"Show Me" and "Tell Me"

In November 1913 a new era in American medicine marched into the Gold Room of Chicago's Congress Hotel behind Franklin Martin, a dynamic, no-nonsense surgical gynecologist. A procession of one thou-

sand blue-and-scarlet-robed surgeons, each a member of the newly organized American College of Surgeons, followed their leader into the vast
hall. They had convened in order to draw other doctors into their specialty
ranks, to impress upon general practitioners the limit of the generalist's
surgical abilities, and to achieve organizational and political dominance
over them.

Martin and his minions argued that a well-organized group of full-
time surgeons could provide sophisticated specialty skills that the public
would come to view as lifesaving and then demand as a right. "Patients
with intelligent judgment in other matters, were cheerfully hopping up
on operating tables and allowing a medical school graduate with one
year of training in an internship to peer and search aimlessly within their
abdominal and other body cavities,"[19] bemoaned a member. For Martin
and his followers such surgical recklessness had to stop.

Conflicts between general practitioners and specialists had reached a
fever pitch early in the twentieth century as scientific and technical breakthroughs made it possible to be a "surgeon" rather than a "generalist."
Before the abdomen, chest, and cranium could be safely opened, any manner of physician had performed most surgical operations—amputations,
lancing abscesses, setting fractures. Surgical operations grew increasingly
sophisticated following the acceptance of antisepsis and the groundbreaking work of Halsted in Maryland and Charles and William Mayo in Minnesota. Inadequately trained or incompetent physicians-cum-surgeons
potentially endangered their patients' lives, as well as the reputation of the
profession as a whole.

Martin had realized the immensity of this problem and the consequent
need for a professional jurisdiction. "A renaissance of surgery was dawn-
ing," he explained. "The wilderness with its jungle was being explored,
and this most perplexing of problems had to be solved."[20] Martin was neither an academic nor a renowned surgeon, but his personal narrative as
a general physician who had restricted his practice to surgical gynecology, combined with his involvement in grassroots medical politics, made
him an ideal spokesman for the specialists. In this capacity, he championed efforts both to prohibit nonspecialists from performing surgeries
and to circumscribe the role of the general practitioner. Martin's biographer described his bearing as severe and "Indian-erect."[21] He was not

just square-jawed and austere in appearance, but stern and unyielding in manner as well.

Martin became a national surgical powerbroker in 1905 at forty-eight years of age when he founded one of the earliest journals devoted to the surgeon as specialist. "I was convinced that the profession needed a practical journal for practical surgeons, edited by active surgeons instead of *littérateurs* only remotely connected with clinical work,"[22] wrote Martin. *Surgery, Gynecology & Obstetrics* succeeded immediately and afforded Martin a direct line of communication with thousands of surgeons.

He exploited this opportunity, sharply demarcating the border between general practitioners who dabbled in surgery, self-professed surgeons who continued to treat nonsurgical patients, and legitimate full-time surgical specialists. He pushed and prodded his peers to understand that simply reading *Surgery, Gynecology & Obstetrics* was not sufficient by itself. Surgeons and surgeons-to-be had to see master surgeons perform operations to truly understand technical complexities. "Show me" and "tell me" became twin clinical imperatives for Martin.

In 1910 he placed announcements in his journal for a clinical meeting in Chicago where physicians could visit the operating rooms of the city's great surgeons. "It was an innovation that the academic orators and medical politicians watched with amusement that they did not conceal, but it stirred in the minds of practical surgeons a hope,"[23] claimed Martin. He expected two hundred attendees. Thirteen hundred doctors showed. The registration booths were underserved and overwhelmed. The operating rooms overflowed. Martin named the affair the Clinical Congress of Surgeons of North America.

A second Congress convened in Philadelphia the following year. Over fifteen hundred surgeons from almost every state attended. Several hundred watched as one local surgeon repaired the hernia of John Coombs, pitcher for the Philadelphia Athletics and hero of the 1910 World Series. Newspapers hailed the operation with banner headlines ("Baseball Player Undergoes Treatment at University Hospital") and provided the Congress widespread publicity ("Over 1,000 Delegates Attend Surgical Clinics").[24] At a third Congress in New York City in 1912, at least twenty-six hundred doctors registered and hundreds more attended without paying. Crowds brought chaos to the surgical sessions, and the evening gatherings, when attendees presented scientific papers, were frenzied. Martin's Congress had turned into a logistical nightmare. His attempt to provide live postgraduate surgical education to medicine's rank and file, to democratize surgical education, and to upgrade the operative skills of physicians had succeeded too much.

In addition, there was a policy dilemma. Many attendees were not interested in restricting their practices to surgery. Instead, they had come to learn new surgical techniques in order to augment their general practice and increase income. These men declared themselves adequately educated and well-trained surgeons based simply on the imprimatur of the Clinical Congress and their presence at the event. Much like the Germanic university-trained American physicians who received "diplomas" for their studies abroad, doctors hung the certificate of attendance from the Congress on their office walls to inform patients that they were specialists. A 1915 survey would later show that over one-third of the country's physicians declared themselves general practitioners who also performed surgery.

Martin and his followers came to believe that surgical education and training transcended upgrading the lowest-common-denominator physician to operate with comparative safety. Too many doctors practiced as part-time surgeons, and Martin shortly dismissed "relative" surgical safety as a goal. When he realized that his Congresses functioned as just another pathway to part-time specialization, Martin searched for ways to limit admission. "There must be a change; there must be a change," he preached. "I formulated my program. It involved a new organization, through which definite qualifications for membership would be established."[25]

The question was how stringent those qualifications should be. In an extraordinary burst of travel beginning in early 1913, Martin visited heads of departments of surgery to determine the answer. He inquired at every prominent medical school and hospital from the eastern seaboard to the Midwest and West Coast. The faculties and surgical chairmen overwhelmingly agreed that if the undergraduate medical education system could be standardized, then the same should apply to postgraduate training of surgical specialists.

After several months of consultations, Martin proposed an organization that would establish minimum requirements for a doctor to perform major surgical operations. The suggested prerequisites included at least two years of specialty training, an additional three years as a surgeon's assistant, mandatory yearly visits to recognized surgical clinics, and a written report detailing at least fifty consecutive major operations that the doctor had completed. The new association—Martin named it the American College of Surgeons—would publish a listing of surgical specialists, award these men the title of Fellow of the American College of Surgeons (FACS), and disseminate their names to hospitals and the public as physicians of note.

Martin's attempt to distinguish surgeons from general practitioners had core supporters, including several state medical societies. "If it holds itself aloof and free from medical politics and politicians, it is destined to become the most potent factor in directing and establishing the standards and requirements for all who desire to devote their life to surgery,"[26] wrote an official from Michigan. Legislators in Martin's home state of Illinois and in New Jersey even attempted to pass bills requiring additional surgical licenses beyond the general medical license.

Despite these efforts, many members of the profession and the public immediately challenged Martin's idea. They belittled him and cursed him. "Do you have in mind the establishment of a glorified surgical union, along labor union lines?"[27] asked one foe. Another general practitioner suggested calling Martin's organization the American Surgical Society so that the "mystic letters" after his name would spell "quite nicely, ASS."[28] Leaders of the AMA claimed that Martin sought to establish class distinctions in the medical landscape, similar to old-world European-style clinical divisions between physicians and surgeons. They also worried that a new organization would usurp the Association's recently improved status. "Sees Flaws in Plan to Mark Surgeons: Organization of New College Evokes Adverse Criticism From Medical Journal—Fears a Monopoly,"[29] announced a headline in the *New York Times*. People questioned, both publicly and privately, who Martin and his associates were to select the surgically qualified and to prohibit the general practitioners from operating.

Neither the relentless ad hominems nor concerns about personal safety—fisticuffs broke out at some meetings—dissuaded Martin. When a thousand fellows of the American College of Surgeons assembled in

Chicago on that chilly autumn day in 1913, they established a standard that changed the course of medicine in America. They defined a surgical specialist to the public for the first time. From that day on, no one could deny the specialization of surgery, that unique branch of therapeutics within the whole of health care. The college emphasized the specialist's professional authority and clinical competence by standardizing the surgeon. Its very existence implied that full-time surgical specialists outperformed general practitioners with their part-time approach to surgery. Equally important, the strength of the college encouraged nonsurgical specialists, including obstetricians, ophthalmologists, pediatricians, and pathologists, to claim their organizational stake in medicine's divided future.

The college established the precedent that the profession, rather than the state, should determine qualifications for medical specialties. Flexnerian-style medical education and stricter state licensing standards had not adequately delineated generalist from specialist. Medicine had begun to police itself, and in doing so introduced a clinical hierarchy into everyday practice that left generalists with unsettled professional prospects. These factors created inevitable animosities and placed general practitioners on the defensive and for good reason. Specialists were on top, and the college had admitted almost thirty-three hundred surgeons by the end of 1915.

The Minimum Standard

Surgery began to dominate clinical service in America's hospitals during the first two decades of the twentieth century, and the majority of hospitals were permitting any practitioner who considered himself a competent surgeon to use the facilities. Administrators, however, seeking to improve financial and managerial efficiency, began to favor controlling surgical standards to weed out operating room incompetents. This was possible since the American College of Surgeons was promising to endorse a discrete group of physicians as capable surgeons. Only "an applicant who can meet all of the college's requirements was fitted to do actual surgery,"[30] assured Martin.

In a classic catch-22 dilemma, however, the college could not evaluate the competency of surgeons independent of the hospitals where they practiced. Martin's scheme required applicants to submit a list of completed major surgical operations along with a description of the hospital where the procedure was performed. "We found evidence that much surgical work was being done in hospitals that lacked many facilities essential in the scientific care of the patient," recounted Martin. "Cases were unsystematically recorded and the professional work was generally without supervision."[31] The fellowship denied over half of the applicants and the rejected physicians were upset. They were troubled not because the college had impugned their surgical skills, but because it was judging their abilities against the management of their hospitals, something outside the control of most clinicians.

Under pressure from rejected doctors, hospital administrators asked the college to furnish examples of acceptable operative records, define standards for laboratories, and outline staff organizational requirements. Leaders of the college soon issued guidelines, known as the "minimum standard," intended to foster an environment that would safeguard patients, enhance the careers of specialist surgeons, and assure professionalism in a hospital's staff. "Any advance in medicine must begin—and end—with the welfare of the patient," wrote a representative of the college. "Just as surely as the patient is benefited, so also will be the doctor and the hospital."[32] In attempting to upgrade the nation's hospitals with its "minimum standard," leaders of the college soon created a national commission on hospital standardization.

In forming this committee the college consolidated twenty years of work by numerous reform-minded groups for greater efficiency and scientific management in the health care industry. The public began to perceive the college as defending its welfare and effectively lobbying for competency in the nation's doctors. Similar to *Good Housekeeping* magazine, whose recently introduced "Seal of Approval" guaranteed the superiority of any product advertised in its pages, the college fashioned the "minimum standard" as its stamp of support to the nation's hospitals. The leaders of the college turned to Ernest Codman, the Boston surgeon who had previously developed the "end results system," to chair the commission.

The "minimum standards" were not demanding by modern standards. The program required that each hospital organize its doctors as a "definite group or staff" and restrict membership to men "competent in their respective fields and worthy in character and in matters of professional ethics."[33] The college's own standards for Fellows already ensured that any surgeon would have adequate technical skills. Moreover, a hospital's medical staff (both physicians and surgeons) had to adopt rules and regulations that would guarantee the best possible service to the public. Doctors had to behave and collaborate with one another and schedule staff meetings once a month to review their clinical work. The program expected that physicians would maintain accurate and complete records of all patients and that these case histories would be accessible to outside inspectors on a moment's notice. Finally, each hospital had to provide laboratory facilities ("chemical, bacteriological, serological, histological, radiographic and fluoroscopic services")[34] under trained supervisors.

Hospital evaluations started in mid-1918, but were hampered by the influenza epidemic that struck the country. The college needed almost eighteen months to complete the survey, although the results were hardly a surprise. Seven out of eight hospitals with over a hundred beds could not meet the standards. Over one-half of the institutions lacked a staff organizational plan and one-third of the facilities did not provide pathology or X-ray services. When the college held a press conference in New York City to report the findings, its representatives named no individual hospitals because many highly regarded facilities had failed to meet the benchmarks. The committee's staff were so concerned about names being leaked to the press that, the night before, they incinerated the printed listings in the furnaces of the Waldorf-Astoria hotel.

The dismal results of the first survey left the leadership of the college in a quandary, uncertain of how to enforce the "minimum standard." Any strong-armed disciplinary action against noncompliant hospitals would be highly unpopular, especially among local physicians who were on the boards of many of the smaller facilities. These hospitals, usually with fewer than fifty beds, dotted the small cities and towns of America, and would face severe financial difficulties if forced to properly equip and staff their institutions.

Martin and other college officials had little choice but to travel throughout the country again, this time promoting standardization to these physicians and hospital administrators. The college's leaders portrayed the "minimum standard" as a means to bring about clinical accountability. They hedged their arguments by assuring their audiences that adoption of the "minimum standard" would engender community support and, in the end, increase the volume of paying patients. "The minimum standard has become to hospital betterment what the Sermon on the Mount is to a great religion,"[35] Martin declared. Many rejected the proselytizing message of Martin, particularly in less populated areas where doctors and hospital executives viewed him as an outside agitator who looked to impose national regulations on a local situation.

The college continued, despite the resistance, to advocate for superior medical care and to emphasize the need for local cooperation. In 1921, Martin and his associates held thirty-one two-day-long state hospital conferences where administrators, physicians, and college officials discussed critical management issues. These gatherings were meant to promote, at least for public consumption, the fact that the profession was democratizing and organizing around the patient as a consumer of sophisticated medical care.

The strategy worked. Newspapers touted the college's efforts. *Harper's Magazine* told of the "new control of surgeons," and how "their adoption of the minimum standard kills the old boarding-house hospital and makes the hospital itself responsible for everything that goes on within its walls."[36] An article in the widely read *World's Work* went even further: "A new era is already here; when the hospitals of America will be institutions for service, from which selfish interest and careless methods have been abolished, and to which the country may look for considerate and efficient treatment, confidently expecting and receiving the utmost that the medical profession is capable of giving."[37] As public support solidified, the college finally published a list of over five hundred approved hospitals in the organization's monthly bulletin in January 1922. Hospital administrators eagerly hung their new certificates of approval in front entranceways and announced their success in local newspapers. By the late 1920s the college had endorsed over 80 percent of the nation's largest hospitals and one-half of moderate-sized hospitals (fifty to ninety-nine beds). Smaller hospitals continued to struggle with the criteria, but strong public condemnation led either to their compliance or closing.

"Broad and firm foundations"

The American College of Surgeons' "minimum standards" helped to standardize hospital care, but they were not the only such measurements employed in the early twentieth century. Several medical colleges and state licensing boards had begun to require that graduates complete an internship or "fifth year"[38] of hospital work to earn their M.D. degree. These medical schools, led by the University of Minnesota and Rush Medical College of the University of Chicago, had been quietly "approving" hospitals for internships. "The hospital internship is no longer for the privileged, but will soon be required of every graduate in medicine," explained an article in the *Journal of the American Medical Association*. "We must be willing to devote ourselves to the long years of patient, grinding tutelage, advancing slowly, under recognized masters, until we have laid broad and firm foundations."[39] These schools were universalizing the educational and training techniques pioneered at Johns Hopkins.

The process to approve hospitals for internships quickly became too burdensome for any individual medical school to handle. The AMA, which had grown uneasy toward the American College of Surgeons and its burgeoning status as a hospital regulator, seized this opportunity to counter the college's influence. The Association planned to introduce a competing hospital standardization program centered on approved internship programs. This work started in 1920, when the Association's Council on Medical Education, the same committee that had assisted Flexner, surreptitiously changed its name to the Council on Medical Education and Hospitals. It then hired a staff of trained inspectors who focused on medical educational standards in hospitals. Later that year the Association published a list of 469 general hospitals with 2,960 "acceptable"[40] internships.

This new hospital listing became one of the AMA's most important and publicized activities. Their *Journal* annually published increasingly detailed hospital statistics, providing the nation's first database for health care planners. These reports included information such as the ratio of hospital beds per an area's population; how the facility was controlled (church, city, county, federal, independent, individual); the type of clinical service (children, general, incurable, industrial, tuberculosis, venereal);

the presence of a training school for nurses; and whether the superintendent was a physician, nurse, or layperson. "The lesson to be learned from these figures is that in the establishing of hospitals hereafter, communities should be selected which are not already abundantly or overabundantly supplied,"[41] cautioned an Association official.

The AMA expanded its involvement in medical education and postgraduate training in 1927, when it published a list of approved residency programs in medical and surgical specialties. "The danger is not from an increasing specialization, but from those who pose as specialists without having secured the essential advanced training,"[42] explained a member of the council. The directory included 270 hospitals with 1,699 approved residencies, including anesthesia, dermatology, gynecology and obstetrics, medicine, neuropsychiatry, ophthalmology, otolaryngology, pathology, pediatrics, radiology, surgery, tuberculosis, and urology. The following year, the council expanded the list to include cardiology, contagious diseases, leprology, metabolic disorders, orthopedics, and tropical medicine. Thus, the Association formally and publicly declared its support for some manner of specialization, a key policy decision that would profoundly impact the future of the country's doctors and health care.

The AMA's efforts to upgrade medical schools, internships, and residencies complemented the American College of Surgeons' promotion of "minimum standards" in hospital organization. The two competing organizations helped hospitals become responsible institutions from the clinical, educational, and organizational perspectives. These early programs of hospital accreditation served as prototypes for all present-day certification systems—in the 1950s, the AMA joined with the American College of Surgeons as well as the American College of Physicians and the American Hospital Association to create the Joint Commission on Accreditation of Hospitals, the precursor to today's Joint Commission on Accreditation of Healthcare Organizations that accredits more than fifteen thousand health care organizations and programs in the United States.

Ambulance Américaine

The initial developments in medical education reform and hospital standardization occurred in the shadow of World War I. The country would not formally enter the conflict until April 1917, but a full two years earlier government officials, with the assistance of civilian authorities, had begun to reorganize and re-equip various military departments, including the medical branch. The military medical buildup utilized the entire range of new technologies, therapies, and health care personnel. The army recruited physicians and nurses as it had done in earlier wars, but the increasing complexity of twentieth-century medicine also necessitated laboratory technicians, nutritionists, pharmacists, sanitary engineers, and X-ray experts. Widespread medical advances meant that, for the first time, American troops would suffer fewer deaths from disease than from battle injuries.

The reformers among the nation's doctors, the same ones who had urged the upgrading of medical schools and hospitals, were now asked to utilize their know-how and develop new military medical strategies for abroad. In particular, the impending conflict would require sophisticated army base hospitals, with a full complement of medical and surgical capabilities. Surgeons, with their interest in hospital standardization and knowledge of trauma care, were the obvious choice to sort out this critical aspect of military preparations. Few among them had the organizational genius, professional credentials, or patriotic fervor of George Crile, a Cleveland surgeon who would help coordinate the nation's military medical preparations and then command the first authorized American army unit sent to Europe, a mobile base hospital.

Martin, the founder of the American College of Surgeons, described Crile as "handsome as a prince," with an "enthusiasm that fairly took your breath."[43] The Clevelander was a popular lecturer and acclaimed writer who extolled the virtues of scientific research and modern medicine. As professor of surgery at Western Reserve Medical School, Crile gained worldwide attention for his work on the treatment of shock and his skill with anesthesia. He performed the country's first successful transfusion of blood from one human to another and later espoused this therapy to treat soldiers with severe injuries. Crile was an honorary Fellow of the Royal

College of Surgeons of England, the second president of the American College of Surgeons, and founder of the renowned Cleveland Clinic. He also hunted big game in Africa, traveled the world extensively, and had a lunar crater named after him. In the two-column editorial that accompanied his *New York Times* obituary in 1943, the writer told of Crile's "restless imagination" and how "there was something about him that recalls the scientific romanticism of the Renaissance."[44]

Crile's war efforts began in 1915, when he went to France with a volunteer civilian surgical unit. He was stationed at the Ambulance Américaine (*ambulance* being the French term for military hospital) in Neuilly-sur-Seine, a northwest suburb of Paris. A Parisian colony of American expatriates had organized the Ambulance at the outset of the war, an attempt to bolster France's initial lack of adequate military medicine. At one point, in September 1914, with the Kaiser's army approaching the outskirts of Paris, a half dozen or so Americans (among them the American ambassador to France as well as his predecessor) had driven their automobiles fifty miles to the Marne battlefields to bring back some wounded. Confusion reigned and no one knows how many injured soldiers returned in these cars, but those who made it to Paris were housed and cared for in a high school building that volunteers outfitted with medical equipment and dubbed the Ambulance Américaine. As the fighting turned into a stalemate, the Americans in Paris looked to their countrymen back home for donations for the Ambulance.

Fund-raising efforts in the United States raised awareness of military medicine, and the work performed at the Ambulance molded military medical preparedness as well. Ambulance administrators decided to staff one of its wards with U.S. civilian surgical teams culled from the nation's elite medical schools and hospitals, the first efforts to bring American-based doctors into the war effort. When the president of Paris's American Chamber of Commerce toured the United States in support of France's war effort and the Ambulance, the first physician he recruited was Crile. "Great as the temptation was, I replied that I would be of no use without my staff," wrote Crile. "Before the evening was over I had evolved the plan of a university [hospital] service."[45]

Crile and his staff of physicians, residents, and nurses from the Lakeside Hospital–Western Reserve University arrived in Paris on New Year's

Day 1915—Crile sailed on the *Lusitania,* which was sunk by a German submarine five months later, turning many Americans against Germany. He took charge of a one-hundred-fifty-bed ward in the Ambulance Américaine as well as the adjacent operating room and experimental laboratory. Crile's team naively assumed they could serve patients in Neuilly like those in Cleveland. But how the day-to-day reality differed. His Cleveland medical team had meager supplies and virtually no trained support personnel—the operating room orderlies included a grand opera singer, a member of a well-known banking family, and a French count.

Although Crile's effort provided only slight medical assistance to France's early war experience, it shaped the development of American military medicine. Crile's duties in Paris ended in April 1915, but on his urging civilian university surgical teams continued working with the Ambulance for another year. These included units from Harvard University, the University of Pennsylvania, Northwestern University, and Washington University. Medical journals widely covered these endeavors, and numerous articles recounted Crile's and others' early encounters with frostbite, gas gangrene, tetanus, and shrapnel injuries. Crile's work at the Ambulance and his frequent inspections of the front also convinced him that his organizational plans could extend to any future military hospitals.

Base Hospitals

Crile returned to Cleveland a vociferous civilian proponent of military medical preparedness. With the United States still two years from a declaration of war, many considered talk of preparedness to be premature if not overtly partisan. Crile's sentiment may have swayed toward France after his volunteer stint, but his newfound passion stemmed from an understanding that a country at war would not have the luxury of medical preparation. He now believed that delivery of frontline medical care required four fundamental practices: imaginative organization, day-to-day adaptability, streamlined clinical services, and coordinated specialty care. Crile informally presented these concepts at an American First Aid Conference that the Red Cross sponsored in late spring 1915. Several months later he provided additional details at the American College of Surgeons annual meeting in Boston. Crile asserted that a lack of military medical preparation in France had initially made "the surgeon more dangerous than the enemy," which could be avoided, he stressed, with "adequate organization in times of peace."[46] An editorial writer in the influential *Boston Medical and Surgical Journal* agreed with Crile's assessment: "Without doubt, hospital units for base hospitals, composed of carefully selected civil surgeons, would be of great value."[47]

The surgeon general of the U.S. Army heard of Crile's proposals. He asked Crile and representatives from the Red Cross to stage an experimental mobilization of a base hospital at the next American College of Surgeons meeting in Philadelphia in late October 1916. Crile located the encampment on the expansive Belmont plateau in Fairmount Park. "The idea of this trial-and-error mobilization was a good one, as it disclosed defects, particularly in the operating-room equipment,"[48] recalled Crile. Army, navy, and Red Cross officials as well as leading surgeons spent several days inspecting the temporary structures and familiarizing themselves with new technologies. The mock medical mobilization fascinated the public, and local newspapers provided prominent coverage: "Surgeons Examine Wartime Hospitals: Unit Demonstrates the Feasibility of Mobilization Methods."[49]

Crile told visitors that a five-hundred-bed unit could be served by the typical base hospital, with its chief surgeon, eight associate surgeons, three anesthetists, two pathologists, two dentists, two radiologists, an internist, a neurologist, an eye specialist, a stenographer, and fifty nurses, along with ancillary support staff and adequate supplies. His scheme allowed each unit to continue research projects that the sponsoring university hospital already had in progress. Crile stressed that the reputation of the parent institution and its physician staff would guarantee the quality of its field hospital. No one would need to screen out incompetent physicians and surgeons. More important, the doctors' familiarity with one another would smooth their transition to military medical service.

War contingency planning ramped up in autumn 1916. President Woodrow Wilson assigned six members of his cabinet to a Council of National Defense. He named a seven-member board of distinguished Americans, including Franklin Martin, to advise this council. In turn, Martin appointed Crile to a Committee of American Physicians for Medical Preparedness and asked him to chair a number of subcommittees. The

Committee represented the country's more than ninety thousand physicians and was, according to one historian, "the crucial step in the linkage of civilian doctors into the military effort."[50] With Martin leading the nation's wartime medical mobilization and Crile organizing the military's field hospitals, the status of surgeons as specialists within the medical profession soared, as did respect for their opinions.

The United States declared war on April 2, 1917, and Crile's group, with its seventy-eight personnel, was the first official American army unit sent to France, where it assumed command of a run-down British field hospital in Rouen. "We disembarked in military fashion and with drums and fifes blaring, marched through the streets amidst throngs of French people cheering lustily *'Vive les Américains!'* "[51] wrote Crile. The U.S. Army had established forty-nine other base hospitals by the war's end, most of them patterned on Crile's plan, a respected American physician commanding each one. Virtually every important medical school in every major city in the country claimed its own base hospital. Hometowns sponsored them with pride. Local businessmen raised money to equip their units, while women volunteered with the Red Cross, hand-making surgical dressings, sheets, pillowcases, and towels.

War has always posed moral dilemmas for doctors. The greater their efficacy, the longer the conflict can endure. Successful surgeries push soldiers back to the front to face the devastating cannonade yet again. Doctors gain unparalleled clinical experience through incalculable human suffering. World War I was no exception, a conflict of attrition, unrelenting bombardment, and deadly new weaponry (flame throwers, poison gas, and tanks). Over the course of forty-eight months, countless millions of the world's sons moved an intricate system of underground trenches little more than a few miles in either direction.

Unlike in earlier wars, however, the treatment of enormous numbers of casualties employing science-based therapies and X-rays advanced wound management considerably. Doctors used newly developed antiseptic solutions to irrigate injuries and refined a fundamental surgical principle, the removal of all devitalized tissue prior to suturing a wound. Surgeons performed a greater variety of complex procedures, including elaborate abdominal and reconstructive head and neck operations. In internal medicine, physicians dealt with new and strange diseases (trench foot, shell shock, traumatic amnesia, and pulmonary distress from gassing) in unprecedented numbers.

The war provided thousands of doctors with a crash course in military medicine that catapulted clinical practice forward. "Every bed, every aisle, every tent, every inch of floor space was occupied by stretchers," wrote Crile. "The operating rooms ran day and night, without ceasing. I had two hundred deaths on one night in my own service. The seriously wounded piled up so fast that nothing could be done with them."[52] Army doctors, using science and modern technologies at base hospitals, increasingly depended on diagnostic tests and meticulous record keeping. The American College of Surgeons' program of minimum standards shortly incorporated these fundamentals.

The war also underscored the importance of specialty practice to the future of American health care. "Segregating 'war surgeons' into specialties was looked upon as an innovation at the beginning of the World War,"[53] wrote Martin. Neurosurgery, orthopedic surgery, plastic surgery, and psychiatry each emerged as stand-alone specialties in the wake of the atrocities that the trench warfare of World War I produced. But the war also revealed that specialists needed strict standards, as enlistment testing of physicians for specialty practice showed that many were grossly undertrained and deficient in clinical skills. For example, at a time when the military wanted every doctor it could get, the army rebuffed over 50 percent of the supposed ophthalmologists and ear, nose, and throat specialists seeking enlistment.

The base hospitals, with fledgling specialists staffing their wards, created a national wartime medical and surgical elite. This cadre of talented doctors, along with their base hospital executives, dominated postwar American medicine. In particular, these men convinced others of the soundness of acute medical care and acute care hospitals (acute care facilities are those intended for short-term medical or surgical treatment, as opposed to institutions for the chronically ill). Following the war, hospital administrators, along with their physician staffs, conspicuously embraced costly technologies and supervised the construction of enormous medical centers to house hundreds, and occasionally thousands, of patients with acute diseases at a time. Thus was born the mammoth and complex hospital that defines present-day American health care.

The ascent of American medicine to a position of international leadership began with the medical triumphs of the war. Prolonged battle had destroyed much of Europe—Germany, in particular, was in economic and scientific ruin. As a result, a vacuum existed globally in both medical research and clinical therapeutics. It was natural and inevitable that physicians from the United States, least affected emotionally and physically by the war's aftermath, would easily fill this void. Few could argue that American medicine was not vastly different and improved from where it had been. "There was never a war in which the medical profession received the authority and won the credit as it did in the last war," wrote a contemporary observer, "and there never was a time when the medical profession had the honor and credit that it has today."[54]

Crile returned to Cleveland a war hero, decorated with the American Distinguished Service Medal as well as honors from France and Great Britain. Martin left his government post with a personal thank-you from President Wilson and a formal congressional citation. As for the other thirty thousand–plus physicians who served in the army and navy, they brought their war tales and clinical skills back home. There they revitalized hospitals, rejuvenated medical schools, and guided the rapidly changing world of American medicine.

Physicians were about to convert their embrace of science, technology, and efficiency into economic power through higher incomes, professional power through specialization, legal power through hospital regulation, and social power through true healing of the sick. The public had never experienced such a fundamental change in medicine, nor had doctors ever received such approbation. Medicine's overriding influence on a person's health was a novel cultural phenomenon and confirmed the diagnostic abilities and therapeutic competencies of the nation's physicians. American medicine and its healers had a newfound enthusiasm and swagger.

❧ Seven ❧

CHALLENGES OF SUCCESS

Diseases of Deficiency

I N THE HALF century between Appomattox and the Treaty of Versailles, the nation's doctors had slowly assimilated the bedrock medical concepts of anesthesia, germ theory, antisepsis, microbiology, pathology, and public health. These foundations were the root of modern medical science, but American medicine immediately after World War I still remained rudimentary in many respects. It was, however, on the cusp of another leap forward, and the two and a half decades between the World Wars would bring such outstanding achievements as X-raying the brain, the kidneys, and the gallbladder, discovering the role of chromosomes in heredity, use of radium to treat cancers, and employing sulfa drugs to combat infections. "Medical progress does not move forward with the even pace of the clock hands," explained a 1937 article in *The New Republic* that summarized recent medical advancements. "It jumps unpredictably, at its own fitting time of ripeness."[1]

Medical research in the forty years before World War I had focused disproportionately on identifying bacteria, a one-sidedness that had hampered medical progress. "It has been maintained," wrote a contemporary medical writer, "that the entrance of bacteriology on the stage, in the last quarter of the nineteenth century, for a time displaced physiological experimentation, and this [bacteriological] interlude had the effect of narrowing the outlook and rendering medicine less rational."[2] Physicians, preoccupied with these external agents of infection, had excluded other possible causes of disease, but the reign of the microbe was coming to an end.

As the scope of medical inquiry widened, investigators found that often the cause of ill health was not the presence of something, like bacteria, but the lack of a substance. This observation opened up new worlds of medical care. Whereas doctors had earlier been classifying diseases based on humoralist speculation or on recognized bacteria, now they also could categorize (and consequently target and treat) diseases into conditions due to an absence of external factors (e.g., rickets or scurvy from vitamin deficiency) and those due to failure to produce substances within the body (e.g., diabetes or goiter from hormone insufficiency).

By the 1930s, American medical scientists had identified and described the effects of vitamins A, B1 (thiamine), B2 (riboflavin), B3 (niacin), B9 (folic acid), C, D, and E. Researchers were able to investigate the consequences of removing specific vitamins from an individual's diet and surmise which vitamin-rich foods could treat disease states. Vitamin deficiency illnesses like beriberi and pellagra stopped tormenting the impoverished as public health administrators learned to supplement their nutritionally inadequate diets.

Once it became known that vitamins were essential to good health, pharmaceutical companies rushed to synthesize the vitamins in laboratories and peddle their product to the nation's consumers. Private drug companies advertised their new creations and convinced the public to consume ever larger quantities of vitamin pills as a panacea toward a long life. "Vitamins partaken of in adequate quantities prolong the span of life," championed a drug industry spokesperson in 1936, "while a lack of them in the human body are responsible for many Winter ills and often directly cause an early death."[3] Thus began America's obsession with megadoses of vitamins.

But vitamins were only part of the story. Endocrinology, the study of hormones, developed in this period as well. By 1940, the country's doctors had investigated most of the body's internal glands—the adrenals, gonads, pineal, pituitary, and thyroid. They extracted from these specialized tissues a group of active factors—internal secretions transported in the blood as invisible chemical messengers that act along with the nervous system to regulate bodily functions—known collectively as hormones. Adrenaline from the adrenal glands was the most well known, but thyroxine from the thyroid became the most fabled. "This pinch of material," proclaimed one researcher, "spells all the difference between complete imbecility and normal health."[4] When biochemists showed that thyroxine contained a high percentage of iodine, this led to the introduction of iodized salt. The use of the reformulated salt lowered retardation rates in youngsters and lessened goiter (an enlarged thyroid) in adults.

The dynamic development in medical research during this period is best illustrated through the efforts to cure pernicious anemia. The investigation, and subsequent diagnosis and therapy, bridged the studies of both vitamins and hormones. Pernicious anemia, like vitamin and hormone insufficiencies, is a disease of deficiency. It is neither common nor rare, but, as its name implies, is a bona fide killer. There is little difficulty recognizing the victims. They have an unnatural lemon-yellow pallor because their bone marrow underproduces red blood cells. They also have prematurely gray hair, walk unsteadily, are short of breath, endure chronically swollen tongues, and suffer from numbness and tingling in their hands and feet.

Shortly after World War I, clinicians began studying pernicious anemia with broader techniques that took advantage of the scientific method, incipient medical technologies, and an understanding that disease was not necessarily the end result of bacterial contamination. They examined blood samples of anemic patients under powerful microscopes and found that these individuals had low red blood cell counts. Initially, following this discovery, doctors treated victims of pernicious anemia with blood transfusions, a recently developed medical technique. Transfusions, however, only transiently increased a patient's red blood cell count and had no effect on the disease's disabling neurological symptoms.

A team of three physicians, who had studied the disease for five years, then determined a simple truth: a dietary defect caused pernicious anemia and it could be overcome through a nutritional regime high in liver. The importance of the breakthrough cannot be understated. "When a new and important fact has been established, the effect is somewhat like that of a bomb falling to earth," explained one contemporary observer. "Those theories that do not admit of being reconciled with it are exploded, being replaced at once by others that can be brought into better harmony with the newly acquired item of factual knowledge. And that has been the case with [pernicious anemia]."[5]

Discovering the cure for pernicious anemia gained America its first Nobel Prize in Physiology or Medicine in 1934. Despite repeated medical triumphs, from Walter Reed's observation that a virus spread by mosquitoes caused yellow fever to Béla Schick's devising a test to determine if a person is susceptible to diphtheria, the country's physicians had been shut out of the highest international prize in medicine. Europeans had walked away with every award since it began in 1901. The 1934 victory was largely unexpected given such history—one of the physicians told the *New York Times* that he was "flabbergasted."[6] The recognition of these American doctors for their work on pernicious anemia validated the nation's medical authority internationally like nothing before. "The United States is no longer a hinterland in physiology and pathology," wrote an impressed newspaper editor. "It takes its place with older countries in alleviating human suffering and making life more useful by systematic exploration of the unknown in laboratories and clinics."[7]

The Nobel Prize–winning research, however, left an important question unanswered: what was stored in liver that cured pernicious anemia? It seemed implausible that patients with the illness simply disliked this particular food. Even if they could tolerate liver, they could not be expected to eat half a pound of raw liver daily for the remainder of their lives.

William Castle, a young doctor from Harvard who worked with the Nobel laureates, picked up where their research left off. He postulated that the stomach of a person with pernicious anemia failed to secrete normal acid-laden digestive juices. Castle reasoned that the stomach contains an active factor that, together with a substance stored in the liver, is necessary to produce red blood cells. To test his theory he organized one of the most repulsive-sounding experiments in American medical history: healthy volunteers ate finely ground lean beef muscle (hamburger), kept it in their stomach just long enough (one hour) for the gastric juices to act on it, and then regurgitated the contents; Castle had his pernicious anemia patients subsequently ingest the partially digested matter. The medical establishment ridiculed Castle's ideas and methods, but his experiment succeeded in curbing the pernicious anemia in his test subjects. The regurgitated stomach contents cured the illness as effectively as liver. When Castle presented his results, he invoked the motto of England's illustrious Most Noble Order of the Garter to quiet his critics *("Honi soit qui mal y pense"*[8]—"Shame upon him who thinks evil of it").

Researchers in the 1940s, using more sophisticated laboratory tools, confirmed the biochemistry and physiology behind Castle's work. They determined that the stomach secretes a protein called "intrinsic factor." This protein brings about the absorption of the mysterious liver substance that the Nobel laureates had stumbled upon. In 1948 scientists isolated this material from the liver and named it vitamin B12. Since then, doctors have treated pernicious anemia with a monthly injection of vitamin B12, effectively bypassing a diseased digestive tract.

The Power of Electricity

The technological revolution in clinical treatment that began with the X-ray, blood transfusions, and the blood pressure cuff continued as the twentieth century progressed. Doctors used the new technologies with increasing frequency in hospitals and their offices. This growing reliance on sophisticated instruments and laboratory tests continued to change how physicians managed their patients. For instance, the development of improved electrical illumination in the 1920s finally allowed doctors to use tools to investigate directly the inner recesses of the body. Medical devices designed to let doctors glimpse inside a patient had been of limited use without sufficient light, and until the commercial availability of special incandescent bulbs, there was no adequate solution. As electric lighting grew more sophisticated, doctors embraced a panoply of essential diagnostic tools: the ophthalmoscope for eyes, the otoscope for ears, the laryngoscope for the larynx, the bronchoscope for the lungs, the proctoscope for the rectum, the cystoscope for the bladder.

Access to improved electrical sources meant doctors could employ increasingly refined diagnostic tools in their everyday practice. The centrifuge—a centuries-old, whirling, rickety apparatus that separated cream from milk to ease butter churning—had evolved from a hand-cranked device into a motorized rotor that spun fluid to concentrate dissolved solids. The modernized centrifuge, dependent on electricity, became crucial to the study of blood and urine—this type of centrifuge was used in the research on pernicious anemia. The more powerful and fast centrifuges became, the more efficiently doctors could use the data that they produced. The way this technology improved medical care is most easily demonstrated by tracing the early history of urinalysis.

Physicians first recognized the importance of urinalysis in diagnosing and treating illnesses during the last half of the nineteenth century. Solid particles are present in urine and their composition reveals much about a person's health. These substances, including blood or pus in some cases, are best seen under a microscope and need to be in a concentrated form. Initially, the only way to examine them was to let the urine stand in a tube for an extended period of time, often a day or more, while the solids gradually settled on the bottom of the tube. Once this separation had occurred, a doctor poured off the fluid and examined the remaining contents under a microscope. The entire process was inefficient and imprecise.

The introduction of the hand-driven, multigeared urinary centrifuge in the 1890s was a clinical boon. It increased a physician's efficiency. "The instrument is a time-saver when compared with old style slow and inefficient apparatus,"[9] claimed a sales brochure. Doctors could perform a urinalysis soon after they obtained the urine specimen and could repeat the test as often as necessary. By observing changes in the urine over time, doctors could monitor the patient's daily clinical status and make accurate diagnoses.

With the increasing use of electric power, an even more efficient, ultra-high-speed bench-model centrifuge became available in 1921 and further streamlined the process. Modern doctors consider urinalysis a routine and unimaginative medical test, but from 1900 to 1930 it epitomized medical progress. A physician who owned a centrifuge and performed same-day in-office urinalyses was considered scientifically sound and medically savvy.

Perhaps the most important and utilitarian medical technology to emerge from the interwar period was the electrocardiogram. Before its arrival, doctors were limited in their diagnosis of heart conditions to the sounds they could glean through a stethoscope, but the electrocardiogram dramatically increased the amount of information available to doctors.

The heart is an intricate muscle that responds to minute electric currents generated from specialized nervous tissue within the organ itself. When the current is released, it causes heart cells to contract. A series of coordinated contractions creates a beat, the celebrated, life-assuring "lub-dub, lub-dub." An electrocardiogram tracing records the electrical action that constitutes each "lub-dub," a series of craggy-shaped waves labeled P, Q, R, S, and T.

During the 1920s, American physicians began to use the electrocardiogram to verify the diagnosis of a heart attack. They correlated the signs and symptoms of a cardiac problem with changes in the patient's P, Q, R, S, and T rhythms on an electrocardiogram. "With the aid of a galvanometer [electrocardiogram], knowledge has been gained concerning the effects of certain drugs in modifying rhythm," explained a physician at the Rockefeller Institute for Medical Research, "and as a result it has been possible to employ these drugs with greatly increased accuracy and efficiency."[10] This deft piece of research led to the routine use of the electrocardiogram in patient care.

The potential of the electrocardiogram fascinated Americans like few medical breakthroughs since the X-ray. Its arrival coincided with the ascendance of heart disease as the leading cause of death for Americans, something that continues to the present. By the mid-1920s, 200,000 people a year were dying of heart diseases. "When the automobile came in the 1920s and the population at large became more prosperous and overnourished," surmised one physician, "the current epidemic of coronary heart disease began and incidentally involved younger and younger men."[11] At the time, this was a novel explanation, but the answer was more complex. Public and private institutions directed increasing amounts of research funds toward the care of the heart in an effort to determine the true cause. Cardiac clinics sprang up as well as specialty training programs in heart diseases.

By the 1930s continuing development of the electrocardiogram, as well as X-ray imaging, helped transform the reasons for which acute care hospitals admitted patients. The management of illnesses and accidents stopped being the sole basis for admission. A new style of medicine evolved, based on the growing complexity and presumed effectiveness of a hospital's ingenious instruments and sophisticated tests. Patients entered an institution specifically to be "worked up." In such a scientifically refined setting, individuals could be studied and diagnosed in detail, not merely evaluated and treated. This established a new paradigm in patient care and proved a transformative juncture in American medicine as doctors and hospitals moved from a strictly reactive attitude to one that included preventive concerns.

The Unassuming Appendix

Clinical practice and surgical technique improved alongside the advances in medical research and medical technology. Nothing encapsulated this progress as well as appendicitis, which burst onto the medical scene in the years surrounding World War I. A confluence of factors—improved surgical technique, greater willingness of patients to undergo invasive procedures, expanded diagnostic capacity—made appendectomies (removal of the appendix) the preeminent surgical procedure in the interwar years. Surgeons oriented their practices around the operation and hospitals adapted as well to meet the enormous clinical demand. Simply put, taking care of the unassuming appendix helped reshape American medicine.

The term "appendicitis" first entered the medical lexicon in the late nineteenth century. For centuries healers had accepted misguided notions concerning bellyaches and their origins. Traditional medicine viewed the ileocecal junction—the area where the end of the small intestine, the ilium, joins the beginning of the large intestine, the cecum—as the root of most abdominal evil. Doctors had myriad expressions for problems in this area, but none of them amounted to anything more than semantics: cecitis, ileocecal abscess, iliac passion, pericecal abscess, typhlitis, or the grandiloquent perityphlitis vermicularis. This muddled vocabulary, indicative only of a lack of understanding, persisted until a generation after the Civil War. No one had considered that bellyaches could originate in a part of the abdomen next to the ileocecal junction.

In 1886 Reginald Fitz, a Harvard professor, turned traditional medicine on its head when he declared that inflammation of the lowly appendix caused many abdominal pains. This assertion shocked his audience, comprising members of the Association of American Physicians. The fast-talking, no-nonsense Fitz explained that he had observed hundreds of dissections of persons who died in various stages of appendiceal disease.

His research convinced him that the ileocecal junction had been mistakenly vilified. The true culprit for much abdominal pain and disease was the appendix. He grouped the various disorders of the appendix together under the term "appendicitis." Fitz sounded to his peers like a wild-eyed clinical extremist, both intemperate enough to define a new, potentially far-reaching disease and confident enough to lecture them on how to make a diagnosis. He even had the audacity to suggest that appendicitis was strictly a surgeon's disease: "Its eventual treatment by appendectomy is generally indispensable."[12] Fitz made appendicitis a recognized pathologic entity and laid the groundwork for the emergence of appendectomies as commonplace.

Until the 1880s, abdominal surgery of any kind had been one of medicine's taboos. Surgeons had an operative death rate in the abdomen that approached 100 percent. This situation changed as doctors began employing antiseptic methods and using anesthetic routines. Operating room mortality dropped to 50 percent in the late 1880s and the death rate from abdominal surgery fell below 5 percent by the turn of the century. "Now there is no organ in the abdominal cavity that is not daily explored," proclaimed Samuel Hopkins Adams, the muckraking reporter, in 1905. "Perhaps the most notable success is in appendicitis. Twenty years ago the sufferer from appendicitis died. Today the death rate in the best equipped hospitals is not two per cent."[13]

The increase in technical skills that surgeons obtained by performing appendectomies accounted for much of this remarkable decline. Surgeons had embraced Fitz's message about who the appendix belonged to: the organ was their domain, appendicitis was their disease, the decision to operate was their choice, and if physicians wished to save patients' lives, then surgeons needed to be consulted sooner rather than later. "American surgeons," according to one admirer, "have done more to show the importance of operative treatment of appendicitis than the rest of the world put together."[14]

Despite high success rates, the diagnosis of appendicitis is a challenging procedure for surgeons because of the appendix's unpredictability. Surgeons thrive on anatomical certainty, and the appendix's varied location is the knife wielder's curse. Most of the abdomen's internal organs— the gallbladder, liver, pancreas, spleen, stomach, and small and large intestines—are attached to their surroundings by ligaments and folds of tissue that provide morphologic consistency. Without this measure of constancy, the surgeon's quest to cure disease would be next to impossible. The appendix's whereabouts, however, can occasionally epitomize all that is uncertain about the human body. The organ is wormlike in appearance and of varying girths—usually three inches in length but occasionally up to ten inches—with its base appended to the right side of the large intestine. The appendix and its problem-producing tip (with appendicitis, where the inflamed tip lies is where the patient's pain is most intense) wander wherever they like, whether upward toward the liver, downward into the pelvis, sideways into the middle of the abdomen, forward toward the abdominal wall, or stealthily tucked behind the large intestine itself.

The myriad locations also made diagnosis a challenge at first. Patients with appendicitis displayed countless symptoms and signs, many of which mimicked other derangements. These included pain, loss of appetite, and vomiting. Doctors who relied on observation alone easily confused the disease with less serious conditions. Many cases also were atypical. Identifying a diseased appendix was more often art than science for the first generation.

The improved diagnostic equipment that emerged after World War I helped doctors to recognize appendicitis at an early stage, before the organ burst. Physicians analyzed the blood and urine with the aid of the centrifuge and microscope and used other devices to count red and white blood cells. A high white blood cell count marked an infection, while the presence of red blood cells in the urine suggested possible appendicitis. The key was to evaluate the appendicitis patient early and follow the ups and downs of the test results. The information that these new medical tools provided, in conjunction with physical indicators like abdominal pain, allowed doctors to recommend appendectomies with a high degree of confidence.

Patients' willingness to undergo appendectomies also increased as physicians improved their diagnostic skills and lowered the operative mortality rates. By 1920, in a large urban medical center, like New York Hospital, surgeons were performing appendectomies on 95 percent of admitted patients with appendicitis. And in a small rural facility like the Watts Hospital in Durham, North Carolina, 286 of the 1,369 procedures completed in their operating rooms during the course of a year were appendectomies. The number of appendectomies steadily rose, consistent with the increasing importance and safety of surgery. "Better to take out a healthy appendix and have a patient recover," justified one devotee, "than [to leave] a diseased one and have the patient die."[15]

The United States was soon in the grip of an appendiceal frenzy. By 1930 10 percent of the patients admitted to the nation's hospitals received a diagnosis of appendicitis and surgeons performed over 100,000 appendectomies annually. "Appendicitis took such a firm hold on the imagination of this country that it became that unhappy object—a fashionable disease," wrote one physician. "People became so fidgety about their appendixes that it only required the consumption of a few green apples to send them pell-mell to the hospital."[16] Another doctor complained: "Appendicitis is a condition which furnishes us with an example of the too-inclusive enthusiasm of the layman toward a surgical condition which he does not fully understand."[17]

The prevalence of the appendectomy in American medicine spilled over into popular culture, becoming something of a fad. There was a well-known musical ditty: "Have you got the new disorder, If you haven't 'tis in order, Midway down in your intestine, Its interstices infestin'."[18] In *Arrowsmith,* the 1924 Pulitzer Prize–winning novel about contemporary medicine, Sinclair Lewis uses the appendix to illustrate a doctor's early ties with his profession. "Look here! Look here! See this?" says the protagonist. "In the bottle? It's an appendix. First one ever took out 'round here. I did it ... did the first 'pendectomy in this neck of the woods, you bet!"[19]

From an ailment that was largely unheard of in the early 1890s, appendicitis became one of the most commonly diagnosed disorders in the interwar years and changed the practice of American medicine as a result. It became the quintessential American disease. Physicians made a substantial portion of their livelihood detecting the disease. Surgery suddenly became an option of first resort for anyone diagnosed with the disease, a boon for surgical specialists. Hospitals grew and prospered on the fees from appendectomy patients. For the first time, institutional treatment in acute care facilities became acceptable and indispensable for large numbers of the general public.

From undersized country hospitals to mammoth city medical complexes, the appendix turned the health care industry into big business. Fledgling pharmaceutical companies, spurred by the seeming epidemic of appendicitis, developed medicines to treat the disease and its complications. They created and marketed antiseptic dusting powders, protein-rich antimicrobial serums, and bacterial antitoxins. This mingling of medical and commercial interests marked the beginnings of modern drug research and helped spark the rise of the pharmaceutical industry.

The treatment of appendicitis shifted the way health care was provided, helped redefine American medicine, and in certain respects revolutionized the way patients were doctored. Among other things, the government and the medical profession became proactive about treatment, sponsoring public awareness campaigns that emphasized early detection of disease. "Don't gamble with appendicitis, don't use a laxative, call a doctor"[20] was one slogan. Such crusades expanded in the 1930s, and included other ailments as well: the March of Dimes and its fight against polio and the National Cancer Institute's promotion of cancer research and cancer control.

As for the appendix itself, the cause of all this excitement: common perception has long been that it is a vestigial organ with no medical purpose. In the mid-1920s, William Mayo, one of the country's most prominent surgeons, proposed that the appendix actually participated in the body's defense against infection. He based his opinion on the discovery that the appendix contains small amounts of lymphatic tissue through adolescence. He argued that these lymph follicles were an individual's first line of defense against bacteria and other foreign invaders, but research has not verified this theory. Present-day research suggests that the appendix's job might include rebooting the intestines with a complement of normal bacteria after illness has decreased their numbers. The ultimate function of the appendix continues to divide physicians. The paradox of the appendix—the frequent need to remove it despite likely immunologic benefits—remains one of medicine's unsolved mysteries.

"His appendix was a long affair"

While the nation's medicine advanced dramatically after World War I, it still remained a threatening environment for many Americans struck down by illness. Medical research, medical technology, diagnostics, and surgical technique had improved but problems persisted. This era lacked intravenous fluids, respirators, even antibiotics. Supposedly conquered diseases like appendicitis continued to pose some degree of risk. And no one would learn that lesson harder than Harry Houdini, clairvoyant, conjurer, escape artist, and one of the biggest celebrities of the 1920s. Houdini had convinced America that nothing could kill him, and he appeared to be right, until the day his appendix acted up.

Much of Houdini's success stemmed from his remarkable strength and stamina. He was one of the country's earliest fitness buffs, and it was essential to his showmanship. The public admired his strongman appearance and well-conditioned abdominal muscles. Though he broke numerous bones and suffered countless injuries during his career, Houdini rarely missed a performance; the aura of invincible health was integral to his act. So when newspaper headlines announced in late October 1926 that the fifty-two-year-old magician was near death after an appendectomy, his supporters were shocked. For days, the nation focused on Detroit's Grace Hospital as Houdini struggled against one postoperative complication after another.

It seemed implausible that one of the country's most famous and health-conscious performers was dying from the ravages of appendicitis, especially given the medical success in treating the disease. Rumors swirled about how so ordinary a medical condition could fell the country's "man of steel." Was it true that a wild fan, wanting to verify the might of Houdini's abdominal muscles, sucker punched the vaudevillian and inadvertently injured his appendix? Or had the performer's pride prevented him from seeing a physician for nagging stomach pains, delaying diagnosis and creating insurmountable medical problems?

The answer was likely a combination of factors. Houdini's busy work schedule (and his strongman's hubris) had barred him from seeing a physician for persistent abdominal distress of several days' duration. True, a zealous fan had recently punched Houdini in the abdomen, but this blow itself did not cause his appendicitis—physical trauma cannot precipitate appendicitis. There is little doubt that Houdini was already suffering from early appendicitis at the time he was struck. He probably ignored his increasing abdominal pain, mistakenly believing that the culprit was severe body blows and not a diseased appendix. Had the punching episode not occurred, Houdini might have realized that his continuing abdominal pain was a sign that something was very wrong and might have sought immediate medical attention.

The suffering Houdini arrived in Detroit from Montreal on Sunday evening, October 24, for a scheduled performance. His physical appearance stunned eager fans. One described him as having a "drawn face and dark shadows under tired eyes."[21] Houdini struggled through the performance (his last show ever). His manager mentioned to a waiting reporter that "the magician complained of severe abdominal pains on the train while going to Detroit," and that "the first twinge of pain was felt last week after he had engaged in a friendly sparring match."[22] Several hours after his appearance, Houdini began vomiting and had a temperature over 104 degrees.

A local physician diagnosed him with acute appendicitis and rushed him to the hospital for an emergency appendectomy. "To delay operation in acute appendicitis is to gamble with death,"[23] proclaimed one expert on the disease. Houdini's surgeon later explained that the performer's appendix was in an especially tricky location: "[It] was a long affair, which started in the right lower pelvis where it normally should, extended across the mid-line and lay in his left pelvis."[24] According to one survey, just 5 percent of appendices traveled such a path. The location of Houdini's appendix had created atypical initial symptoms. His discomfort was not simply confined to the right side of the lower abdomen, and his refusal to consult a physician had eliminated any possibilities of early diagnosis and treatment.

Houdini's appendix soon burst, spilling its fetid contents throughout his abdomen. A fulminating peritonitis—septic inflammation of the colorless, flimsy membrane that lines the abdomen and the internal organs—ensued. Nationwide statistics showed that, in this preantibiotic era, almost 95 percent of patients with Houdini's difficulties at this stage, a perforated appendix with diffuse peritonitis, died. Not only did he have peritonitis, but it had been caused by a particularly virulent strain of streptococci. The situation worsened as blood poisoning set in, the result of the toxic material spreading uncontrollably through his body.

Houdini's team of doctors did their best but the odds were stacked against them at this point. They knew enough about the disease to quickly declare: "Grave doubts are entertained for his recovery."[25] However, they had a somewhat misinformed understanding of appendicitis, and they also set into motion an enduring urban legend when they offhandedly and erroneously remarked, "The playful punches Houdini received were the direct cause of his plight, for one of the blows caused the appendix to burst, saturating his system with poison."[26] In the days following Houdini's appendectomy, telegrams and letters, filled with suggestions and encouragement, flooded the hospital. "If you can squeeze out of boxes and other contrivances," one well-wisher wrote, "you can certainly squeeze out of this job."[27]

In a last-ditch effort to save Houdini, his doctors experimented with novel drugs from Detroit's Parke-Davis Company. The firm, which was known for producing both the highly regarded antiseptic Formidine and the widely used disinfectant Cresylone, had one of the country's first commercial pharmaceutical laboratories. Its scientists had been developing numerous antitoxins, serums, and vaccines in man's battles against bacteria. The *New York Times* reported that one supposedly powerful potion had been "perfected in a Detroit laboratory and used for the first time [on Houdini]."[28] The doctors and Parke-Davis's management refused to divulge the serum's makeup, but according to initial accounts "its effects appear[ed] to be favorable."[29]

They were wrong. In this preantibiotic drug era, no antibacterial medicines were powerful enough to counter a massive infection like Houdini's streptococcal peritonitis. These rudimentary medicines lacked specificity and could not thwart the full array of particular bacterial subtypes. "We have not yet found any chemical substance that is specific for such bacterial infections as tuberculosis, pneumonia, or other forms of the invasion of the body by bacteria," admitted a physician. "We have, of course, such specific therapy as diphtheria antitoxin, or antityphoid and smallpox vaccination, but these are not chemical agents."[30] A terse headline in the *New York Evening Graphic* told it all: "SERUM FAILS."[31] The considerable number of bacteria in Houdini's bloodstream overwhelmed his diminished immunologic defense mechanisms. The physicians were left with a rapidly deteriorating patient.

Houdini was soon in total body failure. The surgeons reoperated in a desperate attempt to stem the streptococcal poisoning. They faced a stinking abdomen filled with yellow-greenish pus and yards of convoluted, inflamed, beet-red intestine. There was little to do. The doctors diplomatically reported Houdini's condition as "less favorable than before the operation."[32] Without antibiotics, intravenous fluids, and respirators, none of which were available, and lots of luck, Houdini had no chance of survival.

On Halloween afternoon, five days after his first operation and forty-eight hours following a second, Houdini died. He joined a long list of famous American appendicitis victims, including George Bellows, Walter Reed, Frederic Remington, and Brigham Young. Houdini's life insurance included an accidental death benefit, but an investigation concluded that the supporter who punched him had not injured Houdini's appendix. "Houdini was already ill when he arrived in Montreal," confirmed a local manager of the insurance firm. "He was not hurt by any stomach-punching demonstrations."[33] Two months after his death, the life insurance company paid his widow $25,000.

A Higher Price Tag

Despite Houdini's death, the extraordinary effort to save him underscored the enormous clinical changes that shaped medicine. Well-intentioned but overzealous physicians and surgeons, profit-driven hospital administrators, aggressive pharmaceutical companies, and a too-quick-to-believe public brought about, for the first time, the triad of unnecessary laboratory tests, ill-advised surgical operations, and uncontrollable health care costs. Medical triumphs exceeded medical failures, and the nation's doctors were benefiting from the profession's coalescing. By the 1930s, medicine had effectively settled many of the thorny political problems of its past. The reforms in medical education and in hospital administration that began in the early years of the century continued advancing. The professional standardization that these reforms helped bring about meant the end of sectarians, incompetent physicians, and poorly run health care facilities and medical schools. State legislatures strengthened licensing laws as well, further ensuring that all American doctors would be held to the same basic standards.

Newly empowered physicians, speaking with a unified professional voice, expanded their influence beyond the confines of clinical medicine. They made demands on the pharmaceutical industry, providing marketing guidelines to mainstream companies. Doctors refused to allow advertisements in medical journals for proprietary drugs and for nonsensical nostrums. The AMA also gave the food industry notice that its products had to meet new nutritional standards if they were to appear in advertisements in the *Journal of the American Medical Association*. In 1937 the inadvertent poisoning and deaths of more than one hundred people from an improperly prepared sulfa drug, "Elixir Sulfanilamide," led to further pressure from the medical profession and hastened the passage of the Food, Drug, and Cosmetic Act, which President Franklin Roosevelt signed into law in 1938. This new legislation significantly increased the government's regulatory authority over drugs. It mandated a premarket review of the safety of new products and banned false therapeutic claims in drug labeling.

As medicine's prestige increased, so did physicians' incomes. In 1938 a study by the U.S. Department of Commerce showed that the average take-home pay for the nation's doctors exceeded $4,000, two and a half times more than a grade-school teacher earned and four times above the national average. Specialists earned almost twice that of general practitioners.

Part of the reason for this earnings increase was that doctors tended to locate their practices in cities and wealthy suburbs. Physicians preferred cities because of the resources for their practice. Urban centers had large numbers of general hospital beds, plentiful accessory facilities for specialty practice, and intellectual communities that promoted the interchange of professional ideas and scientific research. Doctors also tended to live in counties with the highest per capita income. Between 1923 and 1938, the physician–population ratio in the nation's richest counties increased 10 percent while the number declined 27 percent in the poorest. "It becomes increasingly apparent," wrote a contemporary observer, "that wealth is a dominant factor in determining the . . . effectiveness of physician services in different areas."[34]

Better medicine also meant better health for Americans. They lived longer. The average male life expectancy in 1930 was fifty-eight years (up from forty-eight years in 1900), while the average female life expectancy was sixty-one years (up from fifty-one in 1900). Seven percent of the population was sixty-five years of age or older by the 1930s. Markedly fewer women died from pregnancy or childbirth. The infant mortality rate declined almost 40 percent from 1915 to 1935. Leading causes of death shifted from infectious to chronic diseases—a sign of progress in public health administration and clinical care. In 1900 the primary causes of mortality were infectious respiratory diseases (influenza, pneumonia, and tuberculosis) and bacteria-induced diarrhea, accounting for nearly one-third of all fatalities. By 1930, heart disease was number one, making up almost 20 percent of deaths, while deaths from respiratory illnesses and diarrhea declined by one-half.

These improvements in medical care, however, carried a high price tag. The profession, the public, and the government worked to adapt to a new landscape where medical care required heavy capital outlays and medical costs stretched family budgets. In 1935 alone, Americans spent $2.8 billion on health care, approximately 4 percent of the gross national product. While precise records on health care expenditure had not been previously maintained, historians agree that the 4 percent figure was a significant increase from the turn of the century.

The rise of science and technology triggered the end of low-priced medical care. If an individual could not afford a doctor in the nineteenth century, he faced minimal health risk because most therapies were ineffective. The same could not be said of an American after World War I. Effective therapies simply cost more. Few individuals questioned the fact that an appendectomy in a modern hospital operating room should be more expensive than the same procedure performed by a general practitioner on a kitchen table in a patient's home. Acute hospital care required surgeons, anesthesiologists, pathologists, registered nurses, laboratory technicians, X-ray personnel, and pricey equipment. Pharmaceutical companies also drove up medical costs by producing expensive and effective medicines—insulin to treat diabetes became commercially available in the 1920s and sulfa drugs to kill bacteria followed in the 1930s. Furthermore, medical equipment–makers developed elaborate and costly devices for diagnosis and treatment—the sphygmomanometer, or blood pressure meter, was widely used by the 1920s and the iron lung to treat breathing disorders in polio victims became a fixture in hospitals in the 1930s.

Medical and hospital charges were on their way to becoming one of the largest items in a household's budget. Health care expenses consumed one-half of some families' annual earnings. Many Americans found the high fees for physicians' services and the large expenses for hospitalization unreasonable, despite the improved results. "In former years when the range of sickness costs was lower, and few illnesses caused high expenditures, families with middle-class incomes felt financial pinch due to sickness much less frequently than today," wrote a medical economist. "Now, people who are economically secure, humanly speaking, against all ordinary demands, are not secure against the costs of sickness. Thus, the economic problems of medical care now implicate not merely wage-earners but the whole population, except the 5 per cent with the largest incomes."[35]

The social and economic turmoil of the Great Depression in the 1930s exacerbated the situation. Only 3 percent of Americans were unemployed in 1929. Four years later the unemployment rate had octupled nationally and reached 40 percent in some rural states. As the number of American poor swelled, access to medical services decreased. "Everyone knows that the average American family, with more than four persons and an annual income of less than $2,000, cannot afford to pay from $80 to $160 a year for medical service,"[36] complained a writer for *The New Republic* in 1932. Bankrupt farm families, many living far from doctors, hospitals, or other medical facilities, struggled to obtain any level of medical care. In the cities, financially strapped homeowners and landlords failed to pay taxes, depleting the tax-supported relief funds that already covered 15 percent of the national medical bill, primarily for hospital care. Americans in increasing numbers either could not meet the expense of their medical and hospital bills or were denied medical benefits as government-sponsored programs shrank.

The health care situation continued to worsen as the Depression wore on, and politicians began debating the ways to ensure health care for the citizenry. The medical debates were part of a larger reform effort to increase fiscal benefits for all citizens, including unemployment insurance, public relief programs, and Social Security for the elderly. Among the prominent suggestions was the concept of shared risk and the need for federal- and state-sponsored health insurance plans. The content of these debates closely mirrored concepts in President Roosevelt's liberal New Deal (liberal in this era meaning someone who supported government-sponsored social programs, not a proponent of laissez-faire policies). Liberal supporters of the New Deal attempted to convince the public that health care was a social entitlement. Never before had state and federal financing of health services been proposed on such a grand scale.

Physicians largely opposed a heavy-handed government interfering in their day-to-day clinical activities. Most physicians chafed at terms like "governmental control," "welfare state," and "socialized medicine." Doctors generally supported a more conservative or anti–New Deal approach. They clung to the status quo of minimal government involvement, a private medical marketplace, and unimpeded doctor-patient relationships. Like the opponents of fixed-income arrangements, many doctors saw government-managed health care as undermining the status of physicians and the sanctity of the doctor-patient relationship.

"Americanism versus Sovietism for the American people"

Doctors reacted to the medical socioeconomic debates of the 1930s differently from how they had responded to previous public discussions of the internal workings of American medicine (e.g., licensure during the antebellum period; sectarians' rights in the Civil War; and educational and hospital reform at the turn of the twentieth century). Physicians had finally consolidated their scientific, social, and cultural authority into professional power, a process that stretched back to colonial times. American medicine now spoke with a generally unified and forceful voice. Thus, doctors could respond to public discourse in a coordinated and vigorous manner. Not only were physicians organized and acting as one, but they had found an individual to serve as their mouthpiece, their popularizer, and their energizer.

Morris Fishbein was a short, portly man with an unmistakable Hoosier twang. The son of a Jewish émigré glassware retailer, he was born in St. Louis in 1889, raised in Indianapolis, and received his medical education and training in Chicago. In 1924 Fishbein became editor in chief of the *Journal of the American Medical Association*. He held this position for two and a half decades and dominated the profession from this powerful perch. Inexhaustible in his role at the *Journal,* he was the all-seeing, all-knowing, all-consuming overlord of American medicine. A 1937 *Time* story described Fishbein as the personification of American medicine and someone who was "worldly alert."[37]

Fishbein's influence stemmed from his prolific writings and his combativeness as author, editor, and speaker. Rhetoric was his forte and his enthusiasm for the English language was unbounded. "I enjoy verbal fencing," he recalled in his autobiography, "especially the use of a large vocabulary, a fertile imagination, and a sensitivity to semantics."[38] He spewed out fifteen thousand words a week, penned hundreds of editorials for the *Journal,* authored over twenty books, edited dozens more, and composed a health column syndicated to seven hundred newspapers. When Fishbein was not writing, he was delivering speeches—upward of one hundred thirty a year—or recording albums on medical topics for parents and their children.

The AMA that Fishbein represented was a much different, more powerful, organization than the one that had existed in the late nineteenth century and had been obsessed with defeating the sectarians. In 1901 it had reorganized itself by combining its county, state, and national societies into a unified federation, which was colloquially referred to as "organized medicine." The idea had been to enroll an increasing number of physicians until organized medicine represented a majority of the profession. This scheme succeeded because membership in local medical societies, which was linked to mandatory enrollment in the national organization, was increasingly a prerequisite for obtaining hospital privileges and patient referrals. So any doctor who wished to avail himself of hospital privileges or patient referrals ipso facto joined organized medicine. National membership grew from 6 percent of the nation's physicians (eight thousand doctors) in 1901 to half of the profession in 1910. Two decades later the AMA counted almost two-thirds of the country's physicians as its constituents.

During the late 1920s and early 1930s the AMA tested its growing power with a well-publicized campaign against medical self-promoters of all types. Fishbein, serving as the Association's eloquent hatchet man, sharpened his editor's pen and became known as the country's foremost quack buster. He had a "real genius" for it, one colleague said, taking down "reckless and dangerous frauds with a gleam of relish in his eye."[39] Fishbein declared written war on medical bamboozlers, attacking everything from the pseudoscience of sanatology (a system of curing diseases by rectal enemas) to the transplanting of goat testicles underneath an elderly man's skin to rejuvenate him sexually. Quacks, he explained in one of his numerous exposés, "have delayed scientific progress through their attacks on scientific experimentation, and unquestionably have been responsible for the spread of epidemics and for a certain proportion of mortality from disease."[40]

Fishbein's effort to put charlatans out of business was groundwork for his greatest public relations challenge: defending the AMA and its 100,000 members against a growing notion that the medical profession was a conservative, moneymaking monopoly indifferent to cost and the distribution of health care. This view gained strength in the early 1930s, and an increasing number of articles in newspapers and lay magazines stoked the flames of these suspicions. "True, the A.M.A. has no legal authority, no police powers, but it can and does summon its medical squads and battalions to a holy war in defense of their own status, their own emoluments," complained a reporter in *The Nation*. "It does this whenever the pressure of public need fires a group of progressive doctors with the determination to cast off the shackles of the A.M.A.'s pocket-motivated 'ethics' and attempt to give people decent medical care at a price they can afford to pay."[41] An incoming president of the AMA worsened the situation when he ignorantly suggested that the profession decrease the supply of physicians and prevent any attempts to increase the number to meet demands for their services: "Much of the present unrest and anxious emotion about state and socialized medicine is the result of economic fear and uncertainty due to the social dangers that have developed as the result of an overcrowded body of doctors."[42]

The public's concern with medical expenses and delivery of health services prompted the formation of an independent, privately funded commission, the Committee on the Costs of Medical Care. The committee comprised economists, physicians, public health service personnel, social scientists, and lay individuals. It began issuing detailed reports on the state of American health care that included statistics and pertinent financial information. These reports gave Americans access, for the first time, to estimates of their national health care expenditures ($3.65 billion in 1929) and where their money went (30 percent to physicians, 23 percent to hospitals, and 18 percent to drug companies).

The committee's summary report in 1932 was a landmark in the development of medical socioeconomic policy. It combined all the research compiled over five years, provided elaborate statistics, and confirmed the bleak state of affairs. The report included a comprehensive survey of over 8,500 white families. Nearly half of the households with incomes under $1,200 received no medical care, meaning that approximately one-quarter of Americans never saw a physician. Not only was treatment substandard or lacking, but costs were unequally distributed; the less than 4 percent of families with the highest medical bills incurred one-third of the nation's medical expenses.

The report suggested two underlying principles for medical reform: the need for greater cooperation between providers, consumers, and the government; and an insistence that high-quality medical care be made available to all people. The *New York Times* headlined its page-one story on the report: "Socialized Medicine Is Urged in Survey." It said the chairman of the committee declared that the "medical profession was on its way toward some form of community organization, whether it liked it nor not."[43]

The committee offered several recommendations based on the report. Most important, it advocated group medical practices, which it felt would capitalize on both administrative efficiencies and the resources of technology-rich, bureaucratically strong hospitals. Such an approach departed from the inefficient, mom-and-pop business attitude of much of American medicine. The second recommendation was for the use of insurance or taxes to pay for health care. The report emphasized that large expenses were concentrated among a small group of people, those with the most severe medical issues. Since everyone had some risk of becoming seriously ill during their lifetime, the committee suggested that Americans assume a kind of collective responsibility, or health insurance, for each other's medical expenses. The committee also proposed that states and local communities establish health planning agencies to coordinate the delivery of medical care, especially between urban and rural areas. Additionally, the committee called for physicians to devote greater attention to the prevention of diseases and the socioeconomic aspects of clinical practice. To assist doctors in their new medical world, the committee recommended training three types of health care workers in large numbers: nursing attendants, nursing midwives, and hospital and clinical department administrators.

Fishbein and the leaders of organized medicine viewed the report and the committee's recommendations as a radical attack on the essence of American medicine. They abhorred the ideas of yielding clinical decisions to paraprofessionals, bureaucratizing health care planning, and decreasing physician autonomy to reduce economic barriers to medical care. Fishbein assured his readers that the profession would never accept government interference in the practice of medicine, nor would it sacrifice doctors' professional sovereignty to the medical needs of the public: "These invaders will find that there are few physicians indeed so unaware of their obligation to medicine as a profession that they are ready, even in such times as these, to sell their medical birthrights for the promoters' mess of pottage."[44]

Fishbein, a savvy medical politician, had acquired advance copies of the report and worked to contain its impact before the public had an opportunity to digest the findings. This task was daunting even for Fishbein because the committee had an authority of its own to publicize the report, Edward Bernays, a nephew of Sigmund Freud and the country's most renowned public relations expert. "We sent a letter to 25,000 VIPs, to the 2,000-odd editors of daily newspapers, we had radio talks on the National Farm and Home Radio Hour," recalled Bernays. "I was sure the final report would stir the country and bring response in social action."[45]

To counter Bernays, Fishbein wrote a scathing editorial invoking memories of the post–World War I Red Scare with its fears of communist and socialist influence on American institutions. He declared the committee's recommendations to be little more than collectivist propaganda and proclaimed that government and its subsidies must be kept out of medicine. "There is the question of Americanism versus sovietism for the American people," wrote Fishbein. "Let the big business men who would reorganize medical practice, the efficiency engineers who would make doctors the cogs of their governmental machines, give a little of their sixty horse power brains to a realization of the fact that Americans prefer to be human beings."[46]

Fishbein sent copies of his editorial to newspapers in time for them to include the AMA's viewpoints in any coverage of the report. Bernays termed it an "AMA hatchet job on those with whom it disagreed."[47] Fishbein called his ploy "an act in keeping with the best traditions of American journalism."[48] Fishbein had the winning strategy. When the *New York Times* covered the report, it ran an adjacent article with the headline, "Medical Journal Attacks Report, Editorial Declares the Findings of Majority of Committee Incite to Revolution."[49] Fishbein's editorial achieved what he hoped. It sowed confusion in the mind of the public: who should they believe on these important medical issues, the stance of the almost century-old AMA, the authoritative voice of the nation's physicians, or the recommendation of a recently organized commission dominated by nonmedical personnel? Fishbein trusted that the improved status of the medical profession made the answer obvious.

He followed up the editorial with a series of presentations nationwide. The press and public flocked to hear the stump speech of the one-man boss of organized medicine. Fishbein employed a style described as "caustically humorous,"[50] and his audiences responded with a "satisfied titter"[51] when he criticized the proposed hospital-based (also known as corporate) style of practice with its bureaucracy and health insurance schemes. "It's the medical attention that makes a hospital, not the number of girls you have sitting in the waiting room to welcome the guests,"[52] Fishbein told his listeners.

Much as Fishbein anticipated, the sniping between organized medicine and its critics created doubt and discord concerning the report. "Under its present regime the A.M.A. is forehanded," noted a reporter for *Time*. "It anticipates attack against its integrity, cohesion and liberty. With all its mighty might, it protects the interests of the private practitioner."[53]

Fishbein's tactics ultimately overwhelmed his opponents. They tried to smear him as an elitist, an authoritarian, a political reactionary. They colored the AMA as a betrayer of the public's trust. All their efforts failed. The Committee on the Costs of Medical Care failed to create a consensus for political change and its recommendations were left to languish. Several years later, a smug Fishbein noted how the committee's report was "hidden away in the stacks of large libraries," and that "few people indeed pay much attention to it."[54] Bernays was more discerning: "And so medical care of the American people was set back for years, although the committee's report still serves as a guide line to what will inevitably come if the American people are to get the medical care due them."[55]

The AMA's heated reaction to the committee had a chilling effect on national medical politics. The newly elected Roosevelt administration, unwilling to jeopardize passage of the Social Security Act, excluded health insurance from its provisions. The medical lobby also helped defeat other attempts to pass health care legislation, including the federal financing of hospital and medical school construction. Fishbein coordinated virtually all of the opposition to these measures. He had become so influential that when *Time* magazine reported on the political power of organized medicine, it placed him on its cover, along with his prodding quote: "Shall medicine remain a profession or become a trade?"[56]

Despite the AMA's dominant position within the profession, some physicians questioned its policies. In late 1937, four hundred thirty medical academicians, many of whom belonged to the AMA, organized the Committee of Physicians for the Improvement of Medicine. This committee issued a position paper designed to further medical education, medical research, and medical care. The organization's platform acknowledged that the "health of the people is a direct concern of the government"[57] and asked that the federal government establish a department of medicine to coordinate governmental medical activities. The physicians also recommended that the government make available public funds to the indigent for medical care and to medical schools and hospitals for laboratory, diagnostic, and consultative services. The Committee of Physicians did not advocate compulsory health insurance, but instead emphasized hospital-based group practice as a method to improve the delivery of health care. These men were political liberals who disagreed with organized medicine's continued embrace of the traditional, individualistic, fee-for-service, private practice of medicine as the best means to solve cost and distribution problems. In many respects, the platform resembled the recommendations of the Committee on the Costs of Medical Care.

The audacity of these rebellious doctors angered Fishbein. As with his campaign against the report of the Committee on the Costs of Medical Care, Fishbein preempted the Committee of Physicians with a contemptuous editorial. He accused the signatories of being turncoats to the profession: "Such careless participation in propaganda is lamentable, to say the least. Certainly the unthinking endorsers of the principles and proposals owe to the medical profession some prompt disclaimers."[58]

The controversy over the Committee of Physicians was short-lived, as was the group's political influence. The story remains a little-remembered incident in the history of American medicine, but its work damaged the impression of omnipotency that the AMA was trying to protect. The public learned that the Association did not speak for all physicians and that a sizable number of medical men believed the profession needed improvement. "Scores of physicians in good standing are beginning to say openly that medicine must not oppose 'valid experimentation in meeting social needs,'" wrote a reporter in *Harper's*. "These voices will undoubtedly be heard. If they cannot soon prevail sufficiently to end the fruitless, senseless opposition to new types of organization, the loss to everyone concerned will be serious."[59]

These early skirmishes between the AMA, the government, the Committee on the Costs of Medical Care, and the Committee of Physicians for the Improvement of Medicine were the opening salvos in a bitterly fought war over the socioeconomics of health care. A decade later, the ongoing battles resulted in Fishbein being forced to resign as editor of the *Journal of the American Medical Association*. His contentiousness and unalterable belief that government must remain out of medicine grew increasingly at odds with the evolving political philosophy of the AMA.

Bona Fide Specialist or Not

Organized medicine's political struggles in the 1930s provided no solutions for skyrocketing health care costs, but internal bureaucratic battles did settle some of the remaining organizational discord between specialists and generalists. Throughout the twentieth century, specialists had continued to grow in number and, consequently, influence. They comprised 17 percent of the country's physicians in 1930, and the percentage of physicians self-identified as specialists increased 37 percent during the decade. By 1940, full-time specialists comprised 25 percent of the profession.

The ever-broadening specialist corps faced pressures from within and without the profession to define the meaning of a specialist, both in terms of the scope of a specialty and the standards for practice. Voices from within the medical profession pushed for these developments as a way to ensure that specialists maintained their status as elite practitioners. These medical insiders also knew that if the profession did not move to regulate specialists, the state governments would eventually step in to fill this role, a situation that few doctors preferred. There was lay pressure as well. Patients, increasingly dependent on physicians for health care treatments deemed essential and necessary, could not tell who was qualified to do what—licensure only established a floor, and membership in medical societies revealed little about competency. The public needed reassurance from the medical profession that their caregivers had the imprimatur of a respected medical authority. It was simply unsatisfactory that each physician was the sole assessor of his or her own qualifications to practice a specialty.

In response to lay pressure and internal power struggles, specialties began forming organizations to determine who was a bona fide specialist. These self-governing organizations became known as "boards" and evaluated candidates with rigorous written examinations and personal interviews. Successful applicants earned board certification, a designation that specialists highly prized. Board certification indicated clinical competency to the public.

The medical profession, frequently divided over questions of regulation, initially accepted the arrival of specialty boards. The first was created in 1917 for ophthalmology. Eye doctors had practiced their specialized craft since before the Civil War. The profession viewed the new certifying examination as a natural manifestation of ophthalmologists' emerging self-identity, especially the need to separate themselves from the non-M.D. optometrists. General practitioners did not resent or challenge this move as most were neither adept nor interested in eye examinations.

But as the certification process gained momentum across the profession, general practitioners began to oppose these attempts to place limits on who could call himself a specialist and on what he could practice. Each specialty that solidified its identity through board certification appropriated more of medicine for itself and left less for the general practitioner. By 1937, specialties had organized boards for anesthesiologists; colon and rectal surgeons; dermatologists; ear, nose, and throat physicians; obstetricians and gynecologists; orthopedic surgeons; pathologists; pediatricians; psychiatrists and neurologists; radiologists; and urologists.

The AMA agreed with the concerns of general practitioners. The powerful organization insisted that a generalist did not need the consent of a certifying board to term himself a specialist and practice aspects of a specialty. The ever-ready Fishbein set forth the AMA's position in numerous editorials. "The growth in specialization has placed the general practitioner in an inferior position so far as prestige is concerned," he wrote, "even though the general practitioner might well be competent to deal with the majority of patients seeking medical help."[60]

The AMA did not oppose the emergence of free-standing specialty boards, but it attempted to stake its claim to some type of oversight authority. Leaders of the AMA believed that as the most powerful concern within the profession, it should exert control over clinical jurisdictional disputes. Their proposal was to give certification authority to the Council on Medical Education and Hospitals, the suborganization within the AMA that had earlier been involved in regulating medical schools. Once again, Fishbein delivered the message: "The Council on Medical Education and Hospitals of the American Medical Association expresses its approval of various examining boards which conform to standards established by the Council. . . . It is hoped that [we] may begin to establish order in the chaotic condition that now prevails."[61]

That the AMA should manage the growth of specialties made a certain degree of sense. Many viewed the AMA as a fierce protector of all the nation's doctors. This role was constantly reaffirmed by its influential publications, notably the Fishbein-led *Journal of the American Medical Association* and the *American Medical Directory* with its massive registry of the nation's doctors. The organization for many years had also supported educational reform, one of the broadest medical administrative improvements in the early twentieth century; it had been able to invest money and manpower to produce yearly lists of approved hospitals, internships, and residencies for specialty training. Admittedly, many doctors believed that the AMA supported generalist practitioners over specialists (general practitioners made up 80 percent of the Association's membership in 1930), but specialists, particularly academicians, filled the majority of its leadership positions.

Despite the AMA's accomplishments, they could not alter political reality: the specialties had matured without the assistance of the Association and none would go willingly under its control. Fishbein could rail against the specialty boards and the AMA could tout the merits of the Council on Medical Education and Hospitals, but specialists ultimately refused to bow to the AMA's authority.

Without a centralized body like the AMA at the helm, attempts to regulate specialization progressed, but in a confused, desultory manner. An Advisory Board for Medical Specialties was organized to assume jurisdiction over the policies and problems common to the specialty boards. However, it served the interests of academicians and little of those of the private practitioner. Preexisting specialty organizations, like the American Pediatric Society, the American College of Radiology, the American College of Physicians, or the American College of Surgeons, had competing self-interests and failed to unify around board certification. The question of who should control specialization created a complex web of medical organizations rife with infighting and divided loyalties.

Different specialties stood to benefit from board certification in different ways, and consequently leaders in each specialty refused to support one umbrella organization over all of medicine or even over any given specialty. For example, the existing pediatric specialty organization, the American Pediatric Society, only addressed the research aspects of childhood disease and not the day-to-day clinical practice of pediatrics. Pediatricians wanted a separate, independent certifying board to delineate specialist qualifications and promote the growth of general pediatricians. The existing radiology society, the American College of Radiology, provided for organizational cohesion, but members wanted a separate certification board to provide status and emphasize that they were not mere laboratory technicians, but holders of a medical degree.

An additional wrinkle to the entire board certification process came from the further subdividing of medical practices into subspecialties. In certain cases, medicine advanced so rapidly during the early twentieth century that areas that had once been their own specialty became parents to a host of smaller, discrete topics. Internal medicine, for example, a specialty with its own organizational body, the American College of Physicians, had members promoting the inchoate subspecialties of endocrinology, gastroenterology, hematology, infectious disease, nephrology, and pulmonary disease.

Because board certification determined a practitioner's status and expertise, the level of specialization set by the board delineated the boundaries of any given specialty. Internists managed to organize a board to cover the whole of internal medicine, the American Board of Internal Medicine. In doing so, the specialty exerted a degree of control over its budding subspecialties. Surgery followed a different path. Before surgeons had established a board to address the general practice of surgery, subspecialists had organized boards for orthopedic surgery, colon and rectal surgery, urology, and plastic surgery. The presence of the surgical subspecialty boards left an open question: What was to become of the general surgeon?

"Handicraft outruns science"

The concept of "generalism" carried a negative connotation in 1930s medical America. It suggested lack of expertise, unfamiliarity with medical technology, and old-style clinical behavior. General practitioners had been dealing with this stigma for years and now surgeons faced a similar predicament. Many younger general surgeons had trained in multiyear surgical residencies and felt competent with procedures like prostate removals or fracture settings. But in the public's mind, a board-certified urologist was more competent in prostate surgery and a board-certified orthopedist was more competent in fracture repair. Because no general surgery board existed at first, general surgeons could only rely on their membership in the American College of Surgeons to confirm their ability and status to the public.

But the American College of Surgeons was no longer as prestigious in defining a specialist as it had been when Franklin Martin and a thousand surgeons marched into the Congress Hotel in Chicago. The specialist-surgeons who founded the American College of Surgeons in 1913 had hoped both to distinguish surgeons from general practitioners and to raise all surgeons to the highest operative standards. Despite these intentions and the mandates of American College of Surgeons bylaws, the organization had set membership guidelines low in its haste to expand enrollment—by the mid-1920s there were over seven thousand Fellows of the College. The American College of Surgeons emphasized an applicant's ability to perform surgery and was less concerned about the depth of medical knowledge that sustained his surgical judgment. Membership did not depend on examinations or personal interviews. "There is about as much distinction in being a member of the American College of Surgeons as in belonging to the mob in Grand Central Station, New York City," complained a member surgeon from Rochester in 1933.[62]

In the early 1930s a faction of general surgeons decided to distinguish themselves from the College. They were mostly young and well-trained surgical educators from the large cities, men who would ultimately advance surgery through the middle decades of the twentieth century. For now, they were idealists with a steadfast opposition to surgical mediocrity.

Evarts Graham, a man who minced few words, led this breakaway group. It was no surprise that he would serve as the main instigator. Tall, aloof, and patrician in comportment, he never sidestepped a confrontation nor avoided the medical limelight. A series of widely hailed medical firsts had already marked his career. He was the first full-time professor of surgery at Washington University in St. Louis (1919), the first physician to develop an X-ray technique to visualize the gallbladder (1924), the first surgeon to remove a lung for a malignancy (1933), and among the first to demonstrate a link between cigarettes and cancer (1950)—as fate would have it, the chain-smoking Graham died from lung cancer in 1957. He was also the first of a younger generation of general surgeons to challenge the aging founders of the American College of Surgeons over their failure to uphold the academic side of surgery. "The deftness of the operator, the number of operations performed and even the income of the surgeon are often chosen as criteria upon which to measure the greatness of the surgeon," explained Graham. "These are the false standards which lead to unwise operating, too much operating and the commercialism of the profession."[63]

At a series of acrimonious meetings, Graham and his supporters told the leaders of the American College of Surgeons about their plans to organize a certifying body for general surgeons. The college, they said, had allowed "fingers to replace brains" while "handicraft outruns science."[64] Graham's cohorts threatened to turn the college's annual meeting into a "surgical circus"[65] unless the college's leaders cooperated in the founding of the independent board. Representatives of the college, who feared a collapse of their organization, grudgingly agreed to cooperate. The new organization was called the American Board of Surgery.

News of a new surgical board delighted the AMA and Fishbein. They felt the presence of another powerful surgical organization would diffuse the influence of their major political rival, the American College of Surgeons. Fishbein assumed that the new board would be responsible for the "certification of general surgeons," as well as "those practicing in the remaining specialized subdivisions."[66] He was, however, overly optimistic.

Despite high hopes that the American Board of Surgery could formulate a certification procedure that covered all of surgery, its actual effect was limited. Graham, the board's first president, attempted to rein in the surgical subspecialties and tried to broker links between the American Board of Surgery and the already established subspecialty boards. As convincing as he could be, it was to no avail. Established surgical subspecialists pointed to the educational and financial rewards that their own certification represented as reason enough to remain independent of general surgeons. Burgeoning surgical subspecialties, like anesthesiology, neurosurgery, and thoracic surgery, also broke away and organized autonomous certifying bodies. Thus, the American Board of Surgery never gained control of the surgical subspecialties and never established a dominant position in the whole of surgery. To this day, no political commonality exists between general surgery and the various subspecialties. The result is a surgical lobby that functions in a divided manner.

Overall, board certification was a muddled and convoluted process throughout the 1930s, but it did bring about important organizational changes in American medicine. The status and authority that board certification afforded helped to distinguish branches and subbranches of medicine. It also facilitated the growth of specialization. By 1950 almost 40 percent of America's physicians identified themselves as full-time specialists and, of this group, over 50 percent were board certified. In addition, hospitals began to use board certification as a qualification for staff membership and admitting privileges.

While doctors could look back on the 1920s and 1930s as a period of great achievement, they could not ignore the intimidating challenges that this success created. The vast changes that occurred in American medicine during the first decades of the twentieth century, especially the blurring of lines between clinical and public responsibilities, placed a stress on physicians not previously seen. This interplay between internal organizational issues, external political concerns, and startling clinical advances would vex medicine for the remainder of the century. Lay individuals increasingly looked to the government and other agencies, not to the profession, to secure the rights to medical services that they believed were due them. This confusion of allegiance made it appear as if the sophistication and speed of scientific gains had exceeded the capabilities of the profession to handle its political affairs.

Doctors grappled with the perilous questions of how their profession would be organized and regulated in the future. How could the profession provide more modern health care against the backdrop of increasing governmental encroachment on their private practice of medicine? Despite this uncertainty, one thing about medicine was clear: specialty medicine, with its recondite complexities and technologic wizardries, speedily produced staggering clinical triumph after staggering clinical triumph.

Part Three

Triumphs and Trials

⁂ Eight ⁂

ASCENDANCY

Blood for Britain

AMERICAN MEDICINE'S INTERNATIONAL prestige had greatly increased in the interwar years and the United States now led the world in providing many sophisticated medical treatments. Among other things, its doctors were at the forefront of research regarding the preservation and use of blood and its by-products. Acknowledging this expertise, the government of Great Britain reached out to the U.S. medical community for assistance in providing blood for emergency transfusions after Nazi Germany initiated its siege of England—the British Ministry of Health estimated that if the German Luftwaffe's aerial bombardment escalated, 600,000 people could be killed and twice that many injured. Consequently, much like during the First World War with the Ambulance Américaine in France, the country's medical establishment became involved in World War II long before the U.S. government officially declared its participation in any hostilities.

On June 12, 1940, a group of high-ranking physicians who concentrated in blood research met in New York City to discuss how to supply the embattled British with the needed blood. The attendees included a Nobel Prize winner in medicine, administrators of several biological and pharmaceutical firms, and representatives of the surgeons general of the U.S. Army and Navy. The task that the British government had presented them was both straightforward and incredibly complex: organizing a coordinated blood collection effort larger than any the world had ever seen, something not only logistically challenging but pushing the boundaries of medical research.

It was only a quarter century earlier that an American physician first determined how to preserve blood for transfusions. The use of a powerful anticoagulant allowed the blood to be maintained in liquid nonclotted form, which slowed its spoiling and made it available for up to a week. In World War I, a U.S. Army medical officer took advantage of this discovery and set up a rudimentary blood storage facility near the front lines. He completed fewer than two dozen transfusions, but his ice-cooled refrigeration unit, with its supply of anticoagulated blood, was one of the world's earliest blood depots. American medical researchers working in the 1920s and 1930s subsequently identified the A, B, O, and Rhesus (Rh) blood compatibility groups, a discovery that dramatically decreased the threat of fatal mismatch reactions.

As blood transfusions became safe, a physician at Chicago's Cook County Hospital established a laboratory in 1937 that stocked donated blood. He coined the phrase "blood bank," explaining that the term "is not a mere metaphor. . . . Just as one cannot draw money from a bank unless one has deposited some, so the blood preservation department cannot supply blood unless as much comes in as goes out."[1] Blood banking, with its ready availability of blood for transfusions, greatly reduced the time needed to find a matching donor, especially in a medical emergency. Blood banks gradually spread across the nation and led to the development of broad-based donor programs.

Also in this period John D. Rockefeller founded a privately managed blood service in New York, the Blood Transfusion Betterment Association. Despite its quaint name, the organization was as modern as any feature of American medicine. It brought blood researchers together to study the science of blood transfusion as well as to stimulate physician education and training in the specialty field of hematology. The Blood Transfusion Betterment Association also provided the administrative know-how to match hospitalized patients in need of blood with donors, who were on call twenty-four hours a day and paid according to the amount of blood given ($25 for half a pint). In a nod to the philanthropic bent of its major benefactor, the association also raised funds to provide transfusion services to the indigent or, as they were labeled, "impecunious patients."[2]

A good deal of the blood research in the years leading up to World War II focused on how to extend the shelf life of stored blood beyond the seven-day barrier. Investigators began to look into blood plasma as a possible solution. Plasma, a protein-salt suspension with red and white blood cells and platelets, is the liquid component of blood and makes up 55 percent of its total volume (the average person has slightly over five pints of plasma). It is composed mostly of water but contains generous amounts of albumin (the chief constituent of the body's proteins), globulins (mostly antibodies to ward off infections), glucose (the cells' chief energy source), and minerals (calcium, magnesium, potassium, and sodium, among the most well known). Plasma serves a wide variety of functions, from maintaining a satisfactory blood pressure to supplying critical proteins for clotting, hormonal balance, and immunity. To obtain blood plasma, medical technicians first separate freshly drawn blood so that the blood cells settle to the bottom. They then pour off the liquid plasma. Blood plasma could not substitute for a transfusion of whole blood, but would temporarily sustain a victim's blood pressure during transportation to a hospital or, in the case of combat, initially resuscitate casualties at battlefield aid stations.

At the New York meeting to discuss England's medical appeal, the attendees learned that researchers had recently determined how to safely preserve refrigerated blood plasma for almost two months, eight times longer than what was possible with whole blood. Although researchers still considered the use of blood plasma experimental at the time of the New York gathering, the meeting's participants could not ignore its potential usefulness and lengthy shelf life. They decided to organize a Blood Plasma for Great Britain Project—colloquially known as the Blood for Britain plan—which would provide blood plasma to the Allied government on a level never before attempted. The American physicians who started the Blood for Britain project were also acting out of growing concern for the United States' own national defense program and possible military involvement in Asia and Europe.

The Blood for Britain administrators moved quickly to coordinate the collection and delivery efforts. The existence of Rockefeller's Blood Transfusion Betterment Association, particularly its managerial capabilities to procure and service large numbers of donors, led the project organizers to locate their program in New York City. Within several weeks after the initial meeting, they had hired a staff of twenty-two secretaries as well as numerous clerks and telephone operators. Engineers designed a refrigeration truck to carry blood from the various hospitals where it would be donated. The American Red Cross coordinated the public call for volunteer donors, while the Blood Transfusion Betterment Association supervised the actual collection of the blood and the technical separation of the plasma. "Plans Are Laid to Get Blood for British,"[3] declared a boldfaced headline in the *New York Times* in mid-August 1940.

Alongside these technical preparations, the Blood for Britain administrators worked assiduously to garner public support. Radio announcements ran around the clock. Volunteers distributed descriptive pamphlets. Publicity posters appeared on buses and subways. By Labor Day, program staff had registered over one thousand volunteers, and one month later the number climbed to five thousand. Eager donors, acting in support of their across-the-Atlantic ally, filled the collection centers at Presbyterian Hospital, Mount Sinai Hospital, New York Hospital, Long Island College Hospital, Lenox Hill Hospital, Memorial Hospital, and the Hospital for Joint Diseases. "It apparently had a very strong popular appeal," wrote one of the project's managers, "judging by the immediate enthusiastic response from every stratum of society."[4]

Despite Blood for Britain's success in attracting volunteer donors, the program soon encountered technical problems concerning the preparation of plasma on such a large scale. "When we began this work we were led to believe that it would be relatively simple," bemoaned the project's director. "We received the impression that preparing plasma would not be much more difficult than mixing a cocktail."[5] Mass production of plasma for shipment abroad simply differed from the preparation of small quantities of plasma in hospitals for immediate use. Among other concerns, program administrators had to determine how to store plasma (in liquid or dried form), how to design the collection bottle (dumbbell, square straight-sided, or cylindrical), and how to withdraw the volunteer's blood (vacuum versus suction versus simple venous pressure). The first batch of liquid plasma the American team sent to England had a milky appearance. British authorities raised the question of bacterial contamination and rejected it.

Mounting difficulties forced the project's organizers to take what they termed a "radical step,"[6] hiring a full-time, salaried physician to resolve the scientific questions, formulate a standardized collection technique, and better coordinate the cooperating hospitals.

Charles Drew

When executives of the Blood Plasma for Great Britain Project appointed Charles Drew as their mission's manager, they recognized there were few things the thirty-six-year-old could not master. Tall, broad-shouldered, and handsome, he carried himself with an obvious air of authority. "[Drew] was intense," said a friend, "always sticking to anything that needed to be done and not sparing his own energy."[7] He was a highly ambitious, well-organized, multitalented individual, starting with his academic and athletic success at Washington's Dunbar High School, and continuing through his college studies at Amherst College, medical school at McGill University, and surgical fellowship at Columbia University.

The Blood for Britain executives, however, wanted Drew as their director as much for his modern-style medical training as for his personal strengths. Drew represented the new breed of American physician, one who built his clinical expertise upon the knowledge of several specialties as well as an advanced background in scientific research. In Drew's case, this meant the preservation of blood and production of its substitutes. He had spent three years following medical school as a resident in internal medicine and pathology before commencing his surgical training. But the ever-competitive Drew also obtained a second doctoral degree, a doctor of science in medicine (M.D.Sc.), to further distinguish himself.

There was little argument that Drew possessed stellar medical and personal qualifications for the task at hand, but his appointment marked a milestone in American medical history thanks to one further distinction. Drew was African American, and he reached the zenith of the American medical establishment at a time when racial segregation persisted in medical care and racist attitudes defined large segments of the profession. Of the almost twenty thousand doctors who became medical officers in World War II, fewer than six hundred were African American.

Drew's specific training for his eventual stewardship of the Blood for Britain program began in early 1939 when he established Presbyterian

Hospital's first blood bank—he was simultaneously receiving surgical training and working on his doctorate at Columbia. He used this storage facility as the source for his scientific research. Drew's mentor described his protégé's "flare for organization with his attention to detail," and how he "insisted upon adequate controls in his experiments."[8]

Drew's dissertation, an imposing, two-hundred-plus-page encyclopedic compilation of facts and figures about blood banking, established him as one of the nation's most knowledgeable authorities on the latest techniques in blood preservation. By mid-1940, Drew had not only completed his thesis but had authored an additional half dozen papers on various aspects of blood banking, some of which were sponsored by the Blood Transfusion Betterment Association. "Intelligently employed during the first week of storage," he assured both the public and the profession, "[banked blood] need be neither dangerous nor disappointing."[9]

When Drew took control of the Blood for Britain project, he immediately set about remedying the problems that had plagued the early batches of plasma. "The job here is big, hard and important," he explained to his mother. "Mistakes will have international sequelae and must not be made."[10] He swiftly introduced stricter manufacturing criteria for the liquid plasma, including a rigid two weeks' bacterial culture quarantine, random checks to monitor for continued sterility and the presence of toxins, and routine tests of blood samples for syphilis. Drew also standardized and improved the blood collection technique at the participating hospitals, establishing age restrictions (over twenty-one and under sixty years) and blood pressure limits (under 110 systolic and over 80 diastolic). Program staff, under Drew's guidance, instructed donors not to fast in the morning in order to lessen the chance of their having low blood sugar and fainting at the afternoon's bloodletting. Finally, Drew revised record keeping and insisted that donors receive decorative cards from the Red Cross that noted their blood group and recognized their volunteer efforts.

In a few short weeks, Drew transformed the problem-riddled collection effort into the world's first successful mass procurement of blood and production of its by-products. Six weeks after Drew assumed charge, the cooperating hospitals were handling over 200 donors daily, and the Blood for Britain project had shipped 1,575 pints of plasma to England, all of which had tested sterile upon arrival and been given to the Royal

Air Force. Additionally, Drew's program technicians were processing another 3,000 pints they had collected, and were holding a further 1,700 pints of plasma for a final quarantine check before release to the American Red Cross for distribution. As one of the Blood for Britain project's trustees exclaimed, "Since Drew has been in charge, our major troubles have vanished."[11]

The Blood for Britain project under Drew successfully provided the British with the blood that the country desperately needed early in the war. However, the program, which had always been conceived as a short-term commitment, continued for less than a year and officially terminated in mid-January 1941. By that time the British were self-sufficient regarding their own volunteer blood donor programs and production of plasma. Additionally, the German army's much-vaunted land invasion of England never materialized, and the British Royal Air Force had thwarted the Luftwaffe's campaign to gain air superiority in the Battle of Britain.

Drew prepared a final report on the Blood for Britain program and detailed its popular appeal. His account described the 14,556 total donations and how they represented the first effort in the United States to collect large amounts of blood from voluntary civilian donors for wartime use. Drew not only smartly summarized the results of the Blood for Britain project, but he gathered the latest research studies and clinical updates on both sides of the Atlantic regarding blood procurement and its processing.

Now an internationally acclaimed leader in blood studies, Drew rapidly shifted his interests toward America's needs and certain recent medical developments that could further improve wartime blood supplies, specifically, the use of dried blood plasma.

The American Red Cross Blood Bank

The liquid form of plasma had been the mainstay of the Blood for Britain project for several reasons. The urgency of England's appeal favored using liquid plasma, which could be prepared more easily and faster than dried plasma, and liquid plasma was cheaper to manufacture than the dried type, which required expensive specialized equipment. In addition, medical researchers at the time considered the use of dried plasma experimental when contrasted with their growing experience with the liquid form. However, over the course of World War II, scientists learned how to store dried plasma safely for months at a time, far longer than liquid plasma. This dried plasma could be reconstituted into a liquid form with sterile water and be easily administered under battlefield conditions.

Drew first conceived his plan for the mass production of dried plasma as the Blood for Britain project was winding down. He began sending letters to leading blood researchers and pharmaceutical and commercial laboratories around the country to gather information about their dried plasma research and to press for further investigations. He also submitted his ideas to the American Red Cross, including the suggestion that the organization initiate a three-month pilot program for manufacturing dried plasma on a massive scale. Battle-ready containers could be produced with two easily opened tin cans—one containing dried plasma and another holding slightly less than a pint of sterile water used to reconstitute the mixture.

As the country's war footing intensified during this period, high-ranking officials from the armed forces, noting the success of the Blood for Britain program, solicited the Red Cross to create a national blood donor program in January 1941. It would be a massive undertaking, and Red Cross officials considered an experimental pilot project a necessary first step. They looked to Drew, who had already submitted his proposal for such a program, to be its medical director. Numerous Red Cross executives and scientists had collaborated with Drew on the Blood for Britain project and were impressed with his medical knowledge, research capabilities, and work ethic.

One month later the Red Cross appointed Drew director of the first American Red Cross Blood Bank and assistant director of blood procurement for the federally sponsored National Research Council. Soon Drew was sitting in a Red Cross ambulance with a crew of nurses as they hauled a trailer left over from the defunct Blood for Britain project thirty-five miles to a school serving as a blood processing center in Farmingdale, Long Island. It was a symbolic shift for the American medical establishment from the Blood for Britain project to a national blood collection effort, and was also the American Red Cross's earliest attempt at mobile blood collection. Shortly thereafter the organization began installing mobile blood collection units at department stores, government offices, industrial plants, and public schools and universities.

Drew's New York pilot program would pave the way for the Red Cross's nationwide effort to collect blood and provide the armed forces millions of parcels of dried plasma. Eventually, the Red Cross collected, processed, and sent over thirteen million pints of blood overseas, saving tens of thousands of American soldiers from an unnecessary death. By the end of World War II, in 1945, battlefield physicians regarded the shiny tin packets of dried plasma as the war's foremost lifesaving device.

Drew, Racism, and His Death

Despite the success of Drew's pilot program, his tenure with the Red Cross was short-lived, and his resignation corresponded to the start of one of the uglier instances of institutionalized racism in the history of American medicine.

Drew never fully articulated the reasons he resigned from his Red Cross post in April 1941. On the topic of his departure, he cryptically wrote to his wife: "There are some things that I will leave unfinished here which I naturally would like to finish, but I feel that the moment is propitious for pulling out."[12] On the one hand, he had recently completed the final stage of the American Board of Surgery's certification process, and may have wanted to pursue different professional ambitions than those related to blood collection. Additionally, he anticipated possibly being shipped overseas now that he was board certified, though many considered his work with the New York pilot program too important to wartime planning to let him leave the country. On the other hand, the Red Cross failed to offer Drew a managerial position for the nationwide blood program it was about to institute on the heels of his pilot program.

It is unknown if Drew's race factored into the Red Cross's decision. Consequently, historians are uncertain whether Drew resigned out of principle over this apparent affront or out of a desire to pursue other personal goals.

What is definite is that a few months after the Red Cross's national blood donor project began, the organization, under pressure from the military and in an appeasement to prejudice, moved to exclude black donors.

Not until several years later did the Red Cross begin accepting blood from black Americans but rigidly segregated the blood supply.

The black press drew attention to the racist overtones of the policy to prohibit black donors and looked to Drew, among others, for answers. "I feel that the recent ruling of the United States Army and Navy regarding the refusal of colored blood donors is an indefensible one from any point of view," he shortly declared. "As you know, there is no scientific basis for the separation of the bloods of different races except on the basis of the individual blood types or groups."[13]

Black protests grew, while white southern politicians exploited racist fears in the population. A U.S. congressman from Mississippi labeled Drew and his fellow critics "crackpots," "Communists," "parlor pinks," and "fellow travelers," who were attempting to "mongrelize this Nation." The demagogic politician implied that Drew was unpatriotic, endeavoring to destroy the blood donor service and damage the war effort by mixing white and black blood. "They had better remember," the Mississippian warned, "that there is still a Congress of the United States, and that Congress represents the American people and that the American people through their Congress are not going to permit such outrages."[14] The Red Cross's segregation policy would continue throughout the Second World War, finally ending in 1950.

Drew, already a year removed from the national donor program, largely ignored the perverse claims and race-baiting around blood collection that persisted throughout the war. He instead turned his attention to other medical matters. Drew's first love had always been surgery and his military involvement had left little time for the operating room or his favorite role, teaching surgeons. As the most well known of the nation's board-certified black surgeons, Drew considered it an important personal challenge to create a tradition in surgery for black Americans. He became head of the department of surgery at Howard University Medical School and chief surgeon at Washington's Freedmen's Hospital. His influence was so prominent that over half of the black American surgeons who received board certification in the 1940s studied under his direct supervision.

Drew did not allow his teaching responsibilities to impede his commitment to social justice in the medical profession. Though he stayed mainly on the sidelines of the blood collection conflict, he expanded his protests to other forms of discrimination in the medical profession, notably the American College of Surgeons' policy of barring black doctors. He marched in labor parades and gave speeches at public rallies. In early 1944 the National Association for the Advancement of Colored People (NAACP) awarded Drew its Spingarn Medal for his work in blood plasma research. The *New York Times* described this as the "highest achievement of a Negro."[15] The award's prestige further increased Drew's public profile and he used this heightened status to advocate vigorously for racial justice.

Unfortunately, Drew only spent a few years in the medical and public limelight. In the early hours of April 1, 1950, Drew was driving to a medical conference in North Carolina with three colleagues when he fell asleep at the wheel. The car flipped over at more than 70 miles per hour and Drew suffered massive damage to his head and chest. Though he received prompt medical attention, his injuries were too severe for doctors to save his life.

Certain publications speciously reported that Drew, the nation's pioneer blood researcher, had died from blood loss after physicians at a racially segregated hospital refused to treat him. In fact, the white doctors who cared for Drew were well aware of his professional reputation and worked diligently to prevent his death, including giving him a blood transfusion. The racially charged allegations concerning Drew's death likely originated from frustrations with the widespread southern policy of hospital segregation and the denial of medical services that caused the death of countless black accident victims in that era. White hospitals routinely denied admission to black Americans, and black hospitals were underfunded, poorly equipped, and inadequately staffed.

Over time, the circumstances of Drew's death evolved into an emotional urban legend that persists today. The tale of the extraordinarily talented black man, who saved countless lives through his pioneering medical research on blood and was himself refused blood due to his race when he most needed it, continues to resonate in the American racial narrative.

An Incentive to Specialize

One of the great ironies of warfare throughout modern history is that the more brutal and widespread the conflict, the higher the casualty count climbs, the greater are the resulting medical advances.

From a medical standpoint World War II remains the most successful conflict in which the nation's armed forces had ever fought, with accomplishments spanning the entire spectrum of medicine. As discussed, Drew's pioneering blood work into dried plasma, combined with the nationwide donor effort, permitted more effective management of life-threatening combat injuries and made transfusions commonplace. Physicians also applied the lessons of public sanitation first championed by Stephen Smith in the 1870s and strictly enforced measures for the disposal of human waste, curbing a wide variety of illnesses that had arisen in earlier wars. Additionally, doctors used newly developed medicines and vaccines to combat infectious diseases, particularly malaria and yellow fever. Surgeons skilled in orthopedic procedures preserved limbs that would have been lost in previous conflicts, while technical advances in surgery, notably those involving operations on the abdomen and chest, saved countless lives. Psychiatrists diagnosed and successfully treated stress-related disorders—known as "nostalgia" in the Civil War, "shell shock" in World War I, and "combat exhaustion" or "combat fatigue" in World War II. Medical workers tested novel medical evacuation procedures on the battlefields and innovatively organized acute care hospitals.

But to discuss all of these various advances one after another is to ignore what was perhaps the biggest medical distinction between World War II and its predecessors. In both the Civil War and World War I, American medicine leapt forward, largely due to the unparalleled experience that battlefield doctors gained in a short period of time. World War II again gave the nation's physicians intensive practical experience, but the war arrived at a moment when American medicine was in ascendance, a time when the federal government had a newfound faith in the profession and actively worked with its doctors to promote its development.

The federal government's activities during the war, among other things, would put an end to the profession's long-running internecine struggle between generalists and specialists, with specialists triumphant.

Specialization had first emerged in a powerful fashion early in the twentieth century when developments in medical technology, new attitudes about the value of medical research, and changes in the relationship between the public and physicians created space for doctors to focus their training on precise aspects of medical care. Men like Ernest Codman, William Halsted, and Franklin Martin had been at the forefront of this movement, which made occasional demands throughout the 1920s for formal recognition and possible licensure. During the 1930s and the economic downturn of the Depression, medical organizations began organizing specialty boards in response to the public's desire for acknowledgment of specialty services, particularly from a financial standpoint. However, many in the profession still considered medical and surgical specialists technocratic elites who did not represent the mainstream of American medicine, and the triumph of specialists over generalists remained uncertain at the start of the military conflict.

The shift that settled the matter occurred when the U.S. military decided to award higher ranks to certified medical specialists through a points system that explicitly favored doctors with advanced levels of training and localized knowledge. Thus, the military provided doctors with an incentive to specialize that trumped the internal debate within the profession. The press publicized the points system, with the *New York Times* noting in a headline that the military was "aim[ing] to keep the scarce specialists,"[16] and other papers explaining that possession of a specialty diploma indicated a doctor's clinical capabilities—a claim that had been widely disputed throughout the 1930s. "You are holding to the standards of university clinic surgery under fire," claimed an impressed specialist who was observing military physicians, "and in tents with mud floors."[17]

Although the military classification system did not overtly champion the process of board certification, it recognized de facto the importance of such exams, effectively ensuring that they would also become a mainstay of American medicine. The federally backed imprimatur bestowed on those with specialty board diplomas encouraged doctors whose specialties still lacked boards to insist on them. The war's classification system created a sort of virtuous circle of specialization within the profession. Specialties that did not yet have boards—for example, physical medicine and rehabilitation, thoracic surgery, and preventive medicine—quickly moved to implement them and benefit from the military ranking system.

Physicians started treating board certification as an indispensable component of sophisticated health care, especially relative to military medicine, and tens of thousands of physicians vested their professional futures in the success of the board certification process as a result of their wartime experiences. Largely as a result of the military's ranking system, physician specialization became an integral part of the nation's health care delivery system, directly linked to medical education and residency training as well as incorporated into the planning of civilian and military manpower to satisfy needs.

In addition to hastening the triumph of specialization in American medicine, the federal government had begun devoting financial resources to medical research on a grand scale that produced innumerable discoveries throughout the war. As with the debate over specialization, some in the profession resisted this action by the government, as they opposed giving medical research any sort of primacy, favored clinical practice over basic science, and wanted the government to stay out of medicine generally. But the United States invested more funds in medical research than any other country in this period, emphasizing basic science and shortening the lag time between discovery and utilization. The financial commitment to medical research validated its importance as an indispensable science, and the distinction between the utilitarian value of basic and clinical sciences soon disappeared.

With the federal government taking the lead and organizing different groups of investigators, medical researchers could more easily focus their activities and direct them toward a common good. "Never before has there been so great a coordination of medical scientific labor,"[18] noted one observer. Unlike in the Civil War or World War I, where a physician's research or development of surgical techniques was more of an individualistic enterprise, in World War II a wide variety of doctors worked in a coordinated fashion, a process that accelerated the testing and application of a broad range of knowledge.

The development of the bacteria-killing antibiotic penicillin, for example, resulted largely from this new, federally supported approach to medical research. Researchers had first discovered the drug in 1928, but they could not produce adequate quantities for use in clinical practice. Even as late as 1940, the nation only had enough penicillin to treat ten patients. To alleviate this shortage, the federal government in 1941 initiated a coordinated research effort into penicillin production, bringing together the work of investigators in academia, government-funded laboratories, and the chemical, distilling, and pharmaceutical industries.

These disparate researchers began working together to perfect fermentation techniques and soon increased penicillin production exponentially. "No private, uncoordinated procedure could have secured comparable results in anything like the same time,"[19] wrote one participant. By mid-1943 military doctors routinely treated casualties with penicillin thanks to the success of the research efforts. Newspaper articles boasted of "dramatic instances" in which doctors employed penicillin "literally at the last minute"[20] to save the lives of soldiers suffering from blood poisoning, meningitis, pneumonia, and postoperative infections.

The benefits that increased medical research yielded gave the American military a distinct advantage over that of other countries. Just 4 percent of injured American soldiers died during the war, contrasted with 10 percent of wounded German combatants.

John Gibbon and His Heart-Lung Machine

As important as World War II was to developments in American medicine, not every major discovery from that era depended on circumstances that the conflict brought about. The war arguably slowed down some medical breakthroughs by enlisting physicians for the military effort who would otherwise have been pursuing research independently. Coordinated research efforts during the war quickened the development of battlefield saviors like penicillin and blood transfusions, but not every research initiative received federal attention and support. Such was the case with one of the era's most important advances: heart surgery.

By mid-century the nation's surgeons had successfully operated on every bone, muscle, organ, and element of the human corpus, except the heart. This exception was troubling because more Americans died of heart disease than any other medical ailment—in 1940 it accounted for 27 percent of American deaths; by 1953 the figure had increased to 39 percent. Physicians desperately tried to resolve the situation and sought innovative techniques to treat cardiac conditions.

The early methods were often ingenious and occasionally foolhardy. In the 1920s several intrepid surgeons in Boston began blindly inserting scalpels into beating hearts, trying to cut through calcified and scarred valves. The doctors were attempting to open up narrowed apertures and relieve patients of deadly shortness of breath from overtaxed hearts. The results were grim: seven cases and only one short-term survivor. "When a condition is recognized as offering only a fatal or hopeless outlook," explained one of the nation's pioneer heart surgeons, "desperate measures seem less desperate and with application and courage not infrequently can be made safe."[21]

Though the consequences were serious and surgical failure generally meant death of the patient, surgeons continued working to develop techniques to deal with hearts and their diseases. Doctors attempted everything from placing specially designed miniature knives on their fingertips to forging new types of scissors and clamps. But each time, physicians struggled with the same two physiological problems: large quantities of blood flowing through the operative area and the unremitting to-and-fro movement of a living heart.

Doctors first tried to tackle the problem of blood flow. In one dramatic prewar ploy, surgeons tied off all the blood vessels feeding the heart. This provided the physicians a window of three to four minutes to open the organ, complete the repair, sew the tissues back together, and undo the tied vessels before the lack of blood permanently damaged the patient's brain. It was medicine ruled by a stopwatch: nerve-racking and suitable for only a small number of patients (or surgeons for that matter).

Researchers worked to extend the window available to physicians attempting this "total heart inflow occlusion" method. They discovered that cooling a patient's body temperature down to about 85 degrees—normal temperature is 98 degrees—could provide doctors several additional minutes. This reduction in temperature decreased the oxygen demands of the heart and brain and lessened the possibility of stroke. America's operating rooms soon contained anesthetized heart patients immersed in giant ice-filled bathtubs as surgeons went about their business at a more measured pace.

Nonetheless, doctors still had to blindly grope around the inside of the heart, trusting in their experience and knowledge of anatomy, pathology, and physiology. Not unexpectedly, the treatment outcomes remained the same. Physicians could make diagnoses and temporarily ease symptoms, but they could not permanently solve cardiac defects without some method to stop a beating heart and allow a physician sufficient time to repair the organ's problem. Solving this dilemma became something of surgery's holy grail, and one American researcher devoted his professional life to find it.

John Gibbon—his friends called him Jack—came from a long line of physicians, stretching from his father, a professor of surgery at the Jefferson Medical School in Philadelphia, to his great-great-grandfather, a general practitioner with a medical degree from the University of Edinburgh. Gibbon was an intellectual, an independent thinker who considered self-reliance among an individual's most important character traits—and in medical research before World War II, this was undoubtedly true. Some of his colleagues found him self-centered—he was notoriously stubborn, moody, and shy—and labeled him a self-absorbed egoist. But his peculiarities gave him the demeanor necessary to spend a lifetime attempting to devise an artificial heart and lung machine.

As a twenty-eight-year-old research fellow at Harvard in 1931, Gibbon watched a female patient die over the course of an evening from an acute heart and lung condition. Her physicians, like all doctors of the era, could not safely operate on her beating heart. This incident troubled the young Gibbon, and he imagined that surgeons could have saved the patient if they had a device to relieve the heart of work during an operation. "The thought naturally occurred to me," recalled Gibbon, "that the patient's life might be saved if some of the blue blood in her veins could be continuously withdrawn into an extracorporeal [outside] blood circuit, exposed to an atmosphere of oxygen, and then returned to the patient by way of an artery in a central direction."[22] It was an ingenious idea that would allow a surgeon time to lift up the heart and cut into it, without causing a spurt of blood. Thus, the scalpel wielder could see what needed to be accomplished, instead of depending on touch. The concept of performing surgery on the heart in a bloodless "dry field" was a magnificent proposal. It was also absolutely preposterous considering the state of scientific medicine in 1931. For two decades, Gibbon would work to perfect his heart-lung machine.

A brief review of how the heart functions will clarify exactly what Gibbon's machine would need to replace. The heart actually contains two distinct organs, each lying on opposite sides of a shared wall, the septum. Both sections have an upper chamber, or atrium, that receives blood, and a lower chamber, or ventricle, that pumps it out. Although the heart is two separate pumps, they work in a coordinated rhythm that produces the well-known lub-dub sounds of a normal heartbeat. The right side of the heart receives "used" blood from the body and then propels it to the lungs, which remove carbon dioxide and replenish oxygen. From the lungs, the rejuvenated blood heads for the heart's left side, where it is gathered and then pushed out to nourish the body's tissues. Because the heart's left side has to work much harder to accomplish its mission, the pressure within it is markedly higher than that of the right side. Whatever machine Gibbon devised would need to bypass and temporarily replace this entire process mechanically.

He began his quest to engineer his fantastical device independently and with no outside financial support. "The Federal Government," he later remarked, "was not then [in the 1930s] pouring out hundreds of millions of dollars to doctors to perform research. . . . I bought an air pump in a second hand shop down in East Boston for a few dollars."[23] Gibbon made his initial valves out of solid rubber corks and built the circuitry for blood flow from rubber and glass tubing pushed together (plastic was unavailable).

When Gibbon believed his rudimentary prototype would function, he started to perform research trials on animals. He and his wife walked the streets at night with bait and nets hunting for stray alley cats. By 1940, Gibbon had refined his makeshift device into an apparatus that could bypass the heart and lungs of a cat for twenty minutes, with no ill effects and no damage to the animal's nervous system.

World War II interrupted Gibbon's research and clinical work. As a reserve officer in the Medical Corps, he was among the first to enter active service. He shipped out in January 1942 and, the following year, was made chief of surgery at a military hospital in New Caledonia, the French-controlled Pacific archipelago located near the famous Guadalcanal battlefield. He remained stationed in New Caledonia for almost three years. In addition to performing his medical work, he won the chess championship of the South Pacific Theater.

After the war Gibbon became professor of surgery at Jefferson Medical School in Philadelphia, where he resumed researching his heart-lung machine. It was there that he concluded he needed, in his words, "some good engineering advice."[24]

In late 1946 a friend put Gibbon in touch with Thomas Watson, president of International Business Machines, a company that embodied America's postwar economic boom and had a fleet of gifted engineers. Watson immediately supported Gibbon's endeavor and, at their initial meeting, he said, "You name the place and time and I will have engineers there to discuss the matter with you."[25] Subsequent to this get-together, International Business Machines not only provided Gibbon engineering assistance, but the company assumed a large part of the cost of constructing the heart-lung apparatus.

Though Watson ardently supported the effort to develop an artificial replacement for the human heart, he strongly opposed medical research using animals and refused to provide funds for animal experimentation. This proved a conundrum to Gibbon, who lacked sufficient resources to pay for his clinical trials. Then, in 1949, Gibbon received a grant from the federal government for almost $30,000, nearly all of it exclusively for animal research.

With the assistance of Watson's engineers and the federal money, Gibbon improved his device, making it more automatic and versatile. He experimented with various metal screens, plastic and wire meshes, and perforated steel plates to enhance the transfer of oxygen to blood. The new machine was larger than previous ones, had more elaborate control designs, and was filled with a myriad of blood pumps, electrical switches and motors, electromagnets, revolving cylinders, and water baths. Gibbon enclosed the works in an air-conditioned and temperature-regulated metal-and-glass container.

The entire contraption resembled a ridiculous Rube Goldberg–like invention. It damaged blood cells and caused bleeding problems, but his colleagues praised it and the media started to pay attention. *Time* told its readers how Gibbon's mechanical device had taken over the heart and lung functions of dogs for as long as forty-five minutes. The reporter remarked that Gibbon's work would "open 'the last field of surgery.' "[26]

Gibbon believed that the device was ready for humans, but it was one thing to experiment on cats and dogs and another to operate on a living human being. After all, his twenty-year-long quest had begun when he watched a patient die after unsuccessful heart surgery. "Come on, Jack," his friends had started to encourage him, knowing the two decades of time invested in his invention, "when are you going to stop working on dogs and start working on man?"[27]

Around this time Cecilia Bavolek, a college freshman with a worsening heart murmur, was admitted to the Jefferson Medical College Hospital. Doctors diagnosed her condition as an anomalous hole in the shared wall between her heart's two upper chambers. Each minute, several pints of the oxygenated blood returning from her lungs to her heart's left atrium leaked back through the hole and into the right atrium (due to the pressure difference between the atria) instead of being distributed throughout her body. Bavolek's heart was working overtime in an effort to compensate for its own endless cycle of inefficiency. She had been hospitalized multiple times in the prior six months for her severe shortness of breath, palpitations, and fatigue—symptoms of congestive heart failure. It was just a matter of time before the eighteen-year-old would succumb to a massive heart attack.

Gibbon explained the situation to Bavolek and her mother. He also told them of his research on a heart-lung machine and how this apparatus could be the key to Bavolek's leading a normal life. They agreed that experimental surgery with the heart-lung machine was the best medical option.

On the morning of May 6, 1953, with Bavolek anesthetized using sodium pentothal, Gibbon and his three assistant surgeons laid bare her heart. They opened the large veins carrying blood to the heart's right side and slipped in plastic tubes that drained Bavolek's life source away to the heart-lung machine. Inside the device, one pump drew in the blood and a second speeded it to the oxygenation chamber. Electronic controls maintained Bavolek's vital functions, from the blood's flow rate to the oxygen added and carbon dioxide taken away. A third pump sent the refreshed blood back into an artery above the left side of Bavolek's heart, where it was distributed to her body.

Operating on the heart had always been a bloody business, but when Gibbon lifted up Bavolek's heart and opened it, he had a view unlike that of anyone before. He looked into a living but bloodless heart, clearly saw its internal architecture, including the abnormal opening between the atria. He stitched the half-dollar-sized hole shut. "This I did and it went very quickly and easily, giving a secure closure,"[28] explained Gibbon in his operation notes. For twenty-six minutes Gibbon's machine served as Bavolek's heart and lungs. Thus, for the first time in history, man's ingenuity had successfully substituted the heart and lungs given him by nature.

Bavolek awoke without difficulty and showed no signs of brain damage or harm to any of her vital structures. She was home within two weeks and enjoyed a healthy life thereafter.

The publicity-shy Gibbon requested that the operation receive no media hype and refused to pose for a photograph with his device, but the world had other ideas. Newspapers and magazines carried every last detail of the procedure, running headlines like "Heart's Job Done by New Apparatus; Surgeons Close Hole in Empty Organ While Circulation Is Maintained Mechanically."[29] *Time* termed it a "Historic Operation."[30] One newspaper editor wrote: "Surgical history was made the other day in Philadelphia. The accomplishment indicates what we may expect in the future."[31] Gibbon subsequently received numerous awards and was nominated three times for the Nobel Prize.

Gibbon's invention of the heart-lung machine made difficult operations (e.g., valve replacement) comparatively easy to accomplish. It also led to the development of new procedures (e.g., heart bypass) and enabled other high-risk processes (e.g., heart catherization) to become commonplace.

Persuasive, Charming, and Indispensable

Almost a decade of New Deal legislation and five years of hostilities had accustomed Americans to an increasingly strong central government. The considerable expansion of federal influence in health care and medical research that occurred during World War II did not slow down when hostilities finally concluded in August 1945.

In the postwar years America entered a prolonged period of economic prosperity, and the population expected continued improvements in medicine and personal health. The federal government pushed through an unprecedented wave of legislation related to health care that sculpted American medicine in the last half of the twentieth century and made public spending on medical initiatives a permanent component of the federal budget. Government administrators also consolidated and strengthened outdated federal health agencies, like the U.S. Public Health Service, and established new ones, such as the U.S. Department of Health, Education, and Welfare. Using the combined tools of regulatory measures, legislative fiat, or control of budgetary purse strings, federal authorities inserted themselves into a profession that had previously existed with minimal government oversight.

Fate seemed to choose Alabama senator Joseph Lister Hill to champion the legislative offensive. He was the offspring of one of the South's most distinguished physicians, who had named his son after his medical hero, Joseph Lister of antisepsis fame. Though Lister Hill (he never used his first name) was not himself a doctor—he grew queasy at the sight of blood and wounds—he possessed sophisticated views on the medical profession thanks to his father. The older Hill had told his son about his namesake's struggles to introduce the technology of antisepsis to a doubting profession. Consequently, the younger Hill had developed a fundamental belief in the importance of new medical technologies and a conviction in the worth of scientific research.

Lister Hill graduated Phi Beta Kappa from his home state's university at Tuscaloosa, earned a law degree from New York City's Columbia University, and, in 1923, at twenty-eight years of age, was elected to the U.S. House of Representatives. After seven terms as an Alabama congressman, Hill was elected to a vacant seat in the U.S. Senate when President Franklin Roosevelt nominated the state's senior senator, Hugo Black, for the U.S. Supreme Court. Hill would hold the office for five additional terms, serving as longtime chairman of the two Senate committees with jurisdiction over appropriations in medicine and shepherding through almost seventy major pieces of health care legislation.

Hill held sway over the country's health care policies because he oversaw the distribution of federal dollars to state and local governments as well as to public and private institutions. Between 1950 and 1970, the approximate years of Hill's peak political powers, national health care expenditures rose 500 percent, from $12 billion to $69 billion (hospital expenses alone increased from $2 billion to $28 billion). Funds for medical research grew almost 1,000 percent (from under $250 million to $2 billion). By comparison, the country's nominal gross domestic product grew less than 400 percent during those twenty years. The health care workforce also swelled by 225 percent (from 1.2 to 3.9 million people) at a time when the general population increased a mere 34 percent, from 151 million to 203 million.

Hill's medical legislative agenda transformed the delivery of health care, turning it into one of the nation's largest industries. When Hill retired from the Senate in 1968, an editor of the *New York Times* remarked that "Lister Hill has done more for the health of Americans in modern times than any man outside the medical profession."[32]

Early in his senatorial career, Hill set the stage for the federal government to expand health care and medical technology when he began advocating to place the immense power of public finance behind the country's hospitals. He soon cosponsored a bill to allocate federal funds to the individual states for the planning and construction of hospitals. In 1946, Congress passed the Hospital Survey and Construction Act, known by its long-lasting moniker, the Hill-Burton Act. "Of all the legislation for the advancement of care of the sick in the last fifty years," wrote an admiring executive of the AMA, "the Hill-Burton Act was probably the most significant in providing facilities in just about every sizable community in the country."[33] Two decades after the law's enactment, the nation had 9,200 new hospitals, nursing homes, rehabilitation centers, and outreach health clinics, collectively containing more than 416,000 beds.

The passage and implementation of the Hill-Burton Act guaranteed that hospitals would receive the funding necessary to provide high-quality medical services moving forward. Hill, however, recognized that his vision to reshape national health care policy also required large-scale funding for two other components of medicine—scientific research and physician education. Fortunately for the Alabama senator, he had a gift for convincing his colleagues to funnel federal dollars toward medicine. As one of his Senate rivals deadpanned, "[Lister Hill] is so persuasive, so charming, so quietly indispensable, and so personally self-effacing, that we want to give him everything that it is possible to give him."[34]

The federal government had already been sponsoring medical research in some capacity since the late nineteenth century. For instance, the U.S. Public Health Service established a one-room laboratory for bacteriological studies in 1887. The institute's scientists, over the course of four decades, expanded their research to include cancer and mental diseases, and in 1930, Congress rebranded this facility as the National Institutes of Health (NIH). Several years later, the NIH was relocated to an eighty-two-acre plot of land in Bethesda, Maryland, that a philanthropist had donated.

In the period after World War II, however, the federal government would become much more enthusiastic about funding research. The U.S. government, largely as a tactic in the Cold War, began to elevate the importance of the sciences, including medicine, through increased spending and education initiatives. Scientific advancement became, in part, an act of patriotism, a chance for the United States to demonstrate its superiority over the Soviet Union. This was the Space Age and the Atomic Age, a time of astronauts, jet planes, moon rockets, nuclear submarines, and thermonuclear bombs. This jingoistic enthusiasm helped funnel resources to the nation's burgeoning medical research and clinical establishment. The miracles of medicine validated the American way of life, each therapeutic advance a testament to the country's strength and its prosperous future.

Hill advocated an organized national offensive against major diseases through the establishment of federally funded specialty medical research institutes. Each proposed institute would study one group of diseases at a time and constitute a network of research facilities within the preexisting National Institutes of Health.

This postwar national research initiative effectively began with heart disease—the single biggest cause of death in Americans then as now—and a legislative initiative to fund a dedicated research facility. "Fifteen million dollars is needed at once to do for heart disease what is now being done for infantile paralysis [polio]," explained a newspaper editor in the days leading up to the vote in Congress. "If Congress provides the money . . . 9,000,000 who know that they have heart 'trouble' will soon receive better care and the lives of 600,000 graver cases will be extended."[35] Senators and congressmen ultimately appropriated the funds, and President Harry Truman signed a law on June 16, 1948, to create the National Heart Institute as the third research facility in the NIH.

"Continuously and conspicuously palpable"

Hill's alter ego in the medical profession, the man who would eventually steward medical research at the national level, was James Shannon. He was tall and trim and, like Hill, decisive and dispassionate. Shannon earned an M.D. and Ph.D. from New York University, and made his professional mark early with fundamental discoveries in kidney physiology. During World War II, his research in antimalaria drugs, which American troops serving in the South Pacific urgently needed, garnered him the Presidential Medal of Merit. Following the war, Shannon directed the Squibb Institute for Medical Research, where he guided a multidisciplinary endeavor to produce and market the antibiotic streptomycin as well as several blood pressure medicines.

Few physician-administrators rivaled Shannon's broad experience at the intersection of academic, governmental, and industrial medical research, nor were any as visionary or resolute in their actions. Equally important, Shannon had a more nuanced understanding of the federal legislative process than most doctors. In 1949, organizers of the National Heart Institute recruited the forty-five-year-old Shannon to lead the new facility's scientific programs. The appointment allowed Shannon to build from scratch a large-scale research organization.

Shannon proved so effective in running the National Heart Institute's research activities that, in 1955, the surgeon general of the Public Health Service named him overall director of the NIH. Shannon was a hands-on detail-oriented manager, described as "continuously and conspicuously palpable." One of his physician-recruits told of how Shannon "cruised the territory regularly," and "kept everyone abreast of the progress of his efforts to staff up the various labs."[36]

As director, Shannon thrived on the ins and outs of the budget process and intensely prepared for the yearly congressional review of his Institutes' financial plans. He conferred with individual institute and division directors, compiled their requests, and vigorously defended the Institutes' want-list at House and Senate budget hearings. "Medical research in the national interest," Shannon explained, "though costly, should not be restricted by lack of funds."[37]

Shannon and Hill together choreographed the postwar expansion of American medical research. For almost two decades Hill presided over the Senate's annual hearings on appropriations for the NIH while Shannon sat at the witness table. Each year's opening remarks aimed to make lawmakers aware of their own mortality and, consequently, more willing to approve further allocations. Hill would narrate the stories of politicians who had suffered from the sorts of diseases that he felt required additional research funds. This included Secretary of State John Foster Dulles's death from cancer and President Dwight Eisenhower's survival of a heart attack. "There is nothing more important," Hill would remind his colleagues, "than getting the findings and getting them out to the patient's bedside."[38]

Hill performed remarkably year after year, using his detailed knowledge of each proposed bill and his close relationship with Shannon, his star witness, to persuade Republicans and Democrats alike. "The National Institutes of Health owe their extremely flourishing condition to [Lister Hill]," said one of his fellow senators. "He touches the rock of public credit and abundant streams gush forth so that the National Institutes of Health have money running out of their ears, money they do not always know what to do with."[39]

When Shannon retired from the NIH in 1968—the same year that Hill ended his senatorial career—he left behind an organization that had grown into the premier, and largest, medical research institution in the world, operating on a scale inconceivable at the time his work began. He was hailed by his colleagues as the "visionary architect of our nation's biomedical science policy,"[40] a critical thinker who changed the nation's medical research endeavors beyond recognition.

Shannon's influence, however, extended far beyond the NIH's Bethesda campus. He spent less than half of the Institutes' budget on its direct operations. With the remaining funds, he showered the country's hospitals, medical schools, and universities with grants to pursue NIH-sponsored research projects as well as the education and training of biomedical scientists. In fact, one of his first grants, back when he directed scientific research at the National Heart Institute, was the $30,000 that Gibbon received to test his heart-lung machine on animals. It is no coincidence that Shannon's tenure covered a period when researchers unraveled the secrets of genetics, developed scores of protective vaccines, extracted powerful antibiotics from microorganisms in the soil, and synthesized an array of drugs to treat ailments like high blood pressure, diabetes, and failing hearts, not to mention the immunosuppressants. Additionally, thirteen Americans received the Nobel Prize in Physiology or Medicine during the 1960s.

Spheres of Influence

The unprecedented, federally sponsored changes in American medicine following the Second World War divided the profession into several overlapping spheres of influence, updated versions of long-standing conflicts between urban and rural doctors, generalists and specialists, and conservatives and progressives.

The first sphere was the burgeoning empire of increasingly well-funded medical schools with their surrounding cluster of general hospitals, specialty institutions, and schools in dentistry, nursing, pharmacy, and public health. These mostly urban-based, academic medical centers, with their large number of specialists, tended to dominate the profession in their particular locale.

The academic medical centers' influence strengthened throughout the 1950s and 1960s with the continued financial support from Shannon's National Institutes of Health. Twenty-two new medical schools appeared during this period, increasing the nationwide total to one hundred four—these centers, however, still accounted for less than 20 percent of the hospital beds in the country.

As medical schools proliferated, so did the number of academic physicians affiliated with such institutions. The amount of full-time medical faculty doubled during the 1960s to slightly over twenty-three thousand. And half of these individuals received portions of their salary from Shannon's largess with NIH grants (15 percent depended exclusively on his beneficence).

Doctors affiliated with teaching institutions shared similar professional interests that grew out of the nature of the environment in which they practiced. Their daily routines included educating and training physicians as well as conducting research. Academically oriented physicians were typically salaried and depended less on the goodwill of their patients to earn a living. Consequently, academic physicians dealt minimally with the day-to-day pressures of managing a practice, and they had less commitment to the aims of organized medicine to avoid federal and state involvement, especially the key bogeyman, prepaid health insurance plans.

A competing sphere of influence to the academic health care establishment was the growing number of facilities not affiliated with medical schools, so-called community hospitals. These institutions contained the majority of the country's hospital beds. Thanks to the Hill-Burton Act and its successors, community hospitals also received significant federal funding and provided increasingly sophisticated ancillary services. They were generally located in the suburbs and more rural regions, and became health care fiefdoms in their own right as they competed against academic medical centers for patients and revenues.

These community hospitals had their affiliated doctors as well, with a set of concerns widely different from those of the academic physicians. The largest group consisted of office-based, private practitioners. Many of these clinicians, especially the old-style family doctor and other nonspecialists, had lost admitting privileges at hospitals associated with academic medical schools and were forced to attach themselves to what they considered less prestigious community hospitals. Some of these older, poorly trained general practitioners, once the backbone of a school's teaching staff, lost their position as medical educators as well and felt that academics disrespected their less medically sophisticated colleagues.

Through the 1960s community-based private practitioners embodied the organized medical establishment, supporting the AMA. Private practice clinicians, and with them the AMA, opposed government interference in medicine more vocally than their academic counterparts. This group comprised the last vestiges of pre–World War II American medicine in their socioeconomic and political attitudes.

Not surprisingly, the two blocks of physicians—academicians and community-based doctors—often fought over the direction the profession would take. The new wave of post–World War II medical professors considered "local medical doctors"—a common pejorative for community-based nonacademicians—out of step with advances in modern medicine. "The [community] practitioners have lost prestige and they feel it," remarked one medical school professor. "Some of the doctors who were respected in the town are no longer in the same position of authority and respect that they were before we came here. They have lost prestige because they did not have the educational background that the newer doctors now have."[41]

Community-based doctors resented the rise of their academic counterparts and the media attention they received for their research triumphs and therapeutic victories. Most important, private practice physicians regarded their academic counterparts as a Trojan horse that had brought government into medicine. "A lot of us," noted one community-based practitioner, "feel that the medical schools would dominate all of our hospitals if they could. We feel that if it did it would be dangerous for those of us in individual practice."[42]

The spheres of influence that developed in the post–World War II years of economic growth ultimately represent the profession's departure from its earlier exclusive dedication to the care of patients. Instead, American medicine became a conglomeration of diverse branches of medical knowledge, centered on the basic sciences of anatomy, biochemistry, microbiology, pathology, pharmacology, and physiology, each of which was rapidly developing into a wide assembly of clinical and research specialties. The days of turning out standardized family practitioners were gone. The country's medical schools had become federally dominated research institutions intent on educating doctors to assume one of a host of clinical, managerial, or research career choices.

These changes, while creating tension within the profession, helped turn medicine into a prized national asset for a prosperous nation with disposable income. Everyone within the medical establishment benefited from the newfound respect and admiration that Americans had for their caregivers. The postwar economic expansion brought physicians all the patients they could handle, and their salaries rose accordingly. Between the end of World War II and 1970, the consumer price index increased less than 3 percent annually, but physicians' fees grew at 4 percent a year and their incomes 6 percent (income levels reached $35,000 in 1970). In addition, record numbers of students applied to medical school. Applications jumped almost 66 percent in fifteen years, from 14,937 in 1955 to 24,465 in 1970.

In turn, the medical establishment, between the proliferation of hospitals and nursing homes, advances in clinical care, and research triumphs, touched the lives of virtually every American. Hospitals, once considered a depressing final stop before the funeral home, had become gleaming citadels of health care with wide corridors, tempered glass, stainless steel, flashing lights, and astonishing medical equipment. Patients welcomed successful medical treatments once thought possible only as science fiction. The public embraced allergy shots, cancer chemotherapy, hormone replacement, mood-altering drugs, and vaccinations. As doctors applied more sophisticated approaches to diagnosing and treating patients, patients' concerns over complex disease states like hypertension (high blood pressure) and arteriosclerosis (hardening of the arteries) replaced their prior worries over illnesses like tuberculosis and whooping cough.

Medical progress became part of the nation's cultural and social fabric at this point. Magazines and newspapers informed their readers about the recent miracles of scientific medicine. And television brought medicine to the fore of national consciousness. In 1961 tens of millions of Americans watched in evening prime time as Ben Casey, a chief resident in neurosurgery, or Dr. Kildare, a beginning intern, worked in fictional large metropolitan institutions while learning the rudiments of their profession. The following year the networks unveiled *The Doctors* and *General Hospital,* two medical dramas that became staples of daytime soap-opera viewers. Thanks to these programs and the general growth of health care facilities, the country became conversant with coronary care units, emergency rooms, premature nurseries, medical and surgical intensive care units, as well as startling new forms of clinical therapy.

❧ Nine ❧

SUPREMACY

Organ Transplantation

IN LITTLE MORE than fifty years, the United States had transformed itself from a backwater health care province to the unrivaled global leader in medical therapy and operative surgery. American physicians and surgeons grew bolder with each passing decade, trying to erase the line between medical hypotheses and clinical realities. After John Gibbon performed open-heart surgery in June 1953, the barrier became organ transplantation. The conquest of this new frontier captivated the country's physicians and researchers, and the complexity of the objective required doctors to work together across differing specialties, a clinical approach that would come to define American medicine in the last half of the twentieth century.

Like open-heart surgery, organ transplantation started out as a near hopeless field. Technical limitations simply appeared too great, and operative achievements were too few. When doctors diagnosed patients with problems derived from the failure of a specific organ, they were effectively declaring a death sentence.

The initial obstacle was simply figuring out how to suture together blood vessels. Surgeons could not even attempt to transplant organs without the ability to attach them, but they lacked the superfine skills necessary to manipulate such connections. In the early years of the twentieth century, Alexis Carrel, a French surgeon working at New York City's Rockefeller Institute for Medical Research, developed a reliable method of securing blood vessels to one another—he was awarded the Nobel Prize in Physiology or Medicine in 1912 for this achievement. Once this surgical skill was perfected, the field of transplant surgery opened up to greater experimentation as well as to more complex medical challenges.

From an operative perspective, the vital organ easiest for surgeons to detach and reattach was the kidney, which only has three crucial points of connection with the body: the renal artery, the renal vein, and the relatively easy-to-work-with ureter. In comparison, the anatomy of the liver or pancreas is more complex with multiple arteries and veins to care for as well as difficult-to-manipulate secretory ducts. In addition, certain organs, like the lungs and heart, cannot be removed without the use of elaborate temporary measures to sustain life, such as Gibbon's heart-lung machine. Consequently, the thrust of early transplant research focused on the kidney.

These bean-shaped, fist-sized organs, located near the middle of the back, just below the rib cage, are the body's primary filtration system. Every minute, one pint of blood travels to each kidney through its renal artery and spreads to the organ's tiny filtering units, called nephrons. A healthy kidney contains more than one million of these, each with a glomerulus, a ball-like collection of capillaries. These tiny blood vessels function as sieves. They are pockmarked with holes and use a delicate chemical exchange to remove excess water and accumulated waste (known as urea) from blood. The refreshed blood then leaves the kidney via the renal vein and flows back to the heart. The waste, now in the form of urine, exits the kidney through the ureter, which connects to the bladder. In addition to filtering the blood, the kidneys maintain the body's level of vital salts, especially sodium and potassium, thereby regulating blood pressure. Moreover, they control the production of red blood cells and constantly fine-tune the body's acid-base balance.

Problems mount quickly when both kidneys stop working correctly (a person only needs one fully functioning kidney to remain healthy). Individuals in kidney failure grow lethargic. Their hands and feet may swell or feel numb. As unfiltered poisons congregate in the bloodstream, patients become comatose and eventually die. There is no way to repair damaged kidneys, surgically or otherwise. The only long-term solution is replacement with a healthy organ.

At first, surgeons were uncertain what would be the most sensible way to attach a donor kidney. Abdominal surgery was risky and botched operations meant likely death of the patient. Early transplant researchers grappled with a number of questions that seem intuitive in hindsight: Where should a transplanted kidney be placed? What should be done with the ureter? Was it to drain directly to the outside or be reconnected to the bladder? The answers to these questions did not become evident until much later, following a series of animal experiments in the late 1940s and early 1950s demonstrating that a new kidney could be attached in relatively the same manner as the failed one. In the meantime, surgeons in the immediate postwar years tried various creative approaches to save patients in kidney failure. The field was rudimentary at the start, and one famous success story sounds more like a tale taken from a medieval alchemist's diary than a landmark in twentieth-century medicine.

In 1946, a woman was admitted to Peter Bent Brigham Hospital in Boston with acute but recoverable kidney failure that resulted from a botched illegal abortion. Her kidneys were fundamentally sound but needed a period of rest to recover from the trauma they had suffered. Her physician believed that this could be accomplished with a temporary donor kidney, a so-called bridge transplant. He acquired a donor organ from a deceased accident victim and attached it to his patient through blood vessels in her arm. He then taped the external surrogate kidney to her skin, covered it with a moist towel, and kept it warm with heat from a gooseneck lamp. The ureter, which normally connected to the bladder, drained into a laboratory flask. As crude as the solution was, the donor kidney produced urine and, several days later, the patient's own kidneys began to function once again.

The bridge transplant worked admirably, but it could never be a long-term solution (and not simply because patients would have likely refused to walk around with kidneys hanging off their forearms). Subsequent microscopic examination of the donor kidney showed that the patient's body had begun to reject it at a cellular level after only forty-eight hours. A long-term donor kidney (or any organ) perceived as foreign would therefore have no chance of survival. Doctors recognized this problem as the major hurdle in organ transplantation, but they did not yet understand the physiological rationale.

Only in the mid-1940s did medical researchers begin to decode the nature of the immune reaction and the whys and wherefores of organ rejection. The issue turned out to be a dilemma of human individuality. Each person's cells are biochemically unique to that being and foreign to all others. The body's immune system naturally attacks and destroys unfamiliar tissues with an onslaught of killer white blood cells, hostile antibodies, and other antagonistic elements. The researchers concluded that patients' chances for successful transplantations would increase exponentially if doctors could mute immune systems and make them tolerant to foreign tissue—a process labeled "acquired tolerance." But understanding the nature of a problem is not the same as having the solution. Immunosuppression and "acquired tolerance" proved to be incredibly complex research questions.

Nonetheless, American doctors would soon perform a successful long-term kidney transplant in advance of the research, completing one of the greatest medical triumphs of the twentieth century. This unlikely scientific accomplishment was a testament to the vision, cooperation, and courage of the people involved: both the physicians and surgeons and, in this case, the patients.

Francis Moore and George Thorn

Francis Moore, the surgeon who would oversee this revolutionary surgical operation, was a man of grace and warmth, a master of repartee, and a giant of mid-twentieth-century American medicine with an unrivaled knowledge of biological science. According to one colleague, Moore's expertise would "intimidate anyone who disagreed with him or even appeared on the same platform."[1] A journalist, equally impressed, commented: "Men like Francis Moore often seem to be peering even beyond the future."[2] In May 1963, *Time* magazine placed Moore's portrait on the cover, bordered by six words of acclamation: "If they can operate, you're lucky."[3]

Moore was well prepared to be a leader in America's advancement of medicine. He attended Harvard College, where he wrote the Hasty Pudding's 1934 show *Hades! The Ladies!,* which imagined the university as a coeducational institution. He then matriculated to Harvard Medical

School. His initial interest in internal medicine faltered because he found the discipline "[t]oo much talk and theory; not enough action."[4] Instead, Moore shifted his focus to surgery, progressing over the course of a decade from intern to surgical resident to assistant in surgery at Massachusetts General Hospital. In 1948, at age thirty-four, he was appointed to the chairmanship of the surgical department at the Peter Bent Brigham Hospital.

Physicians respected Moore for a wide range of medical achievements. His research contributed to the understanding of how surgical operations altered bodily fluids and chemicals. He also had a reputation for solving difficult scientific puzzles, such as determining the body's normal amount of water, potassium, and sodium, or quantifying the loss of fluids in a burn victim. Admirers claimed that his leadership of the Brigham's surgeons led to major breakthroughs in abdominal operations, heart surgery, and procedures on the blood vessels.

But Moore's influence went beyond his research and clinical accomplishments. He encouraged the interplay between surgeons and physicians, believing that specialists from different fields needed to collaborate when facing modern medical dilemmas. He argued that interspecialty support would hasten medicine's evolution. Although this attitude is commonplace today, it was a minority position at the time.

The doctor with whom he worked most closely in this interdisciplinary respect was George Thorn, the Brigham's brilliant physician in chief and head of the hospital's department of internal medicine. Moore fondly described Thorn as "a surgically minded physician," one who thought of medical developments in surgical terms: "How can it be done, what will be its effect, and when can we get started."[5] Thorn, a gentle and friendly individual, was by all accounts an easy person to collaborate with. "When you were with him," according to his associates, "he was 100% with you, no matter who you were."[6] Eventually, Moore and Thorn would jointly oversee the world's first kidney transplant.

Perhaps the relationship between them thrived because they had much in common, personally and professionally. Like Moore, Thorn was superbly educated and trained, including residency stints at Ohio State and Johns Hopkins. And Thorn had also received his departmental chairmanship at the Brigham at an early age—he was only thirty-six when Harvard offered him the position in 1942. Additionally, the two men were gifted amateur musicians—Moore played piano and Thorn the tenor four-string banjo. They performed together in a small ensemble aptly named the Malady Boys, which frequently entertained the Harvard medical community.

Thorn had built his research career around the kidney and, before the fateful surgery, he was best known for his role in developing the country's first artificial kidney, known as a dialysis machine, in the late 1940s. Although a European doctor had designed the prototype, Thorn improved upon it and made it functionally reliable. For five years he worked in a coordinated fashion with both physicians and surgeons to perfect the device. Like Moore, he relied on interspecialty cooperation to tackle complex problems.

And the dialysis machine had presented plenty of them. Thorn and his band of doctors had to prevent the dialyzed blood from clotting, cooling, frothing, or developing bacteria, challenges similar to those that John Gibbon faced with his heart-lung machine. The finished apparatus looked precarious, with a rotating stainless-steel drum, Lucite hood, warming bath, air traps, clot traps, and myriad motors, switches, thermometers, and control panels. But Thorn had confidence in his machine. "Its use should not be postponed," he urged, "so that it is offered to the patient as a last resort because other methods of treatment have failed."[7]

The dialysis machine was an instant success. It mitigated a number of common kidney ailments, including acute but reversible kidney failure, and, eventually, chronic kidney conditions, such as glomerulonephritis, an irreversible inflammation of the organ. Additionally, the dialysis machine made procedures like the famous Brigham bridge transplant obsolete. Thorn suggested that the device represented the first major step in "a long-range [medical and surgical] program leading to the transplantation of kidneys."[8]

While Thorn is perhaps best known for his kidney-related research, his influence on the profession extended far beyond the laboratory. He was a founding editor of the country's most influential textbook of internal medicine, *Harrison's Principles of Internal Medicine,* which, according to *Time,* had a "humane attitude" and gave doctors "no encouragement to be dogmatic."[9] In his role as a medical writer, Thorn influenced the education, training, and thinking of the country's specialists in internal medicine.

"This sacred kidney"

In late October 1954 twenty-four-year-old Richard Herrick had only a few weeks to live. The reason was severe glomerulonephritis. He was in the final phase of end-stage kidney failure and displayed high blood pressure, convulsions, headaches, vomiting, a weakened heart, and incoherence bordering on all-out madness. His only chance for survival was a kidney transplant, a surgical procedure that had never been successfully performed. The odds didn't favor Richard, but two factors made his case medically unique and would prove lifesaving. First, he had been admitted to Brigham Hospital, home of Moore and Thorn. Second, he was an identical twin.

Although doctors at the time still understood little of organ rejection and "acquired tolerance," they recognized one general exception to the rule of human individuality: identical twins. The different gestation processes of fraternal and identical twins shows why this should be. More than 90 percent of twins are fraternal. At the moment of their conception, two sperm fertilize two different eggs that become two distinct embryos nourished by separate placentas. Fraternal twins can look distinct from one another and be of opposite sexes. They generally have distinct chromosomal profiles as well as dissimilar immune systems. With identical twins, however, the moment of conception occurs when one sperm fertilizes one egg that then spontaneously divides into two embryos joined through a common placenta. Consequently, they have nearly indistinguishable genetic makeups, including the immune systems. One identical twin's immune system will not consider tissue from its sibling to be foreign. Richard, therefore, would not reject a donated kidney from his brother.

Moore and Thorn immediately understood that Richard's identical-twin status made him an ideal candidate for an experimental kidney transplant, but before addressing this possibility, they needed to improve his critical condition. No patient could survive invasive surgery while suffering from high blood pressure, psychotic episodes, and persistent infections. The problem of cleansing Richard's blood would have confounded most hospitals, but the Brigham had Thorn's recently proven dialysis apparatus. The doctors decided to give Richard four hours of blood cleansing using the novel machine. The medical report concluded: "A good chemical response was obtained and 36 hours later the patient's sensorium had cleared and he was cooperative and able to take diet and medicaments by mouth."[10] In other words, Thorn's device accomplished all that was asked of it, efficiently restoring Richard's physical and mental balance. The patient went home to recuperate while Moore and Thorn contemplated a venture into the medical unknown.

The two doctors knew they now had an extraordinary and inimitable opportunity to perform the world's first organ transplant, to save Richard's life, and to make medical and surgical history, but they struggled with the magnitude of the procedure. The possibility of transferring a whole organ from one living being to another was among the most nerve-racking operations ever deliberated. They discussed the issue, but ultimately decided to meet in mid-December for a final decision-making process with their team of anesthesiologists, immunologists, internists, nephrologists, pathologists, and surgeons. With its collective expertise, the interdisciplinary group was better positioned to consider the range of ethical and scientific concerns. Eventually, they concluded that the potential benefits outweighed the risks.

In addition to convincing one another, the Brigham team also had to persuade Richard's brother, Ronald. Part of the final preparations included meetings with him to explain the procedure and answer questions. They were asking him to do something no human being had ever done before: voluntarily allow doctors to remove a major organ for the benefit of another person. Since Ronald only needed one healthy kidney, the short-term clinical risk was minimal, but the long-term effects were less certain. If his one remaining kidney somehow became diseased or injured, he would not have another identical brother to lend him a spare. Ronald, however, did not seem dissuaded by these remote concerns. The two brothers had, according to Moore, "an unusual emotional stake in each other."[11]

Even with Ronald's consent, however, the social and ethical concerns lingered, as they do with contemporary organ donors. There was fear that doctors had unfairly pressured Ronald or that he had felt coerced. Some suggested that using a live donor crossed an ethical threshold and that Ronald should bow out gracefully. But the world's first living organ donor, at least, did not find the situation as ethically treacherous. "They left it up to me to decide," he later recalled. "I was the one who was going to do it; they weren't going to make the decision for me."[12]

Ronald again confirmed his steadfastness the night before the surgery. He was lying in a hospital bed, awaiting the morning's procedure, when his brother passed him a note that said, "Beat it, go home while you can." The guilt over Ronald's sacrifice had apparently grown too strong for Richard to handle. Ronald firmly responded: "I'm here and I'm staying here."[13]

The next morning, December 23, 1954, two surgical procedures began at 8:15. Twin teams of surgeons had to operate on the brothers simultaneously to minimize the amount of time that Ronald's healthy donor kidney was disconnected from a host body. If the organ went without oxygenated blood for a prolonged period, its filtering mechanisms would suffer.

At 9:50 Richard's surgeons called for the new kidney. Moore, who was waiting on the team handling Ronald, carefully walked down the hallway to Richard's operating room. At his waist, he carried a stainless-steel surgical basin swaddled in blue cloth that contained, in his words, "this sacred kidney."[14] Moore handed the organ to a nurse, who passed it to several physicians. They examined the kidney under the shine of overhead lights and pronounced it completely normal. Moore stepped back from the table as a team of his surgeons went about first joining the organ's artery and vein to blood vessels of the anesthetized patient and then connecting the ureter to his bladder.

Shortly after 11:00, the doctors finished securing Ronald's kidney in Richard's lower abdomen, not too far from the appendix. Crystal-clear urine was already flowing copiously through the ureter. Moore later remarked, "Although you may never have developed any affection for urine, if you or your patients are unable to make any, you come to appreciate it."[15] When the surgeons sewed up Richard's abdomen, they had completed what would become the world's first successful long-term kidney transplant.

The operation quickly became major national news. The media began publicizing the accomplishment within days, before the brothers had even left the hospital. "Twin gains in operation, transplanted kidney working 'efficiently,' "[16] read the Associated Press account. A photograph of Richard leaving the Brigham a month after the operation became an iconic image that newspapers distributed widely. It showed Ronald guiding his grinning brother in a wheelchair toward an ambulance to transport him home. *Time* continued to report on Herrick's progress for over a year.

The medical profession took slightly longer to digest the seminal operation, as the Brigham team first submitted the details of the Herrick operation to their peers in early 1956. The article reaffirmed that advanced medicine was moving in an increasingly interdisciplinary direction: Thorn and Moore insisted that the medical and surgical services of the Brigham Hospital be recognized jointly for their efforts. Their report also showed that cutting-edge research required enormous financial resources. An accompanying list of acknowledgments included private foundations, like the John A. Hartford Foundation and the American Heart Association, as well as public sources, like the Office of the Surgeon General and the U.S. Public Health Service. This dual support, particularly from the federal government, followed the financing trend that began in World War II and continued with Lister Hill and James Shannon.

As for the Herrick brothers, they returned to their normal lives. Richard married one of his nurses from the hospital and raised a family. Unfortunately, the glomerulonephritis that destroyed his own kidneys returned to devastate the transplanted one and this, in turn, led to heart problems. He died from a heart attack in 1962. Ronald remains well.

Acquired Tolerance

While the Herrick transplant was a clinical triumph of the highest order, it provided no answers to fundamental questions about organ rejection. The brothers had shared the same genetic structure, circumventing the issue of immunologic intolerance altogether. Thorn, Moore, and their teams of physicians and surgeons still had to resolve the underlying immunologic problem of tissue rejection.

The most promising early research in tissue rejection involved lymphocyte suppression. Lymphocytes are a type of white blood cell that both produce antibodies and attack bacteria and viruses. They are among the most important cellular elements of an immune reaction, and diminishing their numbers reduces immune intolerance. Bone marrow produces lymphocytes, and this tissue is extremely sensitive to radiation.

Consequently, Brigham doctors first tried to solve the dilemma with X-rays. They began exposing test patients to full-body X-rays, hoping to create an environment where a transplanted organ could survive. Inconveniently, irradiation also tended to lower immune defenses so efficiently that a patient could not respond to even a simple infection (e.g., the common cold) and subsequently might die of the most commonplace of illnesses. Of the six patients who received whole-body X-rays and a kidney transplant at the Brigham Hospital between May 1958 and April 1960, only one survived. Moore later commented that the technique's clinical failure gave a new twist to an old cliché: instead of "the operation was a success but the patient died," he quipped, "the graft lived but the patient died."[17] The X-ray technique was a shotgun blast, but doctors needed the precision of a rifle shot.

In the early 1960s they found their ammunition. Chemists had recently synthesized drugs rumored to achieve immunosuppression more safely: 6-mercaptopurine and its close relatives azathioprine and cyclosporine. These new "wonder drugs," like penicillin and streptomycin before them, had potential to resolve a host of medical dilemmas, including organ rejection. Unlike X-ray therapy, which the Brigham doctors usually administered in one irreversible blast, immunosuppressive drugs could be prescribed in small doses, following a daily regimen. Physicians could decrease or suspend dosage levels if a patient's immunological defenses deteriorated too swiftly. The drugs gave the Brigham doctors the clinical control and precision they had lacked with whole-body irradiation.

Almost overnight, the immunosuppressive drugs revolutionized the field of transplant surgery. The Brigham team rapidly transitioned away from the X-ray technique; by mid-1961 they had prepared protocols for a kidney transplant using the new technology. These doctors performed thirteen kidney transplants over the next two years with a success rate above 50 percent, a staggering advance over irradiation therapy with its 17 percent survival. The drugs proved so effective that host bodies could tolerate kidneys that unrelated donors had supplied. The era of identical twins as the only individuals who could undergo a successful kidney transplant was officially over. Kidneys could even come from cadavers.

The Brigham's successful operations provided the model that all subsequent transplants have followed. Their technique first spread to other academic medical centers, and kidney transplants soon became part of the fabric of American and international medicine. "We were no longer unique,"[18] explained Moore with regard to the procedure's proliferation across the globe. His team's prototype, with its impressive cocktail of immunosuppressive drugs, also became a template for more complicated transplants—American doctors performed one of the world's earliest successful heart transplants using this protocol in 1968. Two members of the Brigham kidney transplant team received the 1990 Nobel Prize in Physiology or Medicine for their continuing work with organ and cell transplantation in the treatment of human disease. Currently, over 25,000 Americans receive organ transplants every year—15,000 kidney transplants, 6,000 liver transplants, 2,000 heart transplants, 1,400 lung transplants, 800 combined kidney and pancreas transplants, and 400 pancreas transplants.

The world's first successful kidney transplant changed medicine in even more profound ways. It helped to break a psychological, perhaps spiritual, barrier that viewed the human body as a sacred object able to receive medical care but not designed to provide it. The Brigham team's transplant research showed that the human body was part of the universe of curatives, along with plants, minerals, and synthesized compounds. The research and application of this new concept in medical care—that one person's healthy body could cure another's sickness or that a patient's own tissue could be modified to serve as a source of healing—was a wellspring that helped fuel American medicine's climb to international preeminence.

Whither the General Practitioner

New medical advancements allowed for more complicated treatment options, and these, in turn, necessitated more elaborate clinical care. Doctors had begun routinely employing a multidisciplinary approach to treat patients, similar to the coordinated efforts of Thorn and Moore. Teams of specialized physicians, working in tandem to confront problematic ill-nesses, rapidly became a feature of late-twentieth-century medicine.

This new style of care de facto favored specialists over generalists. Not surprisingly, the percentage of American doctors identifying as special-ists rose dramatically in the postwar period, from 50 percent in the early 1950s to 80 percent by 1970. The shift was especially pronounced in the surgical specialties—general surgeons alone accounted for 10 percent of the nation's physicians.

While the growth of specialism was somewhat inevitable given the advancements in clinical care, several other factors hastened its expansion. For starters, the federal government moved resources toward specialty training. The number of approved residency positions available for spe-cialists rose from about 5,000 in 1940 to 30,000 in 1950 and 65,000 by 1970. In addition, specialism fueled itself. Newly trained specialists inevitably joined their respective specialty societies. These organizations, with their swollen membership rolls and mushrooming treasury coffers, then began to lobby for their own interests.

Specialists had once existed mainly within the confines of academic and urban-based medicine, but their proliferation pushed them outside of teaching centers and large city hospitals, bringing modern medical prac-tice to the nation's quickly expanding suburbs. They constructed outsized office buildings in the neighborhoods surrounding community hospitals. Americans no longer had to travel far to consult specialists, and patients flocked to them to take advantage of the newly accessible expertise.

The general public began shifting away from a long-held view that specialists were merely physicians with distinctive knowledge who only appeared when an illness became serious. Mothers started to take their children to pediatricians, believing that a board-certified doctor knew more about juvenile clinical care than an old-style general practitioner. Pregnant women imagined that obstetricians had greater technical exper-tise in prenatal care and the birthing process than their family's general physician. Adult patients considered internists, with their specialty train-ing in geriatrics, more qualified to handle routine concerns than the family practitioner they had grown up with. A variety of specialties were begin-ning to replace the family doctor for traditional primary medical care, the last refuge of the generalist.

In the past generalists could have rebuffed the advances of specialists through superior political clout. Historically, the AMA, the nation's largest and most powerful medical society, had been a bastion of conservative, generalist attitudes. It had opposed the concept of specialty board certification when freestanding organizations such as the American Board of Surgery first broached the idea in the 1930s. The AMA generally pressed to have oversight authority over specialists. But times had changed. Specialists had infiltrated the AMA as well, and the organization was no longer the monolithic lobby that it had been earlier in the century. Without control of the AMA, general practitioners were politically stranded and lacking a voice.

Even more troubling for these doctors, the medical education system had begun moving away from its traditional support of generalism. The seminal 1910 Flexner Report on medical education had famously opined that medical schools produced generalists and that specialists arose from these ranks. Before World War II, all medical school graduates had completed one year of an internship that prepared them as generalists. Those who desired to specialize had then entered a multiyear, specialty residency that led to board certification. However, following the war, internships changed to accommodate the complexities of modern medicine and moved away from the Flexner perspective. They became less general and more specialty oriented as technology advanced and young doctors abandoned the idea of entering general practice. By 1970 fewer than 12 percent of new medical school graduates became family practitioners.

Generalists had a serious dilemma. Specialists were questioning their level of competency, patients were abandoning them, hospitals were revoking their privileges, young doctors were ignoring them. And the evidence suggested that the situation would only worsen over time. There were few alternatives. General practitioners would have to redefine themselves or go extinct. They chose to employ a timeless strategy: if you can't beat them, join them. General practitioners decided to reinsert themselves into the sociopolitical process of medical professionalization, a path that ironically led toward specialization.

Although they had largely eschewed this process, generalists had taken several steps shortly after World War II to garner some professional cachet. In 1947, a group of generalists had organized the American Academy of General Practice, and three years later, the journal *GP* had begun publication. Several residencies had even appeared by the early 1960s. But these early steps had evinced conflicting attitudes about whether the goal was to professionalize generalism into a medical specialty or simply calcify it. *GP,* at least, had seemed to argue for the latter: "Preserve the general practitioner for ourselves, our children, and the American public. This heritage is, in itself, worth the price asked."[19]

These initial activities had limited impact in strengthening the floundering generalist movement: the only true litmus test for professionalism in modern medicine after World War II was board certification. At first, generalist leaders had attempted to persuade rank-and-file practitioners that an association with the American Academy of General Practice equaled specialty board certification. However, members realized that they would never be accepted as comparable to specialists without an "official" board certificate. Eventually, generalists formed the American Board of Family Practice and quickly launched a public relations campaign to win acceptance. The executive director of the board self-servingly assured the public that "Family Practice IS a specialty."[20] In February 1969 the American Board of Medical Specialties, an accrediting agency that oversees specialty certification, agreed with the executive director and recognized the newly organized board. With that, general practice, now known as family practice, formally became the nation's twentieth principal medical and surgical specialty.

Despite its new status, generalism remained a contentious topic both inside and outside of the profession. Many debated the merits of board certification for something as vague as general practice. On its face, it did not seem to fit the medical dictionary's definition of a specialty: "the particular group of diseases or branch of medical science to which one devotes his time and attention."[21] However, family practitioners now had all the formal trappings of specialists: their own society and journal, residencies, and written examinations for board certification.

Even after board certification, tensions remained between academic medicine and general practitioners. Men like Moore and Thorn could not change their underlying skepticism. To them, general practitioners were community-based clinicians trained in community hospital residencies. Old-line academic medical centers like Harvard, Yale, and Johns Hopkins continued to shun generalists, though this hostility softened once larger urban hospitals, including some established academic medical institutions, began opening family practice programs.

Board certification for general practitioners also left several major questions unsettled. Would the family practitioner, now a self-proclaimed specialist, remain a gatekeeper to a patient's medical care or would physicians in the other primary care specialties continue to usurp this role? If the board-certified family practitioner failed to attract primary care patients, would they have to further subspecialize to compete in areas like pediatrics, obstetrics, and geriatrics? In some respects, board certification created as many questions as it solved, and the answers would depend on how health care developed moving forward.

Nonetheless, the awarding of board certificates to general practitioners was a watershed event in the process of medical professionalization in America. Specialization had triumphed from medical education all the way through clinical care. Patients could no longer seek sanctioned medical advice from anyone but specialists, who were now free to extend their hegemony over the whole of medicine. No other occupation and no other country had such absolute niching of a professional workforce.

The AMA versus National Health Care

While specialists provided more advanced care than the flagging generalists, they charged a higher price for the privilege. Physician and hospital fees skyrocketed during the postwar expansion of health care. From 1940 to 1965, total annual national health care expenditures increased tenfold, from slightly less than $4 billion to $39 billion. The industry's growth rate was outpacing that of the general economy, 34 percent to 25 percent, respectively, in the early 1960s. Medical care had become a vast, uncoordinated industry that consumed almost 6 percent of the country's gross domestic product, double the percentage in the 1930s.

Some Americans were getting priced out of the marketplace, especially those with fixed incomes. The country had the world's most sophisticated health care system, but large sectors of the population could not afford much of it.

From a policy perspective, there were several ways to handle this dilemma. First, the government could simply ignore the problem. This was easy, but politically unpopular. Second, the medical establishment could control cost increases. This was pragmatically difficult. For starters, the fixed costs of health care had risen sharply because of new and seemingly essential medical technologies. In addition, the successful professionalization of medicine meant that doctors wanted to earn incomes commensurate with their social status.

The most feasible solution, at least in the short term, was for the government to provide some form of social insurance for those in need. However, doctors again strongly opposed federal involvement in medicine. They feared that any interference in the privacy of their relationship with patients would trigger a deterioration in the quality of medical care, and they assumed that government control would lead inevitably to a loss of professional independence. While the federal government heavily subsidized medical research and education, it had historically stayed out of the doctor's office and their private practice.

The reason doctors had always been able to bully the federal government on this matter was the influence of the AMA. With its giant membership base, financial resources, and social prestige, it was the most powerful interest group in the nation for much of the first half of the twentieth century. Until World War II, the doctors' lobby had efficiently crushed all calls for greater government involvement, such as that of the Depression Era Committee on the Costs of Medical Care, which advocated making health care available to all people. Roosevelt's expansive New Deal had not even attempted to provide socialized medicine, largely due to the strength of the AMA's lobby.

In the postwar period, however, Democratic presidential administrations began making stronger efforts to break private medicine's hold over health care. President Harry Truman first raised the issue during his 1948 election campaign. After his victory, he continued to criticize organized medicine's "monopoly controls"[22] of the health care system and suggested that the federal government needed to intervene. Eventually, his proposals for a form of national health insurance ended up before Congress.

The AMA reacted swiftly and furiously. It assessed each of its members—almost 75 percent of American physicians—a special $25 fee to fund a coordinated opposition. These contributions allowed it to spend money on a scale that no other lobbying group had ever approached: $1,552,683 in 1949 and $1,326,078 in 1950. The organization hired a public relations firm and sponsored a massive propaganda campaign of pamphlets, press releases, speakers, and radio and television advertising. The strategy was to exploit Cold War–era fears and the message was simple: the president's plan was a dangerous step toward a socialist America.

The AMA also forged political alliances with hundreds of lobbying groups to expand their reach. Many organizations, including the Chamber of Commerce and the Blue Cross, shared a suspicion of big government and its supposed penchant for financial giveaways. Collectively, these allied interests disseminated the message that any government health insurance scheme would lead to overcrowded hospitals, long lines in waiting rooms, and physicians with no incentive to provide superior medical care. In the end, Congress easily defeated any of Truman's health-care-related initiatives.

The AMA's efforts were so potent that nationalized health care became politically treacherous territory for much of the next decade. Historians have suggested that several senior congressmen lost their seats in the 1950 midterm elections because of their firm support for Truman's plan. In 1952 a Republican party platform that criticized federal health insurance programs helped Dwight Eisenhower win the presidency. While he remained in office, the AMA and its political allies easily rebuffed any calls for a government-backed health insurance plan.

In 1960 John Kennedy's Democratic presidential victory renewed the government's efforts, but in a modified form. The idea of national health insurance remained problematic. Kennedy focused specifically on medical care for the aged. Opinion polls showed that his advocacy for this had been among the key issues that differentiated him from his Republican rival, Richard Nixon. Kennedy seemed to have learned from some of Truman's mistakes. His proposals were less capacious and he appreciated that any change to the status quo would produce a serious political fight. Before his administration had even taken office, one of his advisers commented that the AMA subverted the "will of the majority of the people" with "methods of vilification and intimidation of anyone who does not agree with their position."[23]

The AMA again mobilized for an all-out propaganda war. They used tactics similar to the last great battle: print and electronic advertisements combined with grassroots activism. In Operation Hometown, for example, organized medicine provided community doctors with ready-made speeches and gave high school debate teams socioeconomic information. The red-baiting returned as well. In Operation Coffee Cup, Ronald Reagan, then a well-known actor, recorded a message imploring Americans to voice their opposition to nationalized health care: "If you don't, this program, I promise you, will pass just as surely as the sun will come up tomorrow. And behind it will come other federal programs that will invade every area of freedom as we have known it in this country. Until one day . . . we will awake to find that we have socialism."[24]

On May 21, 1962, the AMA attempted its most spectacular public relations gambit. The day before, Kennedy had given a nationally televised speech on health care reform to a rally of twenty thousand senior citizens and labor activists at New York City's Madison Square Garden. The AMA decided that it needed to respond and rented out the same venue the following morning to film a rebuttal. An Association spokesman stood exactly where the president had been and told of how Kennedy's ideas about expanding Social Security to help the aged pay medical bills "were a cruel hoax and a delusion." He warned that in reality the proposals would "wastefully" cover millions of Americans who did not need them and "heartlessly"[25] ignore millions who did—a reference to the three million people over sixty-five years of age without Social Security. The American Medical Association paid $100,000 to broadcast its one-hour response that same night in prime time on one hundred ninety stations of the National Broadcasting Corporation network.

The television attack backfired. The AMA had finally gone too far. It was one thing to argue against socialism, but to disagree with medical care for the aged proved imprudent and unpopular. The *New York Times* coverage of the gambit sided against the doctors—"Senior Citizens' Chief Calls Medical Group's Attack 'Lies and Deceptions.'"[26] Kennedy capitalized on the gaffe as well. At a press conference several days later, he pointedly remarked that in the 1930s the AMA had also led the charge against Social Security, which had subsequently become an incredibly popular program.

The AMA had lost a battle, but it had not yet lost the war. While Kennedy had garnered public support for his proposals, he still lacked a solid liberal Democratic majority in Congress. It was the same problem that had doomed Truman a dozen years earlier. Ultimately, the conservative coalition of Republicans and southern Democrats thwarted much of Kennedy's liberal domestic agenda, including nationalized care for the aged.

However, the situation soon changed. In 1964, following the assassination of Kennedy, President Lyndon Johnson ran for election promising large-scale, government-sponsored reforms, particularly for health care. His opponent, Republican nominee Barry Goldwater, had a conservative, small-government agenda, and his health care proposals consisted of unambitious state, local, and private initiatives. The AMA, not surprisingly, gave its support to Goldwater. Voters, on the other hand, overwhelmingly sided with Johnson and his calls for liberal reform. He won a landslide victory that also swept a liberal Democratic majority into Congress. Suddenly, a Democratic president had enough congressional votes to shepherd in progressive legislation, and health care reform enactment was all but guaranteed.

Once in office, Johnson made health care legislation a centerpiece of the Great Society, his broad collection of progressive initiatives that included the Voting Rights Act of 1965, Volunteers in Service to America (VISTA) (a domestic version of the Peace Corps), Head Start (federal aid for public education), the National Endowment for the Arts, the National Endowment for the Humanities, and the Corporation for Public Broadcasting. His new administration considered medical reform so central that it convinced congressional leadership to give the proposed health care bills—commonly known as Medicare—the numeric symbols of highest priority, H.R. 1 and S. 1, respectively. Congress soon began its hearings on the matter.

When the legislation reached congressional committees for debate, organized medicine and a liberal Congress locked horns in what felt like a winner-take-all battle for the soul of the nation's health care. The AMA spent a staggering $951,570 in just three months of lobbying. Physicians shuttled in and out of the witness seats, fighting a rearguard action against surging public and political support for Medicare. "We physicians care for the elderly and know their health needs better than anyone else," insisted an AMA spokesman. "Doctors cannot be restricted by decisions of untrained Government employees on what services should and should not be performed in medical facilities."[27]

The atmosphere of the hearings was at first businesslike but became contentious. Physicians carped about the socialization of medicine and managed to infuriate committee members hoping to better understand how doctors could work within Medicare's guidelines. A frustrated congressman called the leaders of organized medicine a "little group of cynical men" who considered themselves "would-be czars of the health and welfare of this nation."[28] The situation grew so heated that Congress eventually refused to hear from AMA members altogether.

The congressional ban was the latest affirmation that the organization had lost its political mystique. In less than a generation, organized medicine had gone from dictating the terms of the debate to being banished from it. Two main factors explain this sudden collapse. First, organized medicine had fallen out of touch with shifting political tastes. Its championing of Goldwater and other Republican candidates had proven a political disaster. The nation was demanding change in its medical system, while the leaders of the AMA steadfastly embraced the outmoded fee-for-service, private practice, mom-and-pop business model. Second, the AMA had simply become a weaker organization within medicine. Membership rolls were down to fewer than six of every ten American physicians, and its rigid internal discipline had evaporated. In early 1965 dissident doctors even began holding secret meetings. "Medicare IS going to pass," explained one of them. "The AMA's opposition to the bill would prevent doctors from taking part in planning its administration."[29]

It seems counterintuitive that organized medicine's largest lobbying body would grow less powerful at the exact moment the profession was in ascendance. However, the same factors that helped the profession thrive were marginalizing the influence of the AMA. The backbone of the AMA had historically been the family practitioner, but their numbers were declining with each year as few new doctors became generalists. The other large medical communities—specialists, researchers, and academicians (groups that largely overlapped)—had little interest in the AMA for a variety of reasons. Specialists focused on the goals of their own societies, not organized medicine. Medical researchers depended on their universities and the National Institutes of Health for political support. Academic leaders needed federal funds for medical schools, largely preventing them from participating in the AMA's sociopolitical activities. Organized medicine, by default, had become a reservoir of conservative attitudes within the profession. It had failed to keep up with the transition that physicians needed to make from isolated small-business owners to skilled managers overseeing a team of collaborating health personnel, clinical technicians, nurses, and social workers.

The Battle Over Medicare

In June 1965, with Medicare on the verge of passage, the AMA had its annual convention in New York City. Twenty-five thousand organization members descended on the vast Coliseum at Columbus Circle (now site of the Time Warner Center) to take part in the five-day gathering. To the lay observer it appeared to be an impressive show of strength and unity for organized medicine.

The four-story drug and medical equipment exhibit area resembled a "supermarket of medical products." Attendees strolled around it carrying "shopping bags crammed with pamphlets, boxes and bars of soap, weight-reducing tablets and assorted pills, tubes and bottles,"[30] according to the *New York Times*. Salesmen stood in colorful booths and hawked items with titles like "Help Build Up Run-Down Patients" and "Hear New Facts About the Night Eating Syndrome."[31] At one display, a male model lay on a hospital bed, comfortably reading a copy of *Playboy,* to promote a new product designed to eliminate bedsores.

Doctors gathered in side rooms where they listened to hundreds of scholarly presentations and discussed topics ranging from the latest advances in medicine to the latest advances in quackery. In one panel, the medical director of the Food and Drug Administration gave a lecture on the addictive properties of newly discovered drugs like amphetamines and barbiturates, warning of illegal sales by "vice and crime syndicates."[32] In another colloquium, a psychiatrist worried that an evil, Svengali-like individual would attempt to hypnotize the public en masse through television. He assured attendees that there was a "compelling need" to institute "stringent safeguards and control"[33] over personnel in the broadcast industry.

Among the most serious problems was tension over racial integration within the profession. A daily picket line of one hundred fifty physicians marched at the Coliseum to protest the Association's southern affiliates' discriminatory policies against African-American doctors. An AMA spokesperson unconvincingly explained at a press conference that the organization had urged its member societies "to completely get rid of discrimination," but in view of existing civil rights laws, it "could not order them to do so."[34]

But despite everything happening in and around the Coliseum, the real center of activity for the profession was located six blocks south at the recently completed fifty-story Americana Hotel (now the Sheraton New York at Seventh Avenue and Fifty-third Street). Outside the building, one thousand members of the Congress of Senior Citizens of Greater New York stood chanting, "2–4–6–8, AMA Cooperate—Pass Medicare."[35] Inside the hotel's ballroom, the Association's 235-member House of Delegates, its central decision-making body, met in closed session to discuss the impending Medicare threat.

Almost all the delegates opposed the program. "American people have the most serious misgivings about welfare statism,"[36] an Iowa surgeon told journalists in explanation of his viewpoint. While some cautious delegates suggested that, given Medicare's likely passage, conciliation would be wise, the majority of attendees preferred options like a boycott of the government program or a nationwide doctors' strike. One physician even had the temerity to suggest that "force must be used when reason will not prevail."[37]

The delegates had a difficult choice to make. They could either accept that the government had outmuscled them or they could double-down on their opposition and shift from politicking to insurgency. The future of organized medicine hung in the balance, and the leadership looked to one man: James Appel, the AMA's recently elected president.

Appel's clinical career made him well suited to lead organized medicine's outmoded and conservative House of Delegates. After attending the University of Pennsylvania School of Medicine, he had only completed a general internship before joining his father in private practice. The elder

Appel then tutored his son in an apprentice-like relationship still common in 1930s rural America. With his father as guide, he mastered surgical and obstetrical skills and other rudiments necessary for a family doctor. His father also passed down the view that family practice was a sacred profession: "[Family practitioners] and their patients get to know one another as persons and the rewards are soul-satisfying,"[38] Appel explained. "[They] are infused with the feeling of devotion and humanism."[39] From 1933 until a month before his death in 1981, Appel practiced in the same house in Lancaster, Pennsylvania, where he was born. It is no surprise, perhaps, that a journalist once described the lanky, balding, soft-spoken doctor as "homespun."[40]

Like many general practitioners, Appel felt that his career needed to be defended from the threats of modern medicine and the federal government, and he became involved in local medical politics at a young age. He spent years working his way through the ranks of his county and state medical societies, and in 1962 the AMA appointed him vice chairman of its board of trustees. He ascended to the presidency three years later. As president, he called Medicare's congressional supporters a "flock of misled 'political sheep,'" who ignored the wishes of their constituents and listened only to the "sweet voices of the labor leaders and the ivory towers."[41]

Despite his strong views on the importance of organized medicine, Appel preferred pragmatism to polemics and conciliation to conflict. At the New York City convention, he discouraged physicians from pursuing "unethical tactic[s] . . . such as strike or sabotage."[42] While he resolutely opposed the concept of Medicare, he acknowledged that the legislation had already cleared the House of Representatives and its passage in the Senate was a foregone conclusion. He urged his peers to remember that "[s]ociety depends for its orderly existence upon law. Regardless of our personal opinion, we do not have the right—either as physicians or citizens—to violate a law, or to violate the spirit of the law or its intent. . . . We must make every effort to develop [Medicare's] good points, while working equally hard to eliminate its bad points."[43]

Appel's pacifying rhetoric had little effect on the more ardent of his constituents. Doctors accused him of asking them to "walk like zombies or sheep into involuntary servitude" while the federal government extended "fascist control"[44] over hospitals and medicine. Others sent telegrams to their fellow delegates: "Impeach Appel!"[45]

Going into the final day of the AMA convention, Appel did not know if his pleas would be enough to stave off insurrection. He put the issue of Medicare to a vote in the House of Delegates, while cries of "appeasement" and "surrender"[46] echoed in the ballroom. The options were few, strike or support. The delegates sided with Appel, at least in the interim, and decided to postpone any direct strike action until the Medicare bill became law. They instead requested that Appel and other AMA leaders arrange a final face-to-face meeting with President Johnson to discuss the status of Medicare.

In the end, it didn't matter. An unproductive medical summit took place on July 29, 1965. The following day, Johnson flew to Independence, Missouri, to sign the Medicare bill in the presence of former president Harry Truman. The federal government had finally triumphed over organized medicine.

After Medicare's enactment, the AMA's House of Delegates called a special session. Attendees griped about Appel and the board of trustees' capitulation to outside forces. Talk of a Medicare boycott reached a crescendo. Appel took the podium and calmly suggested that any action resembling a strike was "foolish and petulant."[47] He told the audience that they had done their best to defeat Medicare and failed. "We now are expected by the public, the press and the Congress to act as reasonable and mature men and women."[48] An Association lawyer seconded Appel. He cautioned that an organized boycott would create anticompetition problems and expose any participating physicians to legal penalties under the Sherman Anti-Trust Act, including lengthy jail sentences. Ultimately, the pragmatists prevailed, and the House of Delegates agreed to support Medicare. Organized medicine's quest to remain the arbiter of the nation's health had come to a quiet and definitive end.

Despite organized medicine's official support for Medicare, the early implementation phase was rocky. The AMA tried to prevent expansion of the law, theoretically to protect patients from the constraints of the program. "Doctors seek to set policy and avoid any blame for 'the harmful effects,' "[49] headlined the *New York Times* in November 1965. The Association of American Physicians and Surgeons, a radical splinter group of the

AMA, boasted that fifty thousand doctors had independently "searched their consciences" and agreed not to become "collaborationists in the evil scheme of Medicare."[50]

Over time, however, the medical establishment embraced Medicare. By 1970 most doctors not only accepted the program but considered it a financial pot of gold. Government benefits allowed greater numbers of elderly patients to seek medical care. Since financial considerations had been shifted from the patient to the federal program, doctors were free to provide these patients with fulsome care, especially since Medicare benefits continued to increase throughout the decade.

The passage and successful enactment of Medicare marked a new era in American medicine. The profession was no longer the major decision maker for the nation's health care policies. The term "organized medicine" became something of an oxymoron. The autonomy and authority that doctors had grown accustomed to was gone forever.

Physicians had become but one component in a complex and unruly system. In 1965 there were almost five other health care workers, each with competing interests, for every doctor. New, politically powerful interest groups arose to lobby for consumers, hospitals, insurance companies, medical equipment manufacturers, and pharmaceutical corporations. The most important economic, political, and social forces shaping the character and organization of medicine would now come from outside of the community of doctors.

A Prototypical Modern Disease

Cancer, the prototypical modern disease, is also one of the oldest on record. As far back as ancient Greece, physicians identified its signature malignant swellings. The Romans described these growths as *carcinos,* or "crablike." "Just as a crab's feet extend from every part of its body," wrote one practitioner in antiquity, "so in this disease the veins are distended, forming a similar figure."[51]

The disease defies every rule of biologic sensibility. Malignant cells—autonomous, antisocial, compassionless killers—spontaneously join together in a pact of destruction. They proliferate uncontrollably and often emerge in distant parts of the body, a process known as metastasis. Once cancer arrives, it impedes and suffocates organs and tissues. The disease erodes blood vessels, interrupts hormones, blocks intestines, short-circuits nerves, and destroys vital centers. Over time, the body must mount a battle against itself, but the winner is almost always the same.

Through the centuries, doctors discovered that the disease had hundreds of forms and obeyed few rules; however, modern medicine divides cancer into several broad groups of cellular derivation: carcinomas, sarcomas, leukemias, and lymphomas being the most common. Carcinomas arise in the cells that cover the surface of the body and line organs and glands. They account for over 80 percent of all cancer cases, including the common forms of bladder, breast, colon, lung, pancreas, prostate, and skin malignancies. Sarcomas are much rarer and take hold in supportive tissue cells such as bones, cartilage, ligaments, muscle, and tendons, as well as connective tissue in the blood vessels and brain. The leukemias are derived from the blood-forming cells of the bone marrow, while lymphomas develop in the lymph nodes.

For most of history cancer was the exclusive province of the surgeon. They cut out any tumors visible on the body's surface, providing patients some relief from the pain and stench of their ulcerating sores. Surgery, however, could not excise every microscopic pocket of malignant cells, and new deadly swellings invariably returned. Nor could the knife wielder battle malignancies within the body. The only therapy was a cruel process of watching and waiting.

At the beginning of the twentieth century clinicians stumbled upon a supplemental treatment for cancer: radiation, a newly discovered technology. Tests showed that radiation could reduce the size of tumors. Doctors began to expose postoperative cancer patients to high doses of radiation in an attempt to destroy any residual clumps of malignant cells. Unfortunately, this rudimentary therapy offered little help to the vast number of individuals whose cancer had spread beyond the initial site. The combination of surgery and radium nonetheless remained the best therapy available for the first half of the twentieth century.

In 1947 this changed when a Harvard pediatric pathologist named Sidney Farber discovered that chemical agents could inhibit malignant diseases. His patients were young children with leukemia, an incurable and aggressive cancer characterized by an overgrowth of the white-blood-cell-making tissue of the bone marrow. Farber found that the drug aminopterin blocked the production of the abnormal white blood cells, curbing a patient's out-of-control cancer. After administering this chemical therapy, or chemotherapy, Farber could more easily handle the side effects of the leukemia, including infections and enlargement of the liver, lymph nodes, and spleen. His juvenile patients who received the experimental treatment "began to play" and "run about" with "marked improvements in appearance and interest."[52] "Chemotherapy" soon became a household word and an indispensable tool to treat many malignancies.

"Four-Button Sid"

Farber was prim, proper, and imposing. His associates called him "Four-Button Sid"[53] because he always dressed in custom-made suits with four-button vests. When he entered a room at the Harvard Children's Hospital, those present would often stand as a show of respect. Farber never demanded this. Rather, he had earned such deference through his old-world comportment and his swift advance up Harvard's academic ladder. He had arrived there as a second-year medical student after spending a year in Europe and graduated in 1927. Two years later, after completing his pathology training at the Brigham, he became the first full-time pathologist at Children's Hospital. He was only twenty-five.

Farber shaped his career around the belief that mankind could cure cancer so long as two conditions were met: extensive research and ample support from the public and private sectors. With regard to the first requirement, he led by example. The light in his office never appeared to be off and his dedication to his patients was well known. With regard to the latter, Farber would become the public ambassador for cancer research. He was a stimulating speaker with a flair for the dramatic, and he used these qualities to help channel staggering amounts of money toward finding a cure. Farber described the struggle to defeat cancer as "the greatest mobilization of resources—man, mineral, animal and money—ever undertaken to conquer a single disease."[54]

His fund-raising career began locally, with the civically minded set around Boston. Farber's first major benefactor was the Variety Club of New England, a charitable organization of men in the motion picture and theater business. They had been searching for a medical cause to support and crossed paths with Farber. Few physicians could cajole like him, and the club soon began funding a small cancer clinic that Farber had recently opened at Children's Hospital.

Farber realized that the Variety Club could provide him not only with charitable support but with entertainment industry contacts. He persuaded the club's leadership to help him get a fund-raising appeal before a national audience. They arranged for one of his young cancer patients to appear on the popular radio quiz show *Truth or Consequences* so that he could make his pitch to the entire country. The savvy Farber quickly put together one of the most memorable fund-raising events in American history.

On May 22, 1948, in a nine-minute broadcast, Ralph Edwards, the show's host, introduced the twelve-year-old patient to America. He explained at the opening of the broadcast that "Just like thousands of other young fellas . . . 'Jimmy' is suffering from cancer, but he doesn't know he has it . . ."[55] (Farber, determined to protect the adolescent's identity, had dubbed him "Jimmy.") The youngster told Edwards that he wished for a television set so he could watch his favorite baseball team, the Boston Braves. To Jimmy's great surprise, the entire starting lineup for the team, one-by-one, started walking into his Boston hospital room. The first baseman, Earl Torgeson, handed the child an autographed bat. Next Warren Spahn, one of the greatest left-handed pitchers in history, arrived with a baseball signed by all of the players. Finally, the manager, Billy Southworth, presented the boy a custom-sized uniform and fielder's mitt. Once everyone had crowded into his room, the child and his baseball heroes sang the Tin Pan Alley song "Take Me Out to the Ball Game." The segment ended with Edwards asking listeners to send in "your quarters, dollars, tens of dollars tonight to Jimmy for the Children's Cancer Research Foundation . . . and we'll see to it that Jimmy gets his television set."[56]

Farber had set the initial fund-raising target for the "Jimmy" campaign at $20,000, but the appeal brought in almost a quarter million dollars during its first year. As a result, the Jimmy Fund was born. It soon rivaled the March of Dimes in prominence. Collection canisters, embossed with the Jimmy Fund's slogan "I can <u>DREAM,</u> can't I?," appeared throughout New England, in movie theater lobbies or passed around audiences.

For the real Jimmy, his brush with fame was followed by the remission of his cancer. He returned to his family's farm in northern Maine and lived most of his life in anonymity. The staff at Children's Hospital assumed that Jimmy had died. This made sense since the cure rates for childhood cancers, despite Farber's efforts, were low during that era. At the fiftieth anniversary celebration of the famous broadcast, Jimmy, whose real name was Einar Gustafson, revealed that he was alive. For the next three years, until his death from a stroke, he made guest appearances at numerous Jimmy Fund events.

In 1952 donations to the Jimmy Fund allowed Farber to move out of his small unit in the Children's Hospital and into a four-story redbrick building called the Jimmy Fund Building. It later became the Sidney Farber Cancer Center and is currently Harvard's Dana-Farber Cancer Institute, where the Jimmy Fund serves as its charity branch (the fund remains popular and is the official charity of the Boston Red Sox).

Thanks in part to the success of the Jimmy Fund, Farber's reputation grew. He was becoming one of the most recognized names in American medicine and used his fame and influence to direct the public's attention to the needs of the cancer researcher. He wanted hundreds of cancer centers, patterned after the Jimmy Fund Building, with advanced facilities for research and multispecialty teams of physicians who could attack cancer through surgery, radiotherapy, and chemotherapy. For Farber, it was nothing less than a crusade to establish the control of cancer as a national priority.

He brought his appeals for research directly to Washington, D.C. Beginning in the early 1950s and continuing for a quarter century, Farber acted as a star witness in numerous congressional hearings on medical legislation, often appearing across from Lister Hill. His persuasive testimony convinced Congress to allocate $3 million toward chemotherapy in 1954. Due to Farber's influence, the National Cancer Institute was soon devoting half its budget to chemotherapy research.

But the federal contributions were never enough for Farber. "It is quite clear," he asserted at a meeting of the American Public Health Association in 1960, "that this progress is not sufficient. This effort does not represent the contribution this country should make to these cancer patients."[57]

Over the course of the next decade, Farber appeared to be everywhere in his efforts to push cancer research and treatment into the national arena. The Senate appointed him cochair of a panel to examine the adequacy of funds for cancer research, and the American Cancer Society made him the organization's president. In 1966 he won the Lasker Award for Clinical Medical Research (sometimes referred to as America's "Medical Nobel") in recognition of his 1947 chemotherapy discovery. He also became spokesman for the well-funded Citizens' Committee for the Conquest of Cancer, a grassroots advocacy group whose goal was to initiate an all-out "war on cancer." Like Farber, the Citizens' Committee felt that insufficient federal funding was responsible for the continuing lack of breakthroughs in cancer research.

The National Cancer Act of 1971

Farber's demands were growing bolder, but the era of federal government largess was ebbing rapidly. By the late 1960s politicians and the public began to view total medical expenditures as too high for what the public received back in terms of its health. They no longer equated medicine with "clinical successes" but with "socioeconomic problems." When the word "medicine" appeared in a headline it was paired with "catastrophe" and "chaos." *Time* magazine ran a cover story in February 1969 titled "What's Wrong with U.S. Medicine,"[58] and President Richard Nixon declared several months later that the nation faced a "massive crisis"[59] in health care.

Statistics revealed that this anxiety was well founded. Between 1965 and 1970, total national health expenditures jumped 77 percent to $69 billion annually and now represented over 7 percent of the gross national product. The news was even worse for federal and state governments. In that same five-year period, government spending on health care increased almost 150 percent to nearly $30 billion annually.

This ballooning of government budgets largely resulted from higher-than-anticipated costs for Medicare and its sister program Medicaid, which provided health care coverage for the poor. Part of the problem was that Medicare had never really solved the problem of accelerating health care costs. It had simply shifted them from the consumer to the federal government.

Not only were these health expenditure figures alarming, but they were far above those of other developed countries. Studies suggested that Americans underwent too much surgery in comparison to Canadians and the British. The conclusion was that the American system promoted unnecessary operations, leaving patients overhospitalized and overmedicated. Even worse, although the country had the world's best available medical care, in many health categories it was lagging behind its peers. The United States ranked below Australia, Canada, and many West European countries in infant and maternal mortality, as well as deaths from cancer, heart disease, and pulmonary illnesses.

For the 1970 budget, the Nixon administration confronted these health care problems by attempting to control federal health spending. The medical research community was hit hardest. The budget gave no appropriations increase to the National Institutes for Health and reduced National Cancer Institute funds by 2 percent.

Farber and his supporters were outraged. They felt that Nixon's action in reducing cancer research was a calamitous response to the spiraling costs in health care, and they had statistics to support their side of the argument as well. During the last thirty years, American deaths due to malignancy had increased more than 50 percent, from 11 percent to 17 percent. Cancer was the nation's second biggest killer after heart disease. Even more sobering, Farber's American Cancer Society predicted that during the 1970s cancer would kill three and a half million Americans and manifest itself in almost twice that number. In mid-November 1969, Farber and several other nationally renowned doctors held a news conference to make a last-minute appeal for Congress to reverse the medical research budget reductions. They argued that improvements in patient care were "inseparable from continued progress in research and that both were being jeopardized by the tight budget."[60]

On December 9, 1969, a full-page advertisement appeared in the *New York Times* and the *Washington Post* that declared "Mr. Nixon: You can cure cancer." The Citizens' Committee for the Conquest of Cancer had purchased the ads in an emotional appeal to the masses. The newspapers' broadsides prominently featured commentary from Farber: "[W]e are so close to a cure for cancer. We lack only the will and the kind of money and comprehensive planning that went into putting a man on the moon."[61]

Despite the dramatic tactics, Nixon's 1970 budget went ahead as planned. The newspaper advertisement, however, had not been in vain. Slightly more than a year later, during the 1971 State of the Union address, Nixon announced that he had changed his mind about cancer research. He argued that the "same kind of concentrated effort that took man to the moon should be turned toward conquering this dread[ed] disease."[62] His reference to the moon was an unambiguous sign that the president had heeded Farber's warnings. Nixon subsequently adjusted the budget, added $232 million to the National Cancer Institute, including a special request to allocate $100 million solely for cancer research, and signed the National Cancer Act of 1971.

The government's "war on cancer" finally gave the disease the national attention that Farber had been demanding for over twenty years. It generously supported clinical research, created a network of cancer care institutions, and established clinical trials as a model of modern medical care. Well-funded researchers published hundreds of thousands of insightful scientific papers and devised exotic drugs and therapies to counter the side effects of cancer and its care, which include fatigue, nausea, vomiting, hair loss, diarrhea, constipation, and nerve and muscle difficulties. Laboratories began developing new treatments as well, such as stem cell transplants, immunotherapies, and gene manipulations. Moreover, the government support set a tone for the practice of medicine in America that legitimized extensive laboratory testing and powerful therapies as the preferred pathway to better health. Preventive health care was on the outs.

Unfortunately, the promise of the 1969 newspaper advertisement remains unfulfilled. Cancer is an expensive priority but clinical progress has been uneven during the past four decades. Death rates for breast and colon cancer have fallen, but mortality statistics for brain, liver, lung, melanoma, and pancreatic malignancies have actually risen. Overall, the mortality rate for all cancers, adjusted for the size and age of the population, has decreased only 5 percent over the last half century. In contrast, the death rate for heart disease has fallen over 60 percent in that time, and for influenza and pneumonia, it has dropped 55 percent. Cancer remains a poorly controlled disease even though the federal government, private foundations, and public companies have spent hundreds of billions of dollars on cures since Nixon signed the National Cancer Act.

The disconnect between funds spent and clinical outcomes in cancer care mirrored the larger difficulties that medicine and its physicians faced over the closing decades of the twentieth century. Increases in health care expenditures no longer guaranteed corresponding improvements in health status. And, much like a malignant tumor, the health care industry was threatening to grow out of control and overwhelm the very society that supported it.

❧ Ten ❧

TRANSFORMATION

A Crisis in Manpower

AFTER WORLD WAR II, American medical schools became highly competitive, sophisticated specialty centers bolstered by generous government funding. The learning opportunities and clinical care they provided were unparalleled internationally. Still, the nation was failing to produce enough doctors to match the demand for medical services, which had swelled due to technological advances, lifestyle changes, federal programs, and, most important, population growth. Between 1930 and 1950 the population increased 23 percent (from 123 million to 151 million), but the number of medical schools grew by less than 8 percent (from 76 to 82) and the number of first-year students by only 9 percent (from 6,457 to 7,042). The result was a growing imbalance between the domestic supply of doctors and the demand for health care.

Organized medicine initially denied this looming doctor shortage. Doctors argued that the lack of physicians in many areas of the country resulted from maldistribution rather than true scarcity. They worried that increasing the nation's supply of physicians would compromise the exclusiveness of the profession, something that had taken over two centuries to achieve.

The situation soon reached a crisis level that no amount of semantics could deny. By 1960 the nation's hospitals were seeking fifteen thousand interns annually, more than twice the number of medical graduates. Medical centers could not properly function without a ready supply of young physicians filling the large number of internship and residency positions that had been established in the nation's rapidly expanding health care system. Hospitals had few choices available and began to seek foreign medical graduates to fill their house staff positions.

Traditionally, the situation had been the reverse: American doctors routinely left the country to finish their training abroad. They had traveled to England and Scotland in the eighteenth century and France and Germany in the nineteenth. While the United States had seen limited medical immigration before, it consisted primarily of European physicians escaping Fascist persecution in the 1930s. The nation had never actively incorporated foreign practitioners into the health care system.

In the 1960s a new wave of medical migration changed this. The nation needed doctors to meet rising demand, and foreign doctors wanted to take advantage of the country's robust health care system. The federal and state governments passed legislation that made it easier for international medical graduates to enter and work in the United States. In response, foreign-educated physicians (mainly from India, Korea, Pakistan, and the Philippines) eagerly sought specialty training, scientific research positions, access to medical technologies, and opportunities for private practice. These foreign medical graduates took internships in less desirable hospitals, especially those that provided a disproportionate share of care for the poor, and filled residency programs (e.g., family practice, pediatrics, and psychiatry) that American medical graduates considered less prestigious and less financially rewarding. The flood of foreign doctors during the final decades of the twentieth century also signaled that America had become the new international center for medical education and training as well as the country of overall medical opportunity.

The effect of this migration on physician manpower was, and remains, substantial. By 1975 more than 20 percent of the nation's 380,000 physicians were foreign educated. That same year, international medical graduates constituted 40 percent of all doctors in America receiving their first license to practice. In addition, many foreign medical graduates, though ostensibly in the United States for post–medical school training, decided to remain permanently. They had developed strong links to the nation's cultural institutions as well as its medical structures. International medical graduates currently account for a quarter of the 950,000 physicians in the country.

Statistically, an even greater demographic change was set to occur: the large-scale arrival of women. American medicine had been a grand fraternity of men since its inception, but health care was about to get a makeover.

Although an American woman first earned a medical degree in 1849, the profession had a long history of gender segregation. The reasons for this are varied: parents' reluctance to spend large sums of money to provide their daughter a professional education; social expectations for women to be housewives; attitudes from medical professors who openly declared their aversion to teaching women; concern that women's presence in the profession would lead to declines in the status, autonomy, and earnings of male physicians; men refusing to be treated by women; and existing social norms that directed women toward other areas of health care, specifically nursing. In fact, few woman held any positions of scientific or administrative authority in medicine until the 1940s.

The situation began to change in the late 1960s. Social activists lobbied Congress and sued public institutions to deal with the systemic discrimination against women. These efforts succeeded, resulting in new equal-protection laws that women took advantage of. For example, in 1972, the Title IX Education Amendments of the Higher Education Act banned discriminatory policies in admissions and salaries for any school receiving federal funding. Between 1972 and 1980 medical schools almost doubled the number of females that they accepted, from 15 to 28 percent. By 2005 the number of women entering medical school equaled the number of men, an increase of over 400 percent in thirty-five years. Women currently make up one-third of total physicians in America.

Although females are now well represented in the profession, there remains an unmistakable imbalance within the specialties. Female doctors are concentrated in pediatrics, child psychiatry, obstetrics and gynecology, dermatology, pathology, and public health. Fewer than 10 percent of the nation's surgeons are women, and female physicians are also underrepresented in several procedure-intensive medical fields, such as cardiology and gastroenterology. Some argue that these distinctions stem from lingering sexism within the profession, while others suggest that women gravitate toward specialties that are perceived as being less personally taxing, specifically in response to the pressures of child-rearing and taking care of a home. Studies have found that, on average, female physicians work 10 percent fewer hours per week at their profession and are more likely to seek part-time positions than their male counterparts.

Although the addition of females and foreign doctors to American medicine temporarily addressed the problem of physician shortages, the nation's health care establishment continues to struggle to balance the supply and demand for doctors. The population rose by seventy million from 1980 to 2005, but during that period the number of graduates from United States medical schools remained fairly constant at sixteen thousand a year. Consequently, the number of total physicians has fallen as a percentage of the population. In response, over the last several years medical schools have stepped up annual admissions to eighteen thousand per year. Not only are admissions up at existing institutions but almost twenty new medical schools are in the planning stage, an increase of 15 percent over the one hundred thirty that the country currently has.

A Lump of Porridge

As the face of American medicine changed to include foreign medical graduates and women, it was inevitable that some of the country's most impressive discoveries would come from these groups. In fact, the man who most visibly tackled the nation's leading killer, heart disease, was not originally from the United States, but he would make the country his home. His name was Andreas Grüntzig, and the ailment that he revolutionized treatment for was coronary artery atherosclerosis.

Grüntzig's targeted disease originates with a yellowish white swelling called an atheroma. The name derives from the Greek words *athere,* an expression for a lump of porridge (which is what the Greeks felt the swelling resembled), and *oma,* meaning growth. An atheroma consists of microscopic pieces of cellular debris, including calcium, cholesterol, and fibrous tissue, which create an area of inflammation on a blood vessel's inner wall. As an atheroma matures, it turns craggy and rigid, and, in old age, the growth seeks out the company of neighboring atheromata. The result is a network of crusty, unyielding atheromatous plaques that line and constrict the inner contours of an artery, similar to the rust and mineral deposits that clog old water pipes. It is a degenerative condition, and the collective process of atheroma development, plaque formation, plaque coalescence, and artery deterioration is called atherosclerosis.

Atherosclerosis, a progressive and stealthlike disease, is the leading cause of arteriosclerosis, a general term that is best known colloquially as hardening of the arteries. When an artery is hardened, the flow of blood may be slowed. The tissue that surrounds the narrowed blood vessel gasps for life-preserving oxygen in a condition known as ischemia. Ischemic attacks are harbingers of impending medical disasters, or disasters themselves, and serve as one of the body's most dependable early warning systems.

Atherosclerosis employs a large cast of physiological characters, and ischemic attacks, consequently, take many forms. When the affected artery supplies the heart, the attack is termed angina and is accompanied by chest pain, shortness of breath, and sweating. In a catastrophic scenario the cardiac tissue dies and the victim suffers a myocardial infarction, or heart attack, which can be fatal. When the hardened artery nourishes the brain, the attack is termed a transient ischemic attack and can be accompanied by a myriad of symptoms, including skin numbness, slurred speech, loss of vision, and arm and leg weakness. A transient ischemic attack occasionally concludes in the permanency of a stroke, along with the potential for a coma, paralysis, loss of mental function, and death. Atherosclerosis can also occur in the legs. The insufficient blood supply creates cramping in the buttock, calf, and thigh muscles such that pain occurs when a person walks and, in severe cases, even when he is sitting. As this atherosclerotic-induced leg discomfort or intermittent claudication progresses, the oxygen-deprived skin and underlying tissue become infected and are unable to heal. Among the consequences is amputation. Other sites of atherosclerosis include the kidneys and intestines. In the former case, an atherosclerotic renal artery causes hypertension, or high blood pressure. In the latter case, the patient suffers cramplike abdominal pains, termed chronic mesenteric insufficiency, or "intestinal angina," which accompanies eating.

Despite scientists' persistent investigations, they have still not identified the precipitating cause of atherosclerosis. Researchers, however, have proven that its growth has many catalysts: cigarette smoking, diabetes, a fast-food diet, high blood pressure, lack of exercise, and obesity. When these elements combine with further circumstances, such as advanced age, masculinity, or a genetic predisposition, atherosclerosis can quickly become an efficient killing machine.

For eight decades, atherosclerotic heart disease has been the nation's most proficient medical killer. Almost half a million Americans die of the condition yearly, and fifteen million individuals live with a history of heart attack or symptoms of angina. The annual mortality from atherosclerosis surpasses that of cancer by 40 percent when deaths from atherosclerotic stroke are added to those from heart disease. Not only is atherosclerosis the leading cause of death in the United States but its treatment consumes the largest expenditure for any single class of diseases—over $400 billion annually.

As with other profound medical threats like cancer and hypertension, atherosclerosis intrigued and baffled medical researchers. American physicians began working to defeat the disease early in the twentieth century and were eventually responsible for two key breakthroughs. First, they determined that doctors could introduce a catheter into the coronary arteries without causing the heart to beat out of rhythm and suffer a fatal attack. Second, they discovered that physicians could dilate and reopen clogged arteries in the leg and pelvis by passing progressively larger catheters through the site of the obstruction. Grüntzig, the German physician who pioneered effective atherosclerosis treatment, would eventually wed these two concepts.

Voyage into the Heart

Like many great medical innovators, Grüntzig showed promise from the beginning of his career. He studied medicine in Heidelberg, among the most prestigious German education centers, and continued there with training in cardiology and angiology (the latter is the analysis and treatment of diseases of the blood vessels). In late 1969, when Grüntzig was thirty years old, he moved to Switzerland to assume a residency position at the University Hospital in Zurich. There, his departmental chair commented, "If I asked Andreas to write an article, I'd have it in ten days. If I asked for revisions I'd have them in two. He was quick and absolutely decisive."[1] Grüntzig was not only a gifted academic, but a talented and technically skillful heart specialist. Few physicians could manipulate a catheter and thread a coronary artery as well as he could.

Grüntzig soon turned his attention to the problem of atherosclerosis. He knew about the research advancements the American physicians had made and became convinced that miniature balloons could be used to compress blockages from inside a coronary artery, assuming he could design suitable equipment. Grüntzig imagined that he could take a long thin plastic tube with a tightly folded dachshund-shaped balloon located at its tip and, entering the circulatory system through an artery in the groin, guide the catheter into the curvy toothpick-sized coronary arteries that feed the heart. Once the tube reached an atherosclerotic-induced obstruction, Grüntzig would forcefully inflate the balloon, pushing the atheromatous grume back against the wall of the artery. The blockage would be alleviated, blood flow reestablished, and the patient relieved of his cardiac difficulties. The idea sounded preposterous to many of his colleagues, but the young doctor was convinced that his logic was sound.

Grüntzig began to develop his idea with the same intensity and self-confidence that had earned him the respect of his departmental chair in Zurich. During the day he handled his clinical and administrative duties at the hospital; at night he worked on his idea in his kitchen. He enlisted the assistance of a plastics manufacturer and an organic chemist who had written a textbook on plastics. Grüntzig spent three years trying to design and construct a spaghetti-sized catheter with a miniature balloon at its tip. He tested the hundreds of proposals that his group concocted in a trial-and-error assembly process. It involved adhesives, air compressors, electrical wire insulation, silk mesh, and surgical sutures (usually performed under handheld magnifying glasses). His recollections reveal how tedious the process must have been: "I was able to form a sausage-shaped distensible segment which I tried to reinforce with the silk mesh. When I mounted the material on a normal catheter tubing and applied pressure to distend the [balloon] segment, I suddenly realized that the strength of this material was so great that the silk mesh was not necessary. This was a great breakthrough and enabled me to reduce the size of the catheter."[2] Eventually, Grüntzig developed balloons sturdy enough to compress sizable atherosclerotic lesions and catheters so intricate that, despite their tiny size, they had two lumens, one capable of monitoring arterial pressure and the other of passing fluid into the balloon for inflation. Once Grüntzig was satisfied with the design, he began testing his new device on human cadavers and live animals, and achieved repeated success with dogs.

By 1975 Grüntzig felt that his idea was ready to be shared with the medical community. Despite being German, he decided to exhibit his findings at the annual meeting of the American Heart Association in November. Europe simply had no meetings as authoritative or prestigious. In Germany, for example, several hundred physicians might attend a national cardiology meeting. The American convention, in contrast, would attract thousands, including many from outside the United States. Equally important to Grüntzig was the presence of dozens of medical-device companies looking to funnel funds into the research and marketing of new technologies.

At the convention, more physicians milled around Grüntzig and his exhibit than anywhere else. The sheer outlandishness of his proposal had generated word-of-mouth interest. It also didn't hurt that Grüntzig was a natural showman, who, according to a female admirer, was "Omar Sharif, Clark Gable, and Errol Flynn rolled into one."[3] The visiting doctors gawked at Grüntzig's intricate poster with its bold title, "PERCUTANEOUS DILATATION OF CORONARY ARTERY STENOSIS."[4] The accompanying illustrations and words explained it all, from the anatomy of the heart's coronary arteries to a step-by-step account of how the catheter was steered into these tiny vessels. Grüntzig even provided a histological description of atherosclerosis along with a microscopic study of its component building block, the atheroma. Nonetheless, many remained skeptical. The refrain that "this will never work [in humans]"[5] echoed throughout the exhibit area.

Grüntzig returned to Zurich undeterred and began searching for an appropriate patient with whom to start his human heart trials. He found an ideal candidate in September 1977 when Dolf Bachmann, a thirty-eight-year-old three-pack-a-day smoker, was admitted to the Swiss hospital with unbearable chest pain. Medication could no longer control the patient's bouts of angina, and all clinical indicators pointed to an impending, probably fatal, heart attack. X-rays revealed that Bachmann had a solitary blockage in his heart's main coronary artery, a lesion that physicians dubbed the "widow maker." The obstruction was found near the beginning section of the artery. For Grüntzig, this was a perfect location, an area relatively easy to thread with a catheter. He explained the procedure to Bachmann, noting its experimental status and how it had been refined only in human cadavers and dogs. "What's the big deal?" Bachmann responded. "The difference can't be so great."[6]

The following afternoon, attendants wheeled Bachmann into Grüntzig's catherization laboratory. The hospital's chief of cardiology, chief of cardiac surgery, and chief of anesthesia, as well as cardiology and radiology residents, milled around. Most were bystanders but plainly interested in the goings-on. Bachmann related that the doctors "seemed to be hanging on needles."[7] Thirty years later, he recalled, "I was probably the calmest person there."[8]

The operation began when Grüntzig took hold of his balloon catheter, pricked open Bachmann's femoral artery, and inserted his novel device into the pinhole opening in the patient's inner thigh. For forty-five minutes the surrounding physicians and the patient watched in silent astonishment as Grüntzig guided the tubing toward the heart, passing into the pelvis's common iliac artery and advancing up the great central aorta toward the heart's left ventricle. An adjacent X-ray screen broadcast every twist and turn of the catheter and showed that Grüntzig was only inches and seconds away from the entryway of the diseased coronary artery. He soon pushed the tip of the catheter with its attached balloon into the area of the angina-inducing atheromata. Then Grüntzig grabbed hold of the balloon's inflation system and prepared to start the expansion.

No one was sure what would happen next. Would the inflation of the balloon trigger a fatal coronary event? Perhaps the balloon would burst under the powerful pressure of expansion? And what if the atherosclerotic plaque could not be compressed?

Once, twice, Grüntzig inflated the balloon. Each time he held the peak inflation pressure for several seconds. Bachmann's heart rhythm remained steady, and X-ray images revealed the seemingly impossible: the patient's arterial channel was no longer a rivulet; it was now a wide-open stream.

Grüntzig asked Bachmann how he was doing. Euphorically, the patient answered, "Fine!" Another doctor walked up to Bachmann and told him he was "the luckiest man in the world."[9]

Few events in the history of medicine dramatically alter patient care in a single instant. Grüntzig's success was one. He had managed to relieve heart disease without surgery. When Grüntzig restored blood flow through Bachmann's coronary artery, he achieved the same result as a cardiac bypass operation. The difference was that Grüntzig completed his nonsurgical procedure in less than sixty minutes and with minimal need for an individual to recuperate. Heart bypass surgery, in comparison, involved sawing through a human breastbone and attaching the patient to a heart-lung machine. Then doctors had to suture tiny blood vessels to one another to shunt blood around blocked areas. They next electrically jolted the stilled heart back to life and closed up the gaping wound in the patient's chest. The consequence of such surgery was months of painful recovery filled with a daily regimen of physical rehabilitation and the occasional bout of anxiety and depression. Grüntzig's patient, however, would be able to resume regular activities in days.

The observing doctors in Grüntzig's hospital were stunned by what they saw. Much like the witnesses to the discovery of anesthesia in 1846 in Boston, they had no idea what to say or do. "Everyone was surprised about the ease of the procedure," recalled Grüntzig, "and I started to realize that my dreams had come true."[10] Had the medical world understood beforehand the magnitude of Grüntzig's achievement, physicians would have filled a room the size of Madison Square Garden. Grüntzig, for his part, simply called a friend in California. "I've done it," he said. "You've done what, Andreas?" was the reply. "I have just performed the first angioplasty on the human heart."[11]

Several weeks later, Grüntzig traveled once more to the United States to publicize his discovery at the fiftieth annual meeting of the American Heart Association. He had performed three additional successful procedures in the interim, and had little doubt of the validity of his technique. Sixty of the world's most eminent cardiologists listened to Grüntzig describe his remarkable procedure. The German doctor showed his before-and-after pictures. A chorus of heads nodded along, and the attendees erupted in spontaneous applause before Grüntzig could conclude his presentation. Grüntzig recalled, "I was so surprised that I almost could not proceed with my ten-minute presentation."[12] Overnight, he had become medicine's newest marvel.

In a matter of a few months the European and American media began running stories about balloon angioplasty. "Blowup in the Arteries," headlined *Time* magazine. The article explained that the new procedure "could be used in place of bypass operations . . . at about one-tenth the cost."[13] Walter Cronkite gave a glowing account of angioplasty on the *CBS Evening News*. A report in the *New York Times* presciently suggested that the number of patients who would benefit from the technique was about to "become much larger."[14]

Back in Zurich, Grüntzig tried to handle the flood of attention he received. Medical device makers wanted to manufacture his invention, and physicians wanted to learn his technique. Grüntzig decided that he could reach the largest possible audience through live televised closed-circuit demonstration courses, a testament to his self-assurance. "I saw him as being enormously brave," wrote one spectator. "I thought the fact that he was willing to do those live demonstrations was a tremendous marker of his guts, and his character."[15] Grüntzig performed catheriza-tions, faced complications, answered questions, led discussions, and did his best to convince observers that they were witnessing a revolution in medicine. The visiting physicians cheered after every successful case and marveled at Grüntzig's aplomb.

In July 1979 Grüntzig presented his findings to the wider Ameri-can medical audience in the *New England Journal of Medicine*. The lead article discussed the results of coronary angioplasties in a series of fifty patients. In seven pages filled with illustrations, graphs, tables, and X-rays, Grüntzig detailed his technologic tour de force and explained that there were no deaths nor strokes. "The technique is comparatively sim-ple," Grüntzig wrote. "It has the advantage of providing instantaneous revascularization without the need for open-heart surgery."[16] An accom-panying editorial agreed with his assessment and noted that the promise of coronary angioplasty "remains considerable."[17]

The Medical-Industrial Complex

The year after Grüntzig's article appeared in the *New England Journal of Medicine*, the *Journal* published another influential piece called "The New Medical-Industrial Complex."[18] The feature argued that the nation was facing a new synergy between medicine and American industry akin to the synthesis between the armed forces and domestic manufacturing that President Dwight Eisenhower labeled the "military-industrial complex"[19] in 1961. This ever-expanding "medical-industrial complex" was, and is, composed of, among various disparate elements, proprietary hospitals and nursing homes, insurance companies, diagnostic laboratories, drug manufacturers, medical supply companies, health system consulting and lobbying firms, as well as a wide variety of other health care services enterprises.

This economic transformation leading to the private medical-industrial complex was, ironically, set in motion fifteen years earlier with the passage of the publicly underwritten programs Medicare and Medicaid. Federal funding of health care had made medicine attractive to corporations and its investors by guaranteeing a vast market for medical services.

Doctors initially welcomed industry into health care. The bogeyman had always been publicly funded health care programs that threatened to erode professional autonomy. Many praised this heightened private sector involvement, claiming that free-market competition would be inherently more efficient than nonprofit or governmental competition. Physicians did not generally worry that big business might eventually monopolize ownerships, control pricing, and gain product loyalty.

However, the new medical-industrial complex quickly began to shape American medicine. One of the clearest examples of the new private sector influence was the development of Grüntzig's revolutionary new angioplasty procedure.

The German doctor had initially believed that his discovery had a limited application. At best, he estimated that it would only work on 5 to 10 percent of patients with heart disease stemming from simple blockages that were confined to a single coronary artery. But advances in technology and pharmacology soon made coronary angioplasty a potential treatment for patients with many forms of coronary artery disease, including those with multiple obstructions and those who were in the midst of an evolving heart attack. Within several years, doctors began to consider approximately 75 percent of individuals with heart disease eligible for angioplasty and other catheter-based treatments. The consequent scale of potential angioplasties made it commercially appealing to big business.

It is easiest to understand the probable market for angioplasties by comparing them to the surgical procedure they typically replaced: heart bypass operations. The number of heart bypasses had skyrocketed during the 1970s thanks to safer surgical methods as well as the emergence of the medical-industrial complex. They rose from 14,000 in 1970 to 135,000 in 1980, an increase of almost 900 percent. No other surgical procedure had undergone such an astronomical rise—the closest comparisons were hip replacement, 600 percent; cesarean section, 250 percent; and cataract removal, 100 percent. Hospitals and heart surgeons prospered as the explosion of investment in cardiac bypass technologies created a multibillion-dollar industry built around this one operation. By 1990, annual heart bypass numbers hovered at slightly more than 300,000, and virtually every medium- to large-sized city in the nation claimed one, if not two or three, costly open-heart surgery center(s). At an average hospital cost of $25,000 per case, coronary artery bypass surgery became the single biggest moneymaker in American medicine. Grüntzig and his angioplasty were set to rival this thriving business of repairing sick hearts.

Though Grüntzig was still practicing in Switzerland, he realized that he could profit more from the American market than anywhere else in the world and decided to sell the rights to his catheter to a U.S. manufacturer. American medical companies were themselves eagerly seeking new investment opportunities to capitalize on the profit opportunities that the large-scale public financing of health care had created. Grüntzig eventually settled on C. R. Bard, one of the biggest medical-device makers in the world.

The doctor soon began shuttling back and forth between Europe and America to promote his device in conjunction with his corporate sponsor. The speaking engagements resembled a traveling road show: Grüntzig was the showman while Bard representatives stood at the ready with the catheters for sale. Occasionally, unimpressed heart surgeons in the audience, seeking to defend their trusted bypass procedure, attempted to debunk the discovery, but the unflappable Grüntzig, according to accounts, "would weather every hazard and question . . . with searing honesty."[20] The results were always the same. Grüntzig, the master impresario, gained dozens of new acolytes as he whittled away at his opponents' line of reasoning. Bard could not have asked for a better pitchman.

Grüntzig, quickly becoming an American medical celebrity, grew frustrated with the bureaucratic limitations of European medicine and his bicontinental lifestyle. By early 1980 he decided that his opportunities for advancement in academic medicine were better in the United States. Harvard, Stanford, and the Cleveland Clinic courted him, but he moved to Atlanta's Emory University School of Medicine as director of interventional cardiovascular medicine. The university's affiliated hospital soon constructed several new heart catherization laboratories to meet the demand of patients seeking out Grüntzig's services and physicians looking to learn from the European master.

Emory became Grüntzig's new platform for angioplasty proselytizing. His teaching conferences grew increasingly extravagant, funded by corporate sponsors eager to capitalize on his renown. They offered physicians financial incentives to attend the courses and promised lavish meals and entertainment. During the day, visiting doctors were introduced to state-of-the-art medical equipment. At night, they were feted with formal dress receptions in Atlanta's newly redesigned High Museum of Art. The pure white porcelain-enameled building with its towering atrium that soared upward through four interior levels provided an opulent setting for the nonstop selling of coronary angioplasty.

The marketing of angioplasties proved so successful that Grüntzig began to worry that his technique was spreading too quickly. "I am cautious," he told a reporter in 1983, "because I know that damn balloon catheter; I invented it. It has problems." He felt that the medical establishment was prematurely encouraging the utilization of coronary angioplasty at the possible expense of overall patient safety and welfare. Despite the procedure's popularity, few controlled clinical trials had studied its role in clinical medicine. "You may disrupt the artery. You may close the artery. You may dissect the artery. You may dissect other arteries that were not diseased before," warned Grüntzig. "You can really mess things up."[21]

Grüntzig was not alone in his concerns. The American Heart Association and the American College of Cardiology issued guidelines regarding the use of angioplasty. The highly technical rules essentially advised doctors to be less hasty in their decision to carry out the procedure and stressed that hospitals needed to review success and complication rates.

But appeals for moderation went unheeded. Too many physicians and too many businesses were earning substantial incomes from angioplasties to slow the spread, and the medical-industrial complex continued to facilitate its growth. Bard's successful marketing of Grüntzig's catheter was generating nearly $50 million in annual sales by the mid-1980s. The catheter was the company's most important product. Bard's competition soon moved to reduce this advantage. In 1984 the American pharmaceutical giant Pfizer spent $40 million to take over a small Swiss surgical instrument company that had been selling angioplasty-related equipment that Grüntzig had designed. At the same time, Eli Lilly & Company paid $500 million to purchase a recently organized American manufacturer of angioplasty catheters. Fueled by this corporate competition, American doctors were performing over fifty thousand balloon angioplasties annually by 1985.

The growth was so dramatic that it was even featured in President Ronald Reagan's 1985 State of the Union address. He commented that Europeans were marveling at the "American Miracle" and that "advances in technology [were] transforming our lives." He specifically mentioned several new techniques, including one that "revolutionize[d] heart bypass surgery."[22]

As corporate profits from the sale of Grüntzig-designed catheters increased so did Grüntzig's personal fortune. He became one of the wealthier doctors in the United States. In 1985 alone, Grüntzig received a $3 million payout for consultancy work from Bard. This was in addition to his royalties. Grüntzig spent his money lavishly, most notably in purchasing a multiengine aircraft. "I like flying because it confirms that I have no fear," Grüntzig told his associates.[23]

Unfortunately, this claim proved deadly accurate. On October 27, 1985, Hurricane Juan was drenching the Southeast with pelting rain, and the conditions had grounded most private planes. Grüntzig had only logged fifty-eight hours of air time in his craft (none during inclement weather), but he was convinced that his new plane with its fancy electronic equipment would ferret its way through the storm. He took off from the airport at St. Simons Island, a vacation spot off the Georgia coast, and headed back home to Atlanta. The storm intensified as he approached the DeKalb Peachtree Airport. Fog enveloped Atlanta's metro region and visibility was down to several hundred feet. His orientation impaired, Grüntzig mistakenly flew the plane at full throttle into the ground. It was complete devastation. Authorities found the demolished aircraft in a thirty-eight-foot crater along with its dead pilot, his wife, and their two dogs. The United Press International wire service headline read "Andreas Gruentzig Dies in Air Crash: Developed Technique to Clear Arteries by Using Balloon."[24] In Grüntzig's obituary the New York Times called him a "national treasure."[25]

The death of the nation's biggest proselytizer for angioplasties did little to curb the procedure's growth. In the decade after Grüntzig's fatal accident, angioplasties increased tenfold to 500,000 cases annually, equaling the number of cardiac bypass operations.

Over time, angioplasties grew more complicated and costly as doctors and medical-device companies expanded on Grüntzig's original discoveries with more sophisticated equipment. Heart researchers devised miniature stainless-steel stents to counter the problem that some coronary vessels become reobstructed within the first year after angioplasty. During balloon inflation, the collapsed stent expands and locks in place to form a permanent internal scaffold that keeps the vessel open. These early stents had solved one problem but created another: the device's struts (they embed into the vessel wall to hold it in place) irritated the vessel lining and instigated scar tissue proliferation that also caused a reblockage. To counter this iatrogenic difficulty, researchers began coating stents with a time-released medication designed to interrupt this buildup of new tissue. This innovation effectively eliminated early reobstruction but cost $2,500 per unit. Currently, drug-coated stents generate nearly $6 billion in annual sales for several oligarchic medical equipment companies. It is the richest medical-device market in history.

American doctors now perform almost two million coronary angioplasties annually, making it the nation's top treatment for people having a heart attack or exhibiting worsening symptoms of heart disease. The procedure outnumbers coronary bypasses by four to one. An average angioplasty costs upward of $20,000, a price tag that includes the angioplasty catheter, the drug-coated stent, other medical equipment, and hospital costs. It is estimated that the total costs for angioplasty to the American health care system are over $40 billion annually.

Despite this massive cost, medical opinion is split over the relative effectiveness of the procedure. Studies have shown that in some patients newly developed drugs and a healthier prevention-based lifestyle relieve the symptoms of heart disease as well as stenting. Angioplasty "is doing cosmetic surgery on the coronary arteries," said one outspoken critic of stents. "[It] makes them look pretty, but it's not treating the underlying biology of these arteries."[26] Of course, other investigations have reached the opposite result. "Angioplasty was a true medical breakthrough," claimed the president of the Society for Cardiovascular Angiography and Interventions. "It saves lives—and it preserves and can even improve quality of life. That's its legacy and its future."[27] Shadowing this disagreement is the ongoing dispute between proponents of cardiac bypass operations and angioplasties.

Corporate spending makes the question of whether angioplasties and stents are overused particularly difficult to parse. Medical-device companies spend massive amounts of money on public relations aimed at physicians and the public. Doctors also receive much more money to complete an angioplasty or perform a bypass operation than to prescribe a drug, a factor that numerous critics claim will prejudice a doctor's judgment. Additionally, financial motivations can skew medical research findings.

One of the consequences of the financial motivations and the vast profits found in American medicine is that the medical-industrial complex became so powerful it grew to influence the everyday activities of the individual practitioner to a greater degree than the collective actions of the medical profession itself.

An Interior View

In 1958 forty-seven-year-old Mark Ravitch, an associate professor of surgery at Johns Hopkins, was visiting a hospital in the Soviet Union when he encountered something unusual. "I was startled to see a series of patients who had [surgery] with staples instead of sutures," he recalled, "and saw the extraordinary simplicity and efficiency of the instruments."[28] Although Ravitch was a seasoned surgeon who had graduated Phi Beta Kappa from the University of Oklahoma and completed a general surgical residency at Johns Hopkins, he had never heard of a device that could safely staple together human flesh. The curious medical instrument fascinated him, and, shortly after discovering it, he purchased one for himself at the Surgical Instruments and Apparatus store on Nevskii Prospect in Kiev. When he brought the stapler back to Baltimore, he inadvertently started a process that led to America's multibillion-dollar laparoscopic surgery business several decades later.

Initially, Ravitch's conservative colleagues back in the United States criticized the strange stapler. They felt that the device was an affront to their operative skills. Suturing requires dexterity and patience and has long been the surgeon's trademark. Many knife wielders took delight in their expertise. As Ravitch explained, "Surgeons are proud of their art and reluctant to believe that an automatic instrument can do things as well as they can."[29] More pragmatically, some naysayers warned that if the Russian-designed stapler was useful and supplanted sutures, surgeons would lose their deft finger work abilities and be unable to manually sew in crucial situations where a stapler was not applicable.

Ravitch, however, was a strong-willed and opinionated curmudgeon. He would not let his colleagues' opposition dissuade him, and began to incorporate staplers into his clinical practice. As he imagined, the tool helped him to save time in the operating room and produced results equal to hand-stitched sutures. An intrigued reporter for *Time* wrote that staples were "a stitch to save nine" and that "the new machines have already graduated from stitchwork repairs to performing some of the most important stages of surgery."[30] Ravitch found the tool so effective that he decided to pitch it to American manufacturing companies in the early 1960s.

The companies that he approached showed little interest at first. The medical-industrial complex had not yet formed, and companies were unwilling to invest significant resources to produce novel medical equipment. The feeling among the manufacturers was that "[a] very special instrument of this kind could never recover the enormous costs involved in its development."[31]

Over the course of the next two decades, the financial incentives for medical-device companies began to change. Federally sponsored health care programs and the rise of the medical-industrial complex helped foster a spectacular growth in surgery. During the 1970s, even taking into account the rise in population, gynecologic operations increased 32 percent, orthopedic procedures 26 percent, and urologic surgery 20 percent. As these medical-device companies expanded, they began devoting larger amounts of capital to research, development, and marketing.

Ravitch's stapler suddenly appeared much more appealing to the nation's medical manufacturers. The companies diversified stapler models and offered advanced product lines for operations on the stomach and the intestines in addition to the skin. Thanks to the impact of these companies, the number of individuals who had operations with staples exploded—one manufacturing company, the United States Surgical Corporation, saw its patient base jump from 20,000 in 1969 to 700,000 a decade later.

The remarkable success of the surgical stapler helped convince the medical-device companies to invest more heavily in new technologies. Their product development teams introduced an extraordinary array of new surgical instruments in the 1980s. Among the most important tools was a disposable plastic tubelike device, called a trocar, which a surgeon inserts into a patient's abdomen through a puncturelike incision. This gadget served as a temporary portal into the body for miniature surgical instruments, including graspers, scalpels, scissors, staple appliers, and computer chip television cameras. The internal access and the view of the body's interior that this new medical device gave doctors heralded a revolution in surgical technique that would be known as laparoscopy.

In layman's terms, laparoscopy is called "keyhole," "Band-Aid," or "minimally invasive" surgery. Surgeons use the technique by channeling instruments through the narrow trocar. The most vital of the instruments is a miniature video camera that sends magnified views of the inside of the abdomen to an outside television monitor. A surgeon views the screen and manipulates the tools accordingly. Laparoscopy obviates the time-honored tradition of making lengthy incisions into the abdomen wall. The upshot is less tissue damage, decreased bleeding, fewer infections, diminution in discomfort, and a smaller number of days spent recovering in a hospital. Over time, the technique became quite sophisticated, and doctors began using laparoscopy to complete various abdominal and pelvic operations, including the repair of internal organs, excisions of cancers, and even bypass procedures for obesity.

Corporate money made laparoscopy a possibility and it also assured its popularity. Medical-device companies invested billions of dollars promoting the new technology. High-pressure sales tactics encouraged doctors to adopt the new equipment. Soon, hospitals began constructing operating rooms dedicated to laparoscopy, filling them with new, expensive tools.

By 1994 doctors used laparoscopic techniques to perform almost 90 percent of the 670,000 gallbladder procedures in the United States. By the end of that decade physicians were routinely using laparoscopy for appendectomies, colon removals, hysterectomies, and many other types of abdominal and pelvic surgery.

Notwithstanding laparoscopy's clinical benefits, it is expensive and, consequently, profitable. Corporate and hospital revenues shot up in conjunction with the number of laparoscopic operations. In 1994, for example, the revenue of the United States Surgical Corporation topped $1.2 billion, and 60 percent of this came from laparoscopic products. Other medical-device companies had similarly impressive financial ledgers.

A Mainstay of the Surgeon

Among the biggest potential surgical prizes that laparoscopy could claim was the repair of groin hernias. It is the country's most common abdominal operation—almost a million a year—and the potential for profits is vast. While the procedure has many variations, at its most basic it involves a surgeon repairing a weakening in the lower abdominal wall. Laparoscopic equipment manufacturers focused their massive public relations and advertising campaigns on this ubiquitous operation in an effort to change a century-old operative tradition.

The groin hernia repair is the mainstay of the surgeon. It is a major abdominal operation, yet straightforward enough that surgical professors favor it as a teaching tool for their novitiates. Ravitch, one of his generation's leading experts on hernia surgery, once commented: "If no other field were offered to the surgeon for his activity than hernia repair, it would be worthwhile to become a surgeon and to devote an entire life to this service."[32] He based this observation on the fact that hernia surgery requires all the fundamental elements of a surgical operation: an understanding of functional anatomy; a knowledge of pathophysiology; familiarity with varying techniques of repair; need for gentle handling of tissues; and meticulousness in cutting and separating tissues.

William Halsted, the renowned professor of surgery at Johns Hopkins, first described the modern repair of groin hernias in 1890 and his basic technique endured for most of the twentieth century. The accepted approach required a six-inch incision and numerous sutures to close the rent. Ravitch, along with thousands of other surgeons, advocated Halsted's methods: "It is the simplest operation which will consistently give satisfactory results without extensive dissection."[33]

While the Halsted technique was effective, it triggered severe discomfort in the patient and often required a lengthy period of recovery with weeks of disability. However, surgeons for much of the twentieth century regarded postoperative pain as a minor nuisance. Ravitch's generation paid it little attention. In fact, according to him, the most annoying complications of groin hernia repair were "hemorrhage . . . displacement of the testis . . . [and] infection."[34] He did not even mention discomfort and disability in his description of the operation. But Ravitch was a member of the final generation to hold such an attitude. He died in early 1989, an unremitting champion of Halsted's technique (but with little experience with laparoscopy).

Attitudes about hernia repair changed in the late 1980s. Surgeons conceived of a new generation of hernia repairs that used a smaller incision (two to three inches in length) and a swatch of plastic mesh (instead of sutures) to close the site of the rupture. These mesh-based techniques caused little discomfort, and patients resumed normal activities in a few days. The repair was simplistic and cost-effective. It decreased time in the operating room and eliminated overnight hospital stays. Mesh quickly began to replace sutures for all but the most conservative surgeons.

As mesh-based hernia repairs gained popularity, laparoscopic equipment makers worked to convince surgeons of the advantages of placing the mesh through a laparoscope. They barraged doctors with advertising pamphlets and brochures. Salespeople stressed that a laparoscopic hernia repair left barely visible scars and returned an individual to normal activities in a short time. Of course, simply switching from sutures to mesh had already achieved the bulk of these advantages. Furthermore, although laparoscopy shortened hospital stays for most abdominal operations (e.g., gallbladder removal, appendectomy, colon excision, and hysterectomy), the opposite was true with hernia repairs.

Savvy medical-device makers focused their efforts on the annual convention of the American College of Surgeons, where tens of thousands of surgeons gathered. Corporate salespeople staffed hundreds of booths in the meeting's main exhibition hall. The laparoscopic equipment manufacturers brought twelve-foot-high video screens, sponsored guest lectures, offered giveaways, and provided ample opportunities to use the new hernia-repair devices. They invited surgeons into the booths to test their skills at maneuvering the laparoscope inside the abdomen of a mannequin. Additionally, their video displays included live demonstrations of laparoscopic hernia repairs broadcast through closed-circuit television from operating rooms hundreds and sometimes thousands of miles away.

Unsurprisingly, laparoscopic manufacturers have steadily increased their market share of hernia repairs. Surgeons used the technique for 15 percent of hernia operations in 2003 and at present that percentage has nearly doubled.

While medical-device makers extolled the benefits of laparoscopic hernia repair, they rarely mentioned the cost of the operation. Since doctors can already perform mesh-based hernia repairs on an ambulatory, or in-and-out, basis, laparoscopy cannot possibly provide cost savings through reduced hospital stays. In fact, the laparoscopic approach for mesh hernia repair increased costs due to higher equipment fees. The device manufacturers fail to acknowledge that laparoscopic groin hernia repairs increase both their profits and the nation's health care expenditures, while providing few practical benefits to patients. The emphasis on monetary value for a corporation, hospital, or physician can overshadow the technique's actual medical importance. For some doctors this can cause conflicts of interest that pit the caregiver's personal financial welfare against the clinical concerns of patients.

Uncontrollable Costs

The massive growth of the biotechnology, medical-device, and pharmaceutical industries, along with the vast sums of money spent by federal and state governments on health care, transformed American medicine. It changed from a collection of disparate practices run by individual doctors with few (or no) employees into a conglomeration of hospitals, medical schools, physician offices, corporate enterprises, and ancillary medical agencies. Medicine became profit-driven and inadequately or incoherently regulated. And this new breed of American medicine constituted the largest business component of the nation's economy.

While trillions of dollars in revenues filled the corporate coffers of the medical-industrial complex, the problems of escalating costs that had first appeared in the late sixties began to plague American medicine again. One issue was that innovative and costly medical and surgical treatments were fueling medicine's expansion; prior to World War II, clinical advances did not significantly increase health care costs. The once simplistic, patient-comes-first medical decision had evolved into an often complex situation involving reimbursement issues, lengths of stay, out-of-pocket costs, and monetary restrictions on care. Big medicine meant inefficiencies: overuse of services, overemphasis on technology, and fragmentation of clinical care. At the same time, the freer flow of funds into medicine also increased physicians' incomes. Higher incomes exaggerated financial expectations.

As these problems worsened throughout the 1970s, organized medicine, which might have been able to curtail this spending spiral, grew increasingly weak. Partly, the AMA had lost influence due to political miscalculations and the fracturing influence of specialism. And starting in the late 1970s, a series of judicial decisions removed whatever teeth organized medicine had left. Courts ruled that the AMA and state medical societies could not compel hospital appointments to be contingent on membership in their groups. These decisions also prevented the AMA and its affiliates from punishing physicians who advertised their services. Most conspicuously, the Supreme Court ruled that medical societies were not exempt from antitrust regulations, thereby restricting the ability of medical organizations to coordinate lobbying and work stoppage activities among their members. Stripped of much of its authority, the AMA watched its membership dwindle—it is now made up of less than one in five American physicians. In effect, the AMA no longer speaks for a unified medical profession, and an emboldened organized medicine, as it once existed, does not survive.

With the remnants of organized medicine unable to control health care expenditures, the federal government finally began to enact a series of legislative reforms during the 1980s and 1990s designed to contain the cost increase. The government wanted to control hospital markups and created a program that arranged diagnoses into hundreds of diagnosis-related groups, or DRGs. Hospitals would receive a preset reimbursement for each admission based on a specific DRG, instead of actual monies spent. DRGs were part of the government's attempt to become a more vigilant purchaser of hospital services using so-called prospective payment plans.

The federal government also instituted a convoluted methodology, known as the Resource-Based Relative Value Scale, or RBRVS, that determined how much money physicians should be paid through Medicare and Medicaid. This system calculated doctors' fees using resource costs instead of what a physician deemed his charge should be. Resource costs are based on three components: physician work, practice expense, and medical malpractice premiums. The complex RBRVS tabulates physician payments by multiplying the combined component costs of a service with a conversion factor that Medicare changes annually. Payments are also adjusted by geographic region so a service performed in Manhattan is worth more than one completed in Omaha, for example.

At the same time the government instituted these reforms, it started a move toward managed care for those with private health insurance. The intent of fostering managed care was to reduce the cost of providing health benefits and improve the quality of patient care through a variety of mechanisms, including economic incentives for physicians and patients to select less costly forms of testing and treatment, programs for reviewing the medical necessity of specific services, and controls on hospital admissions and lengths of stay. Critics suggest that it did little besides create an alphabet soup of health care delivery networks, including Health Maintenance Organizations (HMOs), Preferred Provider Organizations (PPOs), Independent Practice Associations (IPAs), and Point of Service plans

(POS). Managed care and its offshoots are now nearly ubiquitous in the United States but they have failed—as did DRGs, the RBRVS, and a host of other reform measures—to control medical costs.

Despite the government's efforts, the rise of for-profit corporate-guided medicine has created an economic tyranny of medical services and scientific technology. The underlying principle that more money expended is better continues to guide the nation's health care system. For procedures like angioplasty, stenting, and laparoscopic hernia repair, the current health care delivery system rewards physicians and hospitals for how much care they provide rather than how cost-effective or clinically valuable it is. The result is that total spending on physicians, hospitals, drugs, tests, and the like is so sizable that it now consumes nearly a fifth of the country's economy and its continued increase threatens America's overall financial stability. Health care will cost the country $2.5 trillion in 2010, and the financial situation will probably worsen with the medical demands of an aging baby boomer generation and the added possibility that tens of millions of uninsured individuals may gain coverage under any new public insurance plan.

Medical Malpractice

One of the consequences of the unwieldy, expensive, and disorganized nature of modern medical care has been a weakening of the physician-patient relationship. In the past, a family physician handled everyday care. If a patient died or suffered illness-related complications, the family assumed that the doctor had done all that was medically possible. The family doctor was considered a friend and confidant, and any discussions concerning an individual's treatment usually ended there. Times have changed. In present-day American medicine, patients often see their physician as one person in a laundry list of unfamiliar and impersonal specialists. A burdensome caseload, dependence on dehumanizing technologies and tests, growing use of paramedical personnel, and financial concerns have reduced medical office visits to perfunctory encounters.

Part of the problem is that primary care giving is currently an underserved practice area in American medicine. Although women and foreigners are well represented in the primary care specialties of internal medicine, family practice, pediatrics, and obstetrics-gynecology, there remains an overall shortage. This deficiency grows even in the face of the four-decades-old strategy of family practitioners to fashion their discipline into an appealing specialty, one that now includes subspecialty training in adolescent medicine, geriatric medicine, hospice medicine, sleep medicine, and sports medicine. In 2009 less than 7 percent of the nation's medical graduates undertook residency training in family practice. "You can't force people into a specialty they don't want," explained a medical school dean. "Let's face it: as long as primary care doctors in this country make a much lower salary than other doctors, it's hard."[35]

The marginalization of primary care and the breakdown of the patient-physician relationship has led to, among other things, a growth in medical malpractice suits. Little trust exists between patients and their multiple specialists. Litigiousness has replaced the faith that earlier generations had in their doctors.

Although malpractice lawsuits have only become a major concern for the medical profession in the last twenty years, they are not a recent phenomenon. They first appeared in the years leading up to the Civil War. At the time, virtually any white male could enter medicine. The lawsuit was a patient's only protection against the lack of medical standards and the clinical misdeeds of suspect caregivers. Attorneys embraced medical malpractice litigation as the newest prospect for career advancement. Of course, given the rudimentary state of medical knowledge and care, it was difficult to prove negligence, and juries rarely awarded significant compensation.

For more than one hundred years, physicians expressed little alarm over the number of lawsuits or the amount of awards, but the situation changed in the 1970s. During the first half of that decade, the number of medical lawsuits filed was four times greater than the number that had been submitted during the preceding three and a half decades. In 1975 alone, patients brought an estimated 14,000 claims. A sizable increase in the average jury award accompanied this rise in medical malpractice claims, from $175,000 in 1975 to $400,000 in 1985 to $575,000 in 1995. The upward trend of malpractice awards continues and multimillion-dollar awards are not even a rarity—in 2003, California had forty-eight medical malpractice awards of more than $1 million.

As lawsuits became more commonplace, malpractice insurance became increasingly onerous. Premiums increased at a pace with jury awards. Litigious states like Florida and New York have annual rates that range as high as $150,000 to $200,000 for high-risk specialties, especially obstetrics and gynecology and neurosurgery. Some physicians have left their practice due to financial considerations, while others have been deprived of malpractice coverage after their insurers abandoned the risky business.

In addition to the insurance dilemma, medical malpractice suits altered the way physicians practiced medicine. Doctors began to intentionally overtest and overtreat patients, a behavior known as defensive medicine. An extra X-ray or additional biopsy ensured that if a lawsuit occurred the physician could prove that he or she had gone beyond what was traditionally required. Doctors have become paranoid from anxiety over potential liability. Many are forced to act first in their own best financial and legal interests and second out of concern for the health and well-being of their patients. Defensive medical practice with its overuse of tests and treatments runs the risk of turning into the new standard, creating a vicious cycle where doctors continually provide unnecessary care to stay ahead of the liability curve.

Of course, no amount of precaution makes a doctor invulnerable to malpractice, and even good physicians can be ruined.

Paul Liebman, effervescent and smiling, was almost everyone's example of a compassionate and skilled physician. He was superbly educated (Georgetown University School of Medicine), well trained (Boston City Hospital), and among the first group of general surgeons in the country to take formal advanced work in vascular surgery (Medical College of Virginia). His vascular practice was among the busiest in south Florida; he presided over the Florida Vascular Society; and he served as vice chief of staff and chief of surgery at his hospital. Over the years his colleagues had honored him with numerous accolades and awards, including a citation in the highly regarded *Best Doctors in America*.

Among other things, vascular surgeons like Liebman deal with problems brought on by varicose veins. These typically occur in the leg and arise when a vein's internal valves are disrupted, causing blood that should flow toward the heart to head in the opposite direction. This malfunction exposes a vein to higher blood pressure than it is designed to withstand. The veins enlarge and turn into unsightly blue, bulging varicosities, visible through the skin of a person's legs. Varicosities are not only cosmetically unappealing but can be a source of pain, skin ulcers, and bleeding.

One of the most common treatments is a surgical procedure called varicose vein stripping. The simple operation was first performed in the 1940s, and several thousand are performed every year in the United States. The surgeon uses a tiny incision near the groin to locate the upper end of the varicosity. He disconnects the enlarged vein from any nearby adjoining vessels, inserts a stiff but flexible wire into its free end, and advances it down and out through a second incision in the mid- to lower calf. Then the surgeon tightly ties the groin end of the vein to the wire and pulls the apparatus downward. As the wire travels through the length of the vein, it turns it inside out and strips the vessel from underneath the skin. The physician then removes the apparatus and the attached vein through the incision in the calf. To control bleeding, the patient's legs are firmly compressed with bandages for several days. Individuals who have had vein removal surgery return home the same day and resume normal activities within two weeks. The risks from vein stripping are few, the most frequent being bruising, blood clots, infection, and numbness in the skin of the leg.

Liebman had performed hundreds, if not thousands, of varicose vein removals during his career. He was thoroughly familiar with the anatomy and physiology of these tortuous veins. Patients in south Florida in need of varicose vein therapy were likely to seek him out. After all, he was widely considered an expert in the region.

In May 2000, Liebman entered an operating room in his hospital and started a routine vein-stripping procedure, but soon something went horribly wrong. He mistook his patient's femoral artery—the largest artery in the leg—for the varicose vein and accidentally stripped it away. Without a functioning femoral artery, the patient's leg quickly turned blue and lifeless. The surgeon recognized his error almost immediately, and he frantically called in a colleague to help reconstruct the artery. The physicians tried to restore blood flow to the leg, but all efforts failed. In the end, the doctors had to amputate the patient's leg above the knee.

There was no disputing Liebman's blunder, though the extent of his culpability is a matter of opinion. On the one hand, the mistake could have stemmed from operative incompetence or negligence. On the other hand, it could have been an unfortunate circumstance of abnormal anatomy (veins can be mistaken for arteries) or extremely bad luck.

Soon the patient filed a malpractice claim against Liebman. His insurance company as well as the hospital's insurance carrier made a monetary offer to settle the case. The patient's lawyers turned down both proposals as not nearly adequate to compensate their client for her suffering and emotional distress. The attorneys requested a jury trial.

While many physicians understand the legal repercussions of medical malpractice suits, they are often unprepared for the emotional ups and downs associated with litigation and the lengthy process of collecting evidence. In seeking just compensation for their clients, lawyers can unintentionally disrupt the personal and professional lives of physicians and set off devastating career setbacks. Physician defendants complain of depression, insomnia, and irritability. And while a malpractice suit is meant to focus on determining compensation and not on a doctor's competency, it implies that the defendant physician is indeed incompetent. The result is many accused physicians feel that they have been caught up in a hostile legal system designed to demonize and malign them.

The time that Liebman spent waiting for his court case was "seven years of torture,"[36] according to one acquaintance. Despite his impeccable professional record, the Florida Board of Medicine moved to sanction him over the varicose vein injury case. The local medical community had held Liebman in such high esteem that it took the board two and a half years to find an expert willing to testify against him. Ultimately, it determined that he had failed to practice medicine with the level of care and skill befitting a reasonably prudent physician. He was fined several thousand dollars and ordered to perform a week's worth of community service. The board also directed him to take additional education and training in varicose vein and vascular management, a humiliating obligation for a thirty-year surgeon who had performed thousands of vascular operations. His punishment additionally required him to give a one-hour public lecture on patient safety called "The Arrogance of Excellence."

Liebman suffered a public pillorying as well. A local paper published a series of front-page stories on the case, generally critical of his professional conduct. "The articles were all highly inflammatory," according to a physician in the community, and showed Liebman "in the worst possible light."[37] In a final insult, an area blog site labeled Liebman its "Knucklehead of the Day" for the "botched" surgery and insisted that the Florida Board of Medicine "pull the guy's license for a year."[38]

The trial finally began in early 2007 and quickly turned into a theater of human emotions. Both sides competed for jury sympathy and sought to exploit every angle of bias. "She has to look at her leg every day," argued the patient's husband. "There has not been justice."[39] Lawyers for the plaintiff described a suffering patient who had waited nearly seven years to have her day in court. The defense argued that their client was a distressed physician whose name deserved to be cleared.

Liebman found the spectacle of the trial even more difficult to tolerate than the seven years that had preceded it. He looked to send a personal message directly to his former patient during the trial: "I'm sorry and I ask your forgiveness."[40] Tragically, he never had the opportunity to speak the words. Liebman complained of chest pains several days into the proceedings. Within hours the sixty-two-year-old surgeon was dead from a massive heart attack.

Almost a thousand mourners attended Liebman's funeral service. At the time of his death, a full-page tribute in the *Palm Beach Post* attested to Liebman's "caring" and healing "many thousands of patients."[41] It was signed by almost four hundred of his peers, coworkers, and friends. "A great doctor died of a broken heart," grieved one of his friends, "while defending himself in court."[42]

A week after Liebman's passing, the trial judge declared a mistrial before a sea of white coats worn by friends who had come to support their fallen colleague. Representatives of Liebman's estate, his lawyers, and the patient's legal counsel then began negotiations toward an eventual settlement. In Liebman's case modern medicine managed to turn both the patient and the doctor into victims.

Ironically, while the sanctity of the patient-physician relationship has suffered in the modern age, public esteem for medicine as an institution remains high and the profession still ranks among the most prestigious of all vocations in America. This standing rests on the remarkable developments in the biomedical sciences. Clinical care, despite the runaway costs and disorganization, is many times improved over that of even thirty years ago. Much of this progress can be attributed to the profession's embrace and defense of rigorous education, training, and specialty expertise.

It is in the steadily shifting balance between the health expectations of the public, the costs of clinical accomplishment, and the aspirations and goals of the profession that conflicts arise. Indeed, the healthier Americans become, the more medicine they seek. One thing is certain, the coming months and years will be a time of momentous decisions for the profession, the public, politicians, and policy makers. How this outcome will be shaped depends on what Americans decide they require for their medical needs. The only thing that is certain is that organized medicine, and consequently America's doctors, will not be dictating the terms.

EPILOGUE

HISTORY IS EASIEST to write when the underlying story has already
finished. But medicine in America continues to evolve. Drawing
tidy conclusions about such material becomes as difficult as tying a pack-
age with a ribbon that stretches forever. Nonetheless, three centuries of
history provide many insights on where medicine has been and where it
may be going.

The relationship that physicians have to the history of their field is
different from that of other professions. The architect continues to find
inspiration in Greek and Roman aesthetics. The engineer looks to early
structural designs to better understand the construction of bridges and
buildings. The lawyer can follow an unbroken chain of case law that pre-
dates the Constitution. But for the American doctor there is little of practical value before World War II and the immediate years that followed.
That period is roughly the hinge between early and contemporary or
modern medicine.

Had *Seeking the Cure* tracked medical history up to the 1940s and no
further it would tell a story that ends decisively in American triumphal-
ism. Science had finally vanquished the bugbears of superstition and tradition. Physicians had organized themselves into a respected profession.
America had achieved a medical prestige commensurate with its economic and political strength. Treatments that we recognize as contemporary first appeared around this time. But beginning in the 1950s, these
manifold victories gave way to a host of distinctly modern dilemmas.

The first challenge that has come to define present-day American
medicine is rising costs. Medicine takes up and affects a larger percentage
of the economy with each passing year. Current estimates put U.S. health

care spending at approximately 16 percent of the gross domestic product, and this figure is expected to continue its historical upward trend, reaching $4.3 trillion, or almost 20 percent, by 2017.

Prior to World War II there had been little of this escalation. Most of the early innovations—Morton's discovering anesthesia, Lister's sterilization procedure, Fitz's defining appendicitis—had minimal material and research costs. But the situation changed in the 1950s due largely to increased investments in science and the rise of the medical-industrial complex. Medical treatments became more powerful and more expensive. New biotechnologies like open-heart surgery, organ transplantation, and coronary artery stenting carried enormous price tags; even everyday diagnostic tools like CAT and MRI scans can cost thousands of dollars. The situation was clear by the late 1960s when President Nixon identified a medical cost crisis, and no sustainable solutions have been found since. If anything, the situation continues to worsen due to a type of feedback loop where investment in research produces remarkable results that set the stage for even more innovative and expensive research and so on. Health care gets better and better, but is affordable by fewer and fewer.

The second most prominent challenge of the modern era is an organizational one. For much of American medical history, the physician was the entire field of health care. Patients had a long-term relationship with a single individual who oversaw all aspects of treatment. Specialists and hospital visits were the exceptions, never the rule. In the modern era, more parties have gotten involved in providing different therapies. Where once there was the "doctor," presently there are multiple physician specialists, a variety of nurses and paraprofessionals, hospital administrators, insurance agents, and quality care personnel, each with their own interests to protect. Physicians no longer set policy, and the doctor-patient relationship has fractured. The system is now a hydra where the heads move as though they do not realize they are attached to the same body. But changing today's status quo requires these parties to act together. As a result, the complicated state of socioeconomics in medicine hampers improvements in health care as well as access to medical advancements.

Patients grow frustrated not only with these logistical and financial difficulties, but also with the fact that modern medicine has fostered a gap between their expectations and realities. Many factors contributed to this phenomenon, but a few stand out. First and foremost, physicians succeeded in transforming themselves from an underappreciated trade full of quacks and charlatans to an esteemed profession. Ironically, doctors solidified their professional status at roughly the same moment when they began to lose their autonomy and control. As they embraced scientific medicine, they learned to cure many common ailments and, in turn, created an illusion that medicine always had the answer. Hospitals also changed from hovels leading the way to the morgue to citadels filled with marvelous technologies. Admission to a modern hospital came to signify better health, not worse. And the advent of Medicare meant that Americans assumed they would have all the tools of the medical complex at their disposal from retirement onward.

While medicine is able to meet some of these expectations, it cannot help but fall short. Protracted battles against diseases like cancer have shown that scientific medicine does not guarantee success. To make matters worse, Americans are bombarded by advertisements for wonder drugs and inundated with stories promising that the next great discovery is about to arrive. There is a message being spread that medicine can solve all the problems a person has, and the gap between expectation and reality grows wider.

But it is not just at the point of clinical treatment where modern medicine has become more problematic. Advances in medical research have muddied the ethical situation as well. For much of American history, medical science triumphed over ethical concerns, which were often rooted in superstition or misinformation. Recall Boylston's fight in 1721 with other Boston physicians who worried that his inoculation treatment would spread smallpox, not lessen its rampage, or the mishandling of President Garfield's care in 1881 and the great debates over the use of Listerism.

The contemporary situation presents conflicts that are more intransigent. Medical science has become so advanced that researchers (and the public) routinely face breakthroughs that touch at the core of what it means to be human: cloning, stem cells, and gene therapy, for example. Perhaps the stage for this modern dilemma was set when Moore and Thorn decided to take a kidney from one twin brother and give it to the other, initiating an era where scientists saw human bodies as the raw material for medical advancement.

Modern medicine has become an arena of trade-offs, a balance between costs, organization, expectations, and ethics. And clinical care hangs in a nearly unadministrable gray area between private service and public good. The question is: How will advancing science and technology relate to these issues?

The most sanguine outlook is that medicine will overcome many of the challenges that we currently face. Imagine walking into a shopping mall where you enter a specialized health care store and deposit samples of blood, hair, saliva, and urine. One hour later, you receive a printout of your health status along with a bag of personalized medicines, matched to your genetic profile. The container also includes digestible computer chips, which will wirelessly relay your medical reports (including your body's reactions to the drugs) to physicians who could be thousands of miles away. This team of doctors will have diagnostic tools that dwarf current technologies—next-generation body scanners will not only have greater resolution and higher magnification, but they will also measure cellular activity in tissues and correlate it with changes in an organ's anatomy, all the way down to the biochemical level.

Once your medical team has processed this diagnostic information, they will have a myriad of new clinical options available. Gene therapy will allow physicians to replace the faulty genes that cause diseases like Alzheimer's, diabetes, and sickle-cell anemia with healthy ones, remedying these illnesses at the most basic of cellular building blocks. Eventually, genetic-based therapies will take the place of operative treatment for cancer and decrease the need for cardiac surgeries or the repair of bodily malformations. In cases where operations are necessary, such as trauma, robotic surgery will handle much of the burden. Robots will also be able to perform procedures that require greater-than-human precision, including face transplants, artificial retinal attachments, and the replacement of body parts once thought impossible.

In this futuristic scenario, living standards will increase dramatically. The celebration of a one hundredth birthday will be commonplace. Women will routinely have babies well into their forties. The need for sleep will be lessened. The bounties of new medicine could transform our everyday experience.

Of course, this is a picture of future life divorced from the realities of contemporary medicine. All of these new biotechnologies—cellular scanners, gene therapies, robotic surgeries, wireless monitoring—will cost much more than the most sophisticated treatments we have currently. Policy makers would have to implement measures to curb runaway health inflation for these breakthroughs to become commonplace. The hypothetical team of health care professionals in this scenario will need to work together to serve the patient. New ideas might encourage better care that is coordinated and efficient or worse care that is bloated and superfluous. The patient will be forced to confront the reality that no matter how advanced medicine becomes, it cannot solve all the problems in life. Finally, society will need to come to terms with where the ethical lines should be drawn on everything from gene therapies to personalized medicine.

If history teaches us anything, it is that medicine will advance and grow inexorably. Americans will be well served to face the economic, political, and social challenges of contemporary medicine directly while acknowledging that it is impossible to predict where the future of medical science will lead us.

ACKNOWLEDGMENTS

I AM UNCERTAIN AS to when I began my research and thinking for this book. Whether it was during my freshman year in medical school in 1971 or while writing my first article on history in 1978 or through the months spent completing a bibliography on American medicine in 1988, I cannot pinpoint the starting date. In truth, it is not an important piece of information, for any comprehensive book on medical history brings together anew a continuum of thoughts that stretch back several millennia.

Acknowledging this, I freely admit to inspiration and guidance from a two-century-old body of writing on the history of medicine in America. Among the most helpful works have been Edward Clarke's *A Century of American Medicine, 1776–1876,* Francis Packard's *History of Medicine in the United States,* Henry Sigerist's *American Medicine,* Rosemary Stevens's *American Medicine and the Public Interest,* Geoffrey Marks and William Beatty's *The Story of Medicine in America,* James Bordley and A. McGehee Harvey's *Two Centuries of American Medicine, 1776–1976,* Paul Starr's *The Social Transformation of American Medicine,* James Cassedy's *Medicine in America, a Short History,* and John Duffy's *From Humors to Medical Science: A History of American Medicine.*

I must also acknowledge the research staff at the New York Academy of Medicine, in particular Arlene Shaner, the academy's assistant curator and reference librarian for historical collections, as well as the personnel of the New York Public Library for their assistance. It is a wonderful pleasure to live in America's greatest town, New York City, and have these two remarkable libraries at one's doorstep.

In 1997 I first spoke with Eric Simonoff. He is the most capable and knowledgeable of literary agents. Eric's wise counsel has allowed me to pursue the career of my dreams, to be a physician who wields both pen and scalpel. At Scribner, my good fortune has been to have Colin Harrison as my editor. This book is far better for his detailed, guiding, and reflective suggestions. To Jessica Manners, thank you for the cheery voice at the other end of the telephone and e-mails. The copyediting, editorial, marketing, production, and publicity departments at Scribner also deserve heartfelt appreciation.

I want to give thanks to my dear friends Laurie and Larry Sussman, who opened their hearts and minds to my desultory writing schedule. To David Oshinsky, historian extraordinaire, goes a special expression of gratitude for his in-depth critique of the manuscript. Barron Lerner, the most competent of medical historians, provided sage advice. And to Eric Carlson, Barnet W. Rider III, Roger Rickard, Brian Phoenix, and Barbara and Jimmy Kusisto for making everything run properly.

My parents, Bea and Al Rutkow, have always been the most vociferous of cheerleaders for my various projects. As they have grown older, I marvel at their zest for life and the equanimity with which they live. This book stands as a tribute to their steadfast support and further validates the enormous sacrifices they made to ensure that I received a splendid education.

There really should be three other individuals listed on the dedication page. To my wife, Beth, and our children, Lainie and Eric, you are omnipresent in the writing of this book. Lainie—lawyer, Ph.D., and public health advocate—is an amazing woman. She lights up a room with her smile and makes everyone feel special. Eric—lawyer and writer—is my private editor within our family. He provides an unmistakable verve and voice to my written words. Beth is my lifelong love and steadfast anchor. I would achieve little without her presence.

NOTES

The major works which shaped my thinking are listed at the beginning of the notes for each chapter.

One Colonial Medicine

Beall, Otho, and Richard Shryock. *Cotton Mather: First Significant Figure in American Medicine.* Baltimore: Johns Hopkins Press, 1954.

Bell, Whitfield. *John Morgan, Continental Doctor.* Philadelphia: University of Pennsylvania Press, 1965.

———. *The Colonial Physician & Other Essays.* New York: Science History Publications, 1975.

Blanton, Wyndham. *Medicine in Virginia in the Seventeenth Century.* Richmond, Va.: William Byrd Press, 1930.

———. *Medicine in Virginia in the Eighteenth Century.* Richmond, Va.: Garrett & Massie, 1931.

Boas, Ralph, and Louise Boas. *Cotton Mather, Keeper of the Puritan Conscience.* New York: Harper & Brothers, 1928.

Fenn, Elizabeth. *Pox Americana, the Great Smallpox Epidemic of 1775–82.* New York: Hill and Wang, 2001.

Finger, Stanley. *Doctor Franklin's Medicine.* Philadelphia: University of Pennsylvania Press, 2006.

Flexner, James. *Doctors on Horseback: Pioneers of American Medicine.* New York: Viking, 1937.

Gordon, Maurice. *Aesculapius Comes to the Colonies: The Story of the Early Days of Medicine in the Thirteen Original Colonies.* Ventnor, N.J.: Ventnor Publishers, 1949.

Kraus, Michael. "American and European Medicine in the Eighteenth Century." *Bulletin of the History of Medicine* 8 (1940):679–95.

Ladenheim, Jules. " 'The Doctors' Mob' of 1788." *Journal of the History of Medicine and the Allied Sciences* 5 (1950):23–43.

Medicine in Colonial Massachusetts, 1620–1820; a Conference Held 25 & 26 May 1978 by the Colonial Society of Massachusetts. Boston: Colonial Society of Massachusetts, 1980.

Pepper, William. *The Medical Side of Benjamin Franklin.* Philadelphia: William J. Campbell, 1910.

Shryock, Richard. *Medicine and Society in America, 1660–1860.* New York: New York University Press, 1960.

Silverman, Kenneth. *The Life and Times of Cotton Mather.* New York: Harper & Row, 1984.

Twiss, John. "Medical Practice in Colonial America." *Bulletin of the New York Academy of Medicine* 36 (1960):538–51.

Viets, Henry. *A Brief History of Medicine in Massachusetts.* New York: Houghton Mifflin, 1930.

1. Zabdiel Boylston, *An Historical Account of the Small-pox Inoculated in New England, Upon All Sorts of Persons, Whites, Blacks, and of All Ages and Constitutions.* (Boston: S. Gerrish in Cornhil, and T. Hancock at the Bible and Three Crowns in Annstreet, 1730) (2nd and corrected edition), p. iv (the preface).
2. Anon., *A Letter from One in the Country, to His Friend in the City: In Relation to Their Distresses Occasioned by the Doubtful and Prevailing Practice of the Inoculation of the Smallpox* (Boston: Nicholas Boone, 1721), pp. 3–4.
3. James Thacher, *American Medical Biography; or Memoirs of Eminent Physicians Who Have Flourished in America* (Boston: Richardson & Lord and Cottons & Barnard, 1828), vol. 1, p. 191.
4. Advertisement in the *Boston Gazette,* Monday, November 21, to Monday, November 28, 1720, p. 4.
5. Boylston, *An Historical Account,* pp. iii and 38.
6. Ralph Boas and Louise Boas, *Cotton Mather, Keeper of the Puritan Conscience* (New York: Harper & Brothers, 1928).
7. John Duffy, *From Humors to Medical Science: A History of American Medicine* (Urbana: University of Illinois, 1993), p. 22.
8. Cotton Mather, *Diary of Cotton Mather, 1709–1724,* vol. 2 (New York: Frederick Ungar, 1957), pp. 620–21.
9. Thacher, *American Medical Biography,* vol. 1, p. 187.
10. Quoted in Otho Beall and Richard Shryock, *Cotton Mather: First Significant Figure in American Medicine* (Baltimore: Johns Hopkins Press, 1954), p. 103.
11. Advertisement in the *Boston Gazette,* Monday, July 10, to Monday, July 17, 1721, p. 2.
12. Mather, *Diary,* p. 632.
13. Ibid., p. 658.
14. Benjamin Colman, *Some Observations on the New Method of Receiving the Smallpox by Ingrafting or Inoculating* (Boston: B. Green, 1721), p. 3.
15. Thacher, *American Medical Biography,* vol. 1, p. 190.
16. Boylston, *An Historical Account.* (London: S. Chandler, at the Cross-Keys in the Poultry, 1726), p. ii (the dedication).
17. Thacher, *American Medical Biography,* vol. 1, p. 190.
18. Quoted in Henry Viets, *A Brief History of Medicine in Massachusetts* (New York: Houghton Mifflin, 1930), p. 64.
19. William Smith, *The History of the Province of New York, from the First Discovery to the Year MDCCXXXII* (London: Thomas Wilcox, 1757), p. 212.
20. Quoted in William Douglas: *A Summary, Historical and Political, of the First Planting, Progressive Improvements, and Present State of the British Settlements in North America,* vol. 2 (Boston: Daniel Fowle, 1751), p. 352.
21. Quoted in ibid., p. 351.
22. *South-Carolina Gazette,* Thursday, May 29, to Thursday, June 5, 1755, p. 3.
23. George Norris, *The Early History of Medicine in Philadelphia* (Philadelphia: private printing, 1886), p. 46.
24. Ibid., p. 58.
25. Benjamin Rush, "An Account of the Late Dr. John Morgan," *American Museum* 6 (1789):354.
26. Quoted in Stanley Finger, *Doctor Franklin's Medicine* (Philadelphia: University of Pennsylvania Press, 2006), pp. 140–41.
27. Quoted in William Middleton, "John Morgan, Father of Medical Education in North America," *Annals of Medical History* 9 (1927):15.
28. Quoted in Whitfield Bell, *John Morgan, Continental Doctor* (Philadelphia: University of Pennsylvania Press, 1965), p. 77.
29. Quoted in Middleton, "John Morgan, Father," p. 17.

30. Quoted in Norris, *The Early History of Medicine,* p. 150.
31. Ibid., p. 155.
32. John Morgan, *A Discourse Upon the Institution of Medical Schools in America* (Philadelphia: William Bradford, 1765), p. 26.
33. Ibid., p. 24.
34. James Flexner, *Doctors on Horseback: Pioneers of American Medicine* (New York: Viking, 1937), p. 21.
35. Morgan, *A Discourse Upon,* p. 18.
36. Ibid., p. 31.
37. Norris, *The Early History of Medicine,* p. 128.
38. Henry Sigerist, *American Medicine* (New York: W. W. Norton, 1934), p. 79.
39. Rush, "An Account of," p. 354.
40. Morgan, *A Discourse Upon,* p. xvii.
41. Ibid., p. xi.
42. Ibid., p. 28.
43. Quoted in Norris, *The Early History of Medicine,* p. 117.
44. Stephen Wickes, *History of Medicine in New Jersey, and of Its Medical Men, from the Settlement of the Province to A.D. 1800* (Newark: Martin R. Dennis, 1879), p. 104.
45. Anon., "Remarks on medical fees," *New York Monthly Chronicle of Medicine and Surgery* 1 (1824–25):25.
46. Joel Headley, *The Great Riots of New York, 1712 to 1873* (New York: E. B. Treat, 1873), p. 58.
47. Morgan, *A Discourse Upon,* p. iii.
48. Rush, "An Account of," p. 354.

Two Democratization of Healing

Calhoun, Daniel. *Professional Lives in America: Structure and Aspiration, 1750–1850.* Cambridge: Harvard University Press, 1965.

Cassedy, James. *Medicine and American Growth, 1800–1860.* Madison: University of Wisconsin Press, 1986.

Fenster, Julie. *Ether Day: The Strange Tale of America's Greatest Medical Discovery and the Haunted Men Who Made It.* New York: HarperCollins, 2001.

Flexner, James. *Doctors on Horseback: Pioneers of American Medicine.* New York: Viking, 1937.

Goodman, Nathan. *Benjamin Rush, Physician and Citizen, 1746–1813.* Philadelphia: University of Pennsylvania Press, 1934.

Haller, John. *American Medicine in Transition, 1840–1910.* Urbana: University of Illinois Press, 1981.

Hawke, David. *Benjamin Rush: Revolutionary Gadfly.* Indianapolis: Bobbs-Merrill, 1971.

Kett, Joseph. *The Formation of the American Medical Profession: The Role of Institutions, 1780–1860.* New Haven: Yale University Press, 1968.

Norwood, William. *Medical Education in the United States Before the Civil War.* Philadelphia: University of Pennsylvania Press, 1944.

Nuland, Sherwin. *Doctors: The Biography of Medicine.* New York: Alfred A. Knopf, 1988.

Pernick, Martin. *A Calculus of Suffering; Pain, Professionalism, and Anesthesia in Nineteenth-Century America.* New York: Columbia University Press, 1985.

Rothstein, William. *American Physicians in the 19th Century: From Sects to Science.* Baltimore: The Johns Hopkins University Press, 1972.

Rutkow, Ira. *Bleeding Blue and Gray: Civil War Surgery and the Evolution of American Medicine.* New York: Random House, 2005.

Shafer, Henry. *The American Medical Profession, 1783–1850.* New York: Columbia University Press, 1936.

Shryock, Richard. *Medicine and Society in America: 1660–1860.* New York: New York University Press, 1960.

———. *Medicine in America: Historical Essays.* Baltimore: The Johns Hopkins Press, 1966.

Warner, John. *The Therapeutic Perspective: Medical Practice, Knowledge, and Identity in America, 1820–1885.* Cambridge: Harvard University Press, 1986.

———. *Against the Spirit of System: The French Impulse in Nineteenth-Century American Medicine.* Princeton, N.J.: Princeton University Press, 1998.

Wolfe, Richard. *Tarnished Idol: William Thomas Green Morton and the Introduction of Surgical Anesthesia; a Chronicle of the Ether Controversy.* San Anselmo, Calif.: Norman Publishing, 2001.

1. James Thacher, *American Medical Biography: Or Memoirs of Eminent Physicians Who Have Flourished in America* (Boston: Richardson & Lord and Cottons & Barnard, 1828), vol. 2, pp. 62–63.
2. Benjamin Rush, *Medical Inquiries and Observations: Containing an Account of the Bilious Remitting and Intermitting Yellow Fever, as It Appeared in Philadelphia in the Year 1794, Together with an Inquiry into the Proximate Cause of Fever; and a Defense of Blood-letting as a Remedy for Certain Diseases* (Philadelphia: Thomas Dobson, 1796), vol. 4, p. 134.
3. Alfred Post, "Curative Effects of Blood-Letting," *Bulletin of the New York Academy of Medicine* 3 (1867):270.
4. John Beck, "On the Effects of Emetics in the Young Subject," *New York Journal of Medicine and the Collateral Sciences* 7 (1846):158.
5. Thacher, *American Medical Biography,* vol. 2, p. 54.
6. Peter Porcupine [William Cobbett], "Birth and Character of Rush," in *The Rush-light* (New York: William Cobbett, 1800 [February 15th]), p. 8.
7. Thacher, *American Medical Biography,* vol. 2, p. 49.
8. Ibid., p. 45.
9. Quoted in David Hawke, *Benjamin Rush: Revolutionary Gadfly* (Indianapolis: Bobbs-Merrill, 1971), p. 220.
10. Letter to the editor in the *Pennsylvania Packet or the General Advertiser,* Saturday, December 9, 1780, p. 3.
11. Thacher, *American Medical Biography,* vol. 2, p. 57.
12. Quoted in Hawke, *Benjamin Rush,* p. 236.
13. Thacher, *American Medical Biography,* vol. 2, p. 54.
14. Ibid., p. 32.
15. Ibid., p. 35.
16. Ibid.
17. James Flexner, *Doctors on Horseback: Pioneers of American Medicine* (New York: Viking, 1937), p. 110.
18. Thacher, *American Medical Biography,* vol. 2, p. 34.
19. T. L. Papin, "Venesection, Its Use and Abuse," *St. Louis Medical and Surgical Journal* 17 (1859):230.
20. Thacher, *American Medical Biography,* vol. 2, p. 34.
21. Nathan Davis, *History of Medical Education and Institutions in the United States, From the First Settlement of the British Colonies to the Year 1850* (Chicago: S. C. Griggs, 1851), p. 84.
22. Quoted in John Warner, *The Therapeutic Perspective: Medical Practice, Knowledge, and Identity in America, 1820–1885* (Cambridge: Harvard University Press, 1986), p. 71.
23. Henry Sigerist, *American Medicine* (New York: W. W. Norton, 1934), p. 132.
24. Quoted in Davis, *History of Medical,* p. 183.
25. Ibid., pp. 117–18.
26. C. C. Cox, "Report of the Committee on Medical Education," *Transactions of the American Medical Association* 14 (1863):77.

27. John Billings, "Literature and Institutions." In *A Century of American Medicine, 1776–1876*, edited by Edward Clarke, Henry Bigelow, Samuel Gross, et al. (Philadelphia: Henry C. Lea, 1876), p. 359.

28. Peter Porcupine [William Cobbett], "The Rushite System of Depletion, with a Statement of Porcupine's Reasons for Opposing It, and a Defense of the Publication for Which He Was Sued by Rush," in *The Rush-light* (New York: William Cobbett, 1800 [February 28th]), p. 49.

29. Post, "Curative Effects," p. 267.

30. F. Campbell Stewart, *The Hospitals and Surgeons of Paris* (New York: J. & H. G. Langley, 1843), p. xvi.

31. James Adams, *History of the United States,* vol. 2: *A Half-century of Expansion* (New York: Charles Scribner's Sons, 1933), p. 163.

32. Quoted in James Cassedy, *Medicine in America* (Baltimore: The Johns Hopkins University Press, 1991), p. 34.

33. John Gunn, *Gunn's Domestic Medicine, or Poor Man's Friend, in the Hours of Affliction, Pain, and Sickness* (Louisville, Ky.: G .V. Raymond, 1840), pp. 12–13.

34. "Remarks Before the State Senate," *Transactions of the Medical Society of the State of New York, 1844, 1845, & 1846* 6 [appendix] (1846):71.

35. Nathaniel Chapman, "Presidential Address," *Transactions of the American Medical Association* 1 (1848):8.

36. "Code of Medical Ethics," *Transactions of the American Medical Association* 10 (1857): 612–14.

37. Daniel Drake, *Discourses Delivered by Appointment, Before the Cincinnati Medical Library Association, January 9th and 10th, 1852* (Cincinnati: Moore & Anderson, 1852), p. 84.

38. Ibid., p. 86.

39. George Norris, Isaac Parrish, John Watson, et al., "Anesthetic Agents," *Transactions of the American Medical Association* 1 (1848):182.

40. Henry Bigelow, "A History of the Discovery of Modern Anaesthesia." In *A Century of American Medicine, 1776–1876,* edited by Edward Clarke, Henry Bigelow, Samuel Gross, et al. (Philadelphia: Henry C. Lea, 1876), p. 80.

41. Advertisement in *Hartford Daily Courant,* Tuesday, December 10, 1844, p. 3.

42. Richard Hodges, *A Narrative of Events Connected with the Introduction of Sulphuric Ether into Surgical Use* (Boston: Little, Brown, 1891), p. 12.

43. Julie Fenster, *Ether Day: The Strange Tale of America's Greatest Medical Discovery and the Haunted Men Who Made It* (New York: HarperCollins, 2001), p. 56.

44. L. J. Ludovici, *The Discovery of Anaesthesia* (New York: Thomas Y. Crowell, 1961), p. 29.

45. Jesse Myer, *Life and Letters of Dr. William Beaumont, Including Hitherto Unpublished Data Concerning the Case of Alexis St. Martin* (St. Louis, Mo.: C. V. Mosby, 1912), p. 229.

46. Letter to the editor in *Hartford Daily Courant,* Monday, December 9, 1846, p. 2.

47. Ibid.

48. Edward Warren, *The Life of John Collins Warren, M.D., Compiled Chiefly from His Autobiography and Journals* (Boston: Tickonor & Fields, 1860), vol. 1, p. 381.

49. Quoted in Hodges, *A Narrative of Events,* p. 35.

50. William Morton, "Dr. Morton's Memoir to the Academy of Sciences at Paris, Presented by M. Arago, in the Autumn of 1847," *Littell's Living Age* 16 (1848):571.

51. "Prizes Awarded by the French Academy for 1847 and 1848," *Boston Medical and Surgical Journal* 42 (1850):278–79.

52. "Inhalation of Ether," *New York Journal of Medicine and the Collateral Sciences* 9 (1847):122.

53. Quoted in Hodges, *A Narrative of Events,* p. 128.

54. "To the Public," *Littell's Living Age* 16 (1848):556.

55. Editorial, "Who Invented Anesthesia?" *New York Times,* Monday, November 15, 1858, p. 2.
56. Quoted in Howard Raper, *Man Against Pain: The Epic of Anesthesia* (New York: Prentice-Hall, 1945), p. 105.

Three Emergence of Modern Medicine

Brieger, Gert. "American Surgery and the Germ Theory of Disease." *Bulletin of the History of Medicine* 40 (1966):135–45.
———. "Sanitary Reform in New York City: Stephen Smith and the Passage of the Metropolitan Health Bill." *Bulletin of the History of Medicine* 40 (1966):407–29.
———. "A Portrait of Surgery, Surgery in America, 1875–1889." *Surgical Clinics of North America* 67 (1987):1181–1216.
Brown, Julie. *Health and Medicine on Display: International Expositions in the United States, 1876–1904.* Cambridge, Mass.: The MIT Press, 2009.
Cavins, Harold. "The National Quarantine and Sanitary Conventions of 1857 to 1860 and the Beginnings of the American Public Health Association." *Bulletin of the History of Medicine* 13 (1943):404–26.
Duffy, John. *The Sanitarians: A History of American Public Health.* Urbana: University of Illinois Press, 1990.
Fisher, Richard. *Joseph Lister, 1827–1912.* New York: Stein and Day, 1977.
Howell, Joel. "Making a Medical Practice in an Uneasy World: Some Thoughts from a Century Ago." *Academic Medicine* 72 (1997): 977–81.
Kramer, Howard. "Agitation for Public Health Reform in the 1870s." *Journal of the History of Medicine and Allied Sciences* 3 (1948):473–88 and 4 (1949):75–89.
Rosenkrantz, Barbara. "Cart Before Horse: Theory, Practice and Professional Image in American Public Health, 1870–1920." *Journal of the History of Medicine* 29 (1974):55–73.
Roses, Daniel. "Stephen Smith, Pioneer of American Surgery and Public Health." *Bulletin of the American College of Surgeons* 76 (1991):11–17.
Rothstein, William. *American Physicians in the Nineteenth Century: From Sects to Science.* Baltimore: The Johns Hopkins University Press, 1972.
Rutkow, Ira. *Bleeding Blue and Gray, Civil War Surgery and the Evolution of American Medicine.* New York: Random House, 2005.
———. *James A. Garfield.* New York: Times Books/Henry Holt, 2006.
Shryock, Richard. "The Origins and Significance of the Public Health Movement in the United States." *Annals of Medical History* 1 (1929):645–65.
———. *Medicine in America: Historical Essays.* Baltimore: The Johns Hopkins Press, 1966.
Sigerist, Henry. *American Medicine.* New York: W. W. Norton, 1934.
Starr, Paul. *The Social Transformation of American Medicine.* New York: Basic Books, 1982.

1. *The Medical and Surgical History of the War of the Rebellion* (Washington: Government Printing Office, 1870–1888), vol. 2, part 3 (Case 1047: William C. Goodell), p. 707.
2. S. Weir Mitchell, "Some Personal Recollections of the Civil War," *Transactions of the Studies of the College of Physicians of Philadelphia* 27 (1905):93.
3. Samuel Gross, "Address of Welcome." *Transactions of the International Medical Congress of Philadelphia, 1876,* edited by John Ashhurst (Philadelphia: printed for the Congress, 1877), pp. xxxiv–xxxv.
4. Samuel Francis, *Biographical Sketches of Distinguished Living New York Surgeons* (New York: John Bradburn, 1866), p. 67.
5. Frank Hamilton, "Discussion of Dr. Hodgen's Paper," *Transactions of the International Medical Congress of Philadelphia, 1876,* edited by John Ashhurst (Philadelphia: printed for the Congress, 1877), p. 532.

6. Joseph Lister, "Presidential Greetings," *Transactions of the International Medical Congress of Philadelphia, 1876,* edited by John Ashhurst (Philadelphia: printed for the Congress, 1877), p. 517.

7. Joseph Lister, "Antiseptic Surgery, Report of Remarks Made Before the Surgical Section, During the Adjourned Discussion on Dr. Hodgen's Paper," *Transactions of the International Medical Congress of Philadelphia, 1876,* edited by John Ashhurst (Philadelphia: printed for the Congress, 1877), p. 538.

8. Ibid., p. 537.

9. "Letter from Philadelphia," *Boston Medical and Surgical Journal* 95 (1876):366.

10. "Meeting of the International Medical Congress," *Boston Medical and Surgical Journal* 95 (1876):327.

11. Hamilton, "Discussion of Dr. Hodgen's," p. 533.

12. Samuel Gross, "Surgery." In *A Century of American Medicine, 1776–1876,* edited by Edward Clarke, Henry Bigelow, Samuel Gross, et al. (Philadelphia: Henry C. Lea, 1876), p. 213.

13. Joseph Lister, "The Antiseptic Method of Dressing Open Wounds, a Clinical Lecture by Prof. Joseph Lister of Edinburgh," *Medical Record* 11 (1876):696.

14. George Shrady, "The New York Hospital," *Medical Record* 13 (1878):113.

15. Daniel Cathell, *The Physician Himself and What He Should Add to His Scientific Acquirements,* 2nd ed. (Baltimore: Cushings & Bailey, 1882), pp. 55–56.

16. John Wheeler, *Memoirs of a Small-Town Surgeon* (Garden City, N.Y.: Garden City Publishing, 1935), p. 19.

17. M. A. Rust, "Evolution of Antisepticism (Unconscious Asepticism—Listerism—Iodoformisation)," *Virginia Medical Monthly* 11 (1884):502.

18. Edward Churchill, ed. *To Work in the Vineyard of Surgery: The Reminiscences of J. Collins Warren (1842–1927)* (Cambridge, Mass.: Harvard University Press, 1958), pp. 138, 146.

19. Editorial, "Science," *Atlantic Monthly* 32 (1873):760.

20. George Napheys, *Modern Surgical Therapeutics: A Compendium of Current Formulae, Approved Dressings and Specific Methods for the Treatment of Surgical Diseases and Injuries* (Philadelphia: D. G. Brinton, 1878), p. 113.

21. G. W. Topping, "Report of Communication from the W.C.T.U. to Michigan State Medical Society, June 8th, 1881," *Transactions of the Michigan State Medical Society* 8 (1881):32.

22. Smith Townshend, "President Garfield's Wound and Its Treatment," *Walsh's Retrospect* 2 (1881):624.

23. Ibid.

24. Doctor Bliss, "Report of the Case of President Garfield, Accompanied with a Detailed Account of the Autopsy," *Medical Record* 20 (1881):393.

25. John Ridpath, *The Life and Work of James A. Garfield, and the Tragic Story of His Death* (Cincinnati: Jones Brothers, 1881), p. 522.

26. Quoted in Kenneth Ackerman, *Dark Horse: The Surprise Election and Political Murder of President James A. Garfield* (New York: Carroll & Graf, 2003), pp. 402–403.

27. Ibid., p. 403.

28. *New York Times,* Tuesday, July 5, 1881, p. 5.

29. Robert Reyburn, "Clinical History of the Case of President James Abram Garfield," *Journal of the American Medical Association* 22 (1894):463.

30. Ibid., p. 460.

31. Quoted in Ridpath, *The Life and Work,* p. 552.

32. "President Garfield's Wounds," *Medical and Surgical Reporter* 45 (1881):83.

33. Quoted in Ackerman, *Dark Horse,* p. 411.

34. *New York Times,* Saturday, July 9, 1881, p. 1.

35. Silas Boynton, "President Garfield's Case," *American Observer Medical Monthly* 18 (1881):493.

36. *New York Times,* Monday, August 1, 1881, p. 1.
37. Ibid., Tuesday, August 23, 1881, p. 2.
38. Ibid., Friday, September 16, 1881, p. 1.
39. Frank Hamilton, "The Case of President Garfield," *Medical Gazette* 8 (1881):334.
40. Moritz Schuppert, "A Review of the Wound, Treatment, and Death of James A. Garfield, Late President of the United States of America," *Gaillard's Medical Journal* 32 (1881):498.
41. John Warren, "Case of President Garfield," *Boston Medical and Surgical Journal* 105 (1881):464.
42. Arpad Gerster, *Recollections of a New York Surgeon* (New York: Paul B. Hoeber, 1917), p. 206 (annotated copy in author's collection).
43. Quoted in R. H. Alexander, *The Life of Guiteau and the Official History of the Most Exciting Case on Record: Being the Trial of Guiteau* (Philadelphia: National Publishing, 1881), p. 138.
44. Frank Hamilton, *Conversations Between Drs. Warren and Putnam on the Subject of Medical Ethics with an Account of the Medical Empiricisms of Europe and America* (New York: Bermingham, 1884), p. 120.
45. Frank Hamilton, *The Principles and Practice of Surgery,* 3rd ed. (New York: William Wood, 1886), pp. 957, 959.
46. John Girdner, "The Death of President Garfield," *Munsey's Magazine* 26 (1902):547.
47. George Shrady, "The Late President Garfield's Case," *Medical Record* 20 (1881):410.
48. Cathell, *The Physician Himself,* 1st ed. (1882), p. 9.
49. Ibid., 10th ed. (1892), p. 25.
50. Ibid., 11th ("twentieth century") ed. (1902), pp. 22–23.
51. Ibid., 13th ("crowning") ed. (1922), p. 38.
52. Ibid., 10th ed. (1892), p. 94.
53. "Recent Literature—*The Physician Himself,*" *Boston Medical and Surgical Journal* 107 (1882):230.
54. Cathell, *The Physician Himself,* 1st ed. (1882), p. 89.
55. Ibid., p. 48.
56. Ibid., p. 127.
57. Ibid., p. 13.
58. Ibid., pp. 122–23.
59. Stephen Smith, *Doctor in Medicine: and Other Papers on Professional Subjects* (New York: William Wood, 1872), p. 132.
60. Frank Hamilton, "Hygiene, Being the Substance of a 'Charge' Given February 1859 to the Graduating Class in the Medical Department of the University of Buffalo," *New York Journal of Medicine* 7 (1859):60, 62.
61. Stephen Smith, *The City That Was* (New York: Frank Allaben, 1911), p. 81.
62. Ibid., p. 102.
63. Ibid., p. 116.
64. Editorial, "The Health of the City," *New York Times,* Monday, January 16, 1865, p. 4.
65. Smith, *The City That Was,* p. 158.
66. Henry Bowditch, "Address on Hygiene and Preventive Medicine," *Transactions of the International Medical Congress of Philadelphia, 1876,* edited by John Ashhurst (Philadelphia: printed for the Congress, 1877), p. 29.
67. Stephen Smith, "History of Public Health, 1871–1921." In *A Half Century of Public Health, Jubilee Historical Volume of the American Public Health Association; in Commemoration of the Fiftieth Anniversary Celebration of Its Foundation, New York City, November 14–18, 1921,* edited by Mazÿck Ravenel (New York: American Public Health Association, 1921), p. 10.

68. Editorial, "Public Health Association," *New York Daily Tribune,* Friday, November 22, 1878, p. 4.
69. Samuel Osgood, "Health and the Higher Culture." In *Public Health, Reports and Papers Presented at the Meeting of the American Public Health Association, in the years 1874–1875* (New York: Hurd and Houghton, 1876), p. 207.

Four Consolidation of Power

Aldrich, Mark. "Train Wrecks to Typhoid Fever: The Development of Railroad Medicine Organizations, 1850 to World War I." *Bulletin of the History of Medicine* 75 (2001):254–89

Brieger, Gert. "A Portrait of Surgery: Surgery in America, 1875–1889." *Surgical Clinics of North America* 67 (1987):1181–1216.

Gevitz, Norman, ed. *Other Healers: Unorthodox Medicine in America.* Baltimore: The Johns Hopkins University Press, 1988.

Gillespie, Robert. "The Train Doctors: A Detailed History of Railway Surgeons." http://railwaysurgery.org/HistoryLong.htm (viewed on November 23, 2006).

Haller, John. *Medical Protestants: The Eclectics in American Medicine, 1825–1939.* Carbondale: Southern Illinois University Press, 1994.

———. *Kindly Medicine: Physio-Medicalism in America, 1836–1911.* Kent, Ohio: Kent State University Press, 1997.

———. *The People's Doctors: Samuel Thomson and the American Botanical Movement, 1790–1860.* Carbondale: Southern Illinois University Press, 2001.

———. *History of American Homeopathy: The Academic Years, 1820–1935.* Binghamton, N.Y.: Haworth Press, 2005.

Hsu, Chi-yuan. *Orificial Surgery: A History.* [Thesis] Department of the History of Science, Harvard University, 1993.

Kaufman, Martin. *Homeopathy in America: The Rise and Fall of a Medical Heresy.* Baltimore: The Johns Hopkins Press, 1971.

Rosen, George. *The Specialization of Medicine.* New York: Froben Press, 1944.

Rothstein, William. *American Physicians in the 19th Century: From Sects to Science.* Baltimore: The Johns Hopkins University Press, 1972.

Rutkow, Ira. "Railway Surgery: Traumatology and Managed Health Care in 19th-Century America." *Archives of Surgery* 128 (1993):458–63.

———. "Edwin Hartley Pratt and Orificial Surgery: Unorthodox Surgical Practice in 19th-Century United States." *Surgery* 114 (1993):558–63.

———. "William Tod Helmuth and Andrew Jackson Howe: Surgical Sectarianism in 19th-Century America." *Archives of Surgery* 129 (1994):662–68.

Shryock, Richard. *Medical Licensing in America, 1650–1965.* Baltimore: The Johns Hopkins Press, 1967.

Starr, Paul. *The Social Transformation of American Medicine.* New York: Basic Books, 1982.

Stevens, Rosemary. *American Medicine and the Public Interest.* New Haven: Yale University Press, 1971.

1. W. James Bushrod, "Annual Address," *Transactions of the Thirty-sixth Session of the American Institute of Homeopathy* [no volume number] (1883): 33.
2. Quoted in William King, *History of Homeopathy and Its Institutions in America,* 4 volumes (New York: Lewis Publishing, 1905), vol. 1, p. 24.
3. Quoted in ibid., p. 27.
4. G. R. Starkey, *An Introductory to the Fifteenth Annual Course of Lectures in the Homeopathic Medical College of Pennsylvania* (Philadelphia: A. M. Spangler, 1862), p. 9.

5. Editorial, "The Homeopathic Examiner," *Boston Medical and Surgical Journal* 22 (1840):82.

6. Oliver Holmes, *Medical Essays, 1842–1882* (Boston: Houghton Mifflin, 1883), pp. 40, 101–2.

7. Worthington Hooker, *Lessons from the History of Medical Delusions* (New York: Baker & Scribner, 1850), p. 86.

8. Editorial, "The Philosophy of Homeopathy," *Boston Medical and Surgical Journal* 24 (1841):97.

9. Editorial, "Homeopathy in the Army," *New York Times,* Saturday, January 11, 1862, p. 4.

10. *The Congressional Globe: The Official Proceedings of Congress* (Washington: John C. Rives, 1862,) p. 996.

11. Starkey, *An Introductory to,* p. 12.

12. Lainie Rutkow and Ira Rutkow, "Homeopaths, Surgery, and the Civil War: Edward C. Franklin and the Struggle to Achieve Medical Pluralism in the Union Army," *Archives of Surgery* 139 (2004):790.

13. *Congressional Globe,* p. 997.

14. Editorial, "Medical Union," *New York Times,* Friday, February 7, 1873, p. 4.

15. King, *History of Homeopathy,* vol. 3, p. 178.

16. Louisa May Alcott, *Jo's Boys, and How They Turned Out: A Sequel to "Little Men"* (Boston: Roberts Brothers, 1886), p. 13.

17. Edwin Pratt, "A Surgical Talk Upon the Orifices of the Body," *Medical Era* 3 (1886):270.

18. C. Weirick, "Clippings and Comments," *Journal of Orificial Surgery* 5 (1897):525.

19. Pratt, "A Surgical Talk," p. 268.

20. *A Biographical History, with Portraits, of Prominent Men of the Great West* (Chicago: Manhattan Publishing, 1894), p. 508.

21. Edwin Pratt, "A Report on Orificial Surgery, Based on Analyses of 1,000 Cases, Prepared for the World's Congress of Homeopathic Physicians and Surgeons Assembled in Chicago, May 29th, 1893," *Journal of Orificial Surgery* 1 (1893):781.

22. Charles Sawyer, "Orificial Philosophy." In *Orificial Surgery, Its Philosophy Application and Technique,* edited by Benjamin Dawson (Newark, N.J.: Physicians Drug News, 1912), p. 123.

23. Erastus Marcy, "On Homeopathic Surgery," *North American Journal of Homeopathy* 1 (1851):150.

24. Charles Thomas, "Address of the Bureau of Surgery—Subject: 'The Year's Progress in Surgery,'" *Transactions of the Forty-third Session of the American Institute of Homeopathy* [no volume number] (1890):630.

25. H. R. Hopkins, "Is It a Profession or a Trade?" In *An Ethical Symposium: Being a Series of Papers Concerning Medical Ethics and Etiquette from the Liberal Standpoint* (New York: G. P. Putnam's Sons, 1883), p. 184.

26. Abraham Flexner, *Medical Education in the United States and Canada* (New York: Carnegie Foundation, 1910), p. 156.

27. Henry Piffard, "The Status of the Medical Profession in the State of New York," *New York Medical Journal* 37 (1883):402.

28. William Ely, "The Questionable Features of Our Medical Codes." In *An Ethical Symposium,* p. 19.

29. "Philadelphia—Homeopaths for the Army and Navy of the United States," *Journal of the American Medical Association* 30 (1898):1430.

30. Ibid.

31. John Wyeth, "The Presidential Address," *Journal of the American Medical Association* 38 (1902):1555.

32. Daniel Cathell, "Was It Wise for the American Medical Association to Change Its Code of Ethics?" *American Medicine* 6 (1903):618–20.

33. Daniel Cathell, *Book on the Physician Himself and Things That Concern His Reputation and Success* (Philadelphia: F. A. Davis, 1908 [20th-century ed.]), p. 257.
34. William Green, "Sphincteral Dilatation as a Resuscitant in Chloroform and Ether Narcosis and Asphyxia Neonatorum," *Medical Century* 4 (1896):414.
35. "Hom. Med. Soc. of Albany Co.," *Homeopathic Times* 5 (1878):238.
36. Fred Robinson, "M.D., Indianapolis," *Journal of the American Medical Association* 16 (1891):864.
37. John Rauch, "Address in State Medicine," *Journal of the American Medical Association* 6 (1886):648.
38. Quoted in John Apperson, "Report on Advances in Practice of Medicine," *Transactions of the Seventeenth Annual Session of the Medical Society of Virginia* [no volume number] (1886):91.
39. D. Humphreys Storer, "Presidential Address," *Transactions of the American Medical Association* 17 (1866):64.
40. Nathan Davis, "Address on the Present Status and Future Tendencies of the Medical Profession in the United States, Delivered at the Annual Meeting of the American Association of Medical Editors in Cleveland, June 5, 1883," *Journal of the American Medical Association* 1 (1883):38.
41. Samuel Gross, "Address of Welcome," *Transactions of the American Surgical Association* 1 (1883):xxii.
42. Quoted in Thomas Bonner, *The Kansas Doctor; a Century of Pioneering* (Lawrence: University of Kansas, 1959), p. 68.
43. Clinton Herrick, *Railway Surgery: A Handbook on the Management of Injuries* (New York: William Wood, 1899), p. 3.
44. R. Harvey Reed, "Railway Surgery—Its Present Status and Importance," *Railway Age and Northwestern Railroader* 18 (1893):522.
45. Christian Stemen, *Railway Surgery, a Practical Work on the Special Department of Railway Surgery: For Railway Surgeons: and Practitioners in the General Practice of Surgery* (St. Louis, Mo.: J. H. Chambers, 1890), p. 300.
46. Ibid., p. 305.
47. F.S.D., "The Missouri Pacific Hospital at St. Louis," *Railway Surgeon* 3 (1897):514.
48. Herrick, *Railway Surgery,* p. 17.
49. Reed, "Railway Surgery," p. 522.
50. "Report of the Committee on Railroad Practice," *Journal of the American Medical Association* 18 (1892):815.
51. F. H. Davenport, "Specialism in Medical Practice; Its Present Status and Tendencies," *Boston Medical and Surgical Journal* 145 (1901):82.

Five Scientific Advancement

Bonner, Thomas. *American Doctors and German Universities: A Chapter in International Intellectual Relations, 1870–1914.* Lincoln: University of Nebraska Press, 1963.
———. *Becoming a Physician: Medical Education in Britain, France, Germany, and the United States, 1750–1945.* New York: Oxford University Press, 1995.
Chapman, Carleton. *Order Out of Chaos: John Shaw Billings and America's Coming of Age.* Boston: Boston Medical Library in the Francis A. Countway Library of Medicine, 1994.
Chesney, Alan. *The Johns Hopkins Hospital and the Johns Hopkins University School of Medicine, a Chronicle,* 3 vols. Baltimore: The Johns Hopkins Press, 1943, 1958, and 1963.
Courtwright, David. *Dark Paradise: Opiate Addiction in America Before 1940.* Cambridge: Harvard University Press, 1982.
Fleming, Donald. *William H. Welch and the Rise of Modern Medicine.* Boston: Little, Brown, 1954.

Flexner, Simon, and James Thomas Flexner. *William Henry Welch and the Heroic Age of American Medicine.* New York: Viking, 1941.

Garrison, Fielding. *John Shaw Billings, a Memoir.* New York: G. P. Putnam's Sons, 1915.

Heuer, George. "Dr. Halsted." *Bulletin of the Johns Hopkins Hospital* 90 (February 1952): supplement.

Holman, Emile. "Halsted Centenary." *Surgery* 32 (1952):443–550.

Howell, Joel. *Technology in the Hospital: Transforming Patient Care in the Early Twentieth Century.* Baltimore: The Johns Hopkins University Press, 1995.

Kaufman, Martin. *American Medical Education: The Formative Years, 1765–1910.* Westport, Conn.: Greenwood Press, 1976.

Ludmerer, Kenneth. *Learning to Heal: The Development of American Medical Education.* New York: Basic Books, 1985.

MacCallum, William. *William Stewart Halsted, Surgeon.* Baltimore: The Johns Hopkins Press, 1930.

Mallon, William. *Ernest Amory Codman: The End Result of a Life in Medicine.* Philadelphia: W. B. Saunders, 2000.

Nuland, Sherwin. *Doctors: The Biography of Medicine.* New York: Alfred A. Knopf, 1988.

Nunn, Daniel. "Dr. Halsted's Addiction." *Johns Hopkins Advanced Studies in Medicine* 6 (2006):106–8.

———. "William Stewart Halsted: Transitional Years." *Surgery* 121 (1997):343–51.

Olch, Peter. "William S. Halsted's New York Period, 1874–1886." *Bulletin of the History of Medicine* 40 (1966):495–510.

———. "William S. Halsted and Local Anesthesia: Contributions and Complications." *Anesthesiology* 42 (1975):479–86.

Reverby, Susan. "Stealing the Golden Eggs: Ernest Amory Codman and the Science and Management of Medicine." *Bulletin of the History of Medicine* 55 (1981):156–71.

Rosenberg, Charles. *The Care of Strangers: The Rise of America's Hospital System.* New York: Basic Books, 1987.

Rosner, David. *A Once Charitable Enterprise: Hospital and Health Care in Brooklyn and New York, 1885–1915.* Cambridge: Cambridge University Press, 1982.

Rothstein, William. *American Medical Schools and the Practice of Medicine: A History.* New York: Oxford University Press, 1987.

Rutkow, Ira. "William Stewart Halsted and the Germanic Influence on Education and Training Programs in Surgery." *Surgery, Gynecology & Obstetrics* 147 (1978):602–6.

———. "How American Surgeons Introduced Radiology into United States Medicine." *American Journal of Surgery* 165 (1993):252–57.

———. "William Halsted, His Family, and 'Queer Business Methods.'" *Archives of Surgery* 131 (1996):123–27.

Stevens, Rosemary. *American Medicine and the Public Interest.* New Haven: Yale University Press, 1971.

Thompson, Roger. *Glimpses of Medical Europe.* Philadelphia: J. B. Lippincott, 1908.

Turner, Thomas. *Heritage of Excellence: The Johns Hopkins Medical Institutions, 1914–1947.* Baltimore: The Johns Hopkins University Press, 1974.

Vogel, Morris. *The Invention of the Modern Hospital, Boston, 1870–1930.* Chicago: University of Chicago Press, 1980.

1. Abraham Flexner, *I Remember: The Autobiography of Abraham Flexner* (New York: Simon & Schuster, 1940), p. 174.
2. William Ayres, "Post-Graduate Study in Europe," *New York Medical Journal* 37 (1883):204.
3. Rodney Glisan, *Two Years in Europe* (New York: G. P. Putnam's Sons, 1887), p. 379.
4. John Wheeler, *Memoirs of a Small-Town Surgeon* (New York: Garden City Publishing, 1935), p. 116.

5. Henry Hun, *A Guide to American Medical Students in Europe* (New York: William Wood, 1883), p. 15.
6. Ibid.
7. Quoted in Simon Flexner and James Flexner, *William Henry Welch and the Heroic Age of American Medicine* (New York: Viking, 1941), p. 99.
8. William Welch, "Report of the General Secretary," *Proceedings of the American Association for the Advancement of Science* 57 (1907):620.
9. "Patriarch's Party," *Time,* Monday, April 14, 1930, p. 32.
10. Remarks of Herbert Hoover, President of the United States, in *William Henry Welch at Eighty, a Memorial Record of Celebrations Around the World in His Honor,* edited by Victor Freeburg (New York: Milbank Memorial Fund, 1930), p. 35.
11. Hugh Young, *Hugh Young, A Surgeon's Autobiography* (New York: Harcourt, Brace, 1940), p. 65.
12. Quoted in Flexner and Flexner, *William Henry Welch,* p. 91.
13. Ibid., pp. 112–13.
14. Ibid., pp. 106–7.
15. Ibid., p. 112.
16. John Billings, "Higher Medical Education," *American Journal of the Medical Sciences* 76 (1878):184.
17. Quoted in Flexner and Flexner, *William Henry Welch,* p. 128.
18. William Welch, "Johns Hopkins Historical Club; Special Meeting, May 26, 1913, in Memory of Dr. John Shaw Billings," *Johns Hopkins Hospital Bulletin* 25 (1914): 252.
19. Quoted in Flexner and Flexner, *William Henry Welch,* p. 151.
20. Quoted in ibid., p. 159.
21. William Welch, "Biology and Medicine," *American Naturalist* 31 (1897):764.
22. Quoted in Flexner and Flexner, *William Henry Welch,* p. 220.
23. William Welch, "In Memoriam—William Stewart Halsted," *Bulletin of the Johns Hopkins Hospital* 36 (1925):38.
24. William Halsted, "The Training of the Surgeon," *Bulletin of the Johns Hopkins Hospital* 15 (1904):271.
25. Quoted in Donald Bates and Edward Bensley, "The Inner History of the Johns Hopkins Hospital—William Osler, MD, FRCP, FRS," *Johns Hopkins Medical Journal* 125 (1969):189.
26. Welch, "In Memoriam," p. 37.
27. William MacCallum, *William Stewart Halsted, Surgeon* (Baltimore: The Johns Hopkins Press, 1930), p. 42.
28. Welch, "In Memoriam," p. 37.
29. MacCallum, *William Stewart Halsted,* p. viii.
30. Peter Olch, "William S. Halsted and Local Anesthesia: Contributions and Complications," *Anesthesiology* 42 (1975):483.
31. Quoted in Flexner and Flexner, *William Henry Welch,* p. 159.
32. Quoted in Peter Olch, "William Stewart Halsted: Legendary Figure of American Surgery," *Review of Surgery* 20 (1963):87.
33. Bertram Bernheim, *The Story of the Johns Hopkins, Four Great Doctors and the Medical School They Created* (New York: Whittlesey House, 1948), p. 14.
34. Harvey Cushing, *The Life of Sir William Osler* (Oxford: At the Clarendon Press, 1925), vol. 1, p. 325.
35. Welch, "In Memoriam," p. 38.
36. Bernheim, *The Story of,* p. 21.
37. Ibid.
38. MacCallum, *William Stewart Halsted,* p. x.
39. Halsted, "The Training of," p. 273.

40. Ibid.
41. Walter Burket, *Papers and Addresses by William Henry Welch* ("The advancement of medical education") (Baltimore: The Johns Hopkins Press, 1920), vol. 3, p. 43.
42. Halsted, "The Training of," p. 272.
43. Bernheim, *The story of,* pp. 43–44.
44. Abraham Flexner, *Medical Education in the United States and Canada* (New York: Carnegie Foundation, 1910), p. 174.
45. Halsted, "The Training of," p. 275.
46. William Welch, "The Hospital in Relation to Medical Science," *Journal of the American Medical Association* 59 (1912):1668.
47. William Keen, "Address in Surgery," *Journal of the American Medical Association* 28 (1897):1107.
48. William Keen, *Medical Research and Human Welfare; a Record of Personal Experiences and Observations During a Professional Life of Fifty-seven Years* (Boston: Houghton Mifflin, 1917), pp. 27–28.
49. Quoted in Armond Goldman, "What Was the Cause of Franklin Delano Roosevelt's Paralytic Illness?" *Journal of Medical Biography* 11 (2003):234.
50. Quoted in Ira Rutkow, "The Letters of William Stewart Halsted and William Williams Keen," *Surgery* 100 (1986):558.
51. William Keen, *Medical Research and Human,* pp. 159–60.
52. *New York Times,* Thursday, January 16, 1896, p. 9.
53. William Hering, "A Year of the X Rays," *Popular Science Monthly* 50 (1897):654.
54. William Keen, "The Use of the Röntgen or X Rays in Surgery," in *System of Surgery,* edited by Frederic Dennis (New York: Lea Brothers, 1896), vol. 4, p. 947.
55. Ibid. p. 955.
56. William Morton, *The X Ray or Photography of the Invisible and Its Value in Surgery* (New York: American Technical Book, 1896), p. 161.
57. Maurice Richardson, "The Practical Value of the Roentgen Ray in the Routine Work of Surgical Office Practice," *Medical News* 69 (1896):719.
58. Thomas Edison, "Photographing the Unseen, a Symposium on the Roentgen Rays," *Century Magazine* 52 (1896):130.
59. Charles Leonard, "The Past, Present, and Future of the Röntgen Ray," *American Medicine* 10 (1905):1083.
60. Keen, "The Use of the Röntgen," p. 953.
61. Morton, *The X Ray or Photography,* p. 160.
62. Quoted in J. William White, "Report of the Committee of the American Surgical Association on the Medico-Legal Relations of the X-Rays," *American Journal of the Medical Sciences* 120 (1900):32.
63. J[ohn] H[omans], "Obituary—Ernest Amory Codman, 1869–1940," *New England Journal of Medicine* 224 (1941):299.
64. Ernest Codman, "Case-Records and Their Value," *Bulletin of the American College of Surgeons* 3 (1917):24.
65. Frederic Washburn, *The Massachusetts General Hospital: Its Development, 1900–1935* (Boston: Houghton Mifflin, 1939), p. 433.
66. Ernest Codman, "The Analysis of End-Results, Joint Discussion," *Surgery, Gynecology & Obstetrics* 36 (1923):140.
67. Eugene Pool, "The Analysis of End-Results, Joint Discussion," *Surgery, Gynecology & Obstetrics* 36 (1923):139.
68. Ernest Codman, *A Study in Hospital Efficiency, as Demonstrated by the Case Report of the First Five Years of a Private Hospital* (Boston: np, nd, probably 1916), p. 175.
69. Ernest Codman, *The Shoulder: Rupture of the Supraspinatus Tendon and Other Lesions In or About the Subacromial Bursa* (Boston: private printing, 1934), p. xxii.

70. Philip Hale [drawn for Ernest Codman], In the Codman papers located at The Francis A. Countway Library of Medicine, Boston.
71. J[ohn] H[omans], "Obituary," p. 298.
72. Codman, *The Shoulder,* p. xxv.

Six Professional Authority

Berliner, Howard. "A Larger Perspective on the Flexner Report." *International Journal of Health Services* 5 (1975):573–92.

Bonner, Thomas. *Iconoclast: Abraham Flexner and a Life in Learning.* Baltimore: The Johns Hopkins University Press, 2002.

Crile, Grace. *George Crile: An Autobiography,* 2 vols. Philadelphia: J. B. Lippincott, 1947.

Davis, Loyal. *Fellowship of Surgeons: A History of the American College of Surgeons.* Springfield, Ill.: Charles C. Thomas, 1960.

Duffy, John. *From Humors to Medical Sciences: A History of American Medicine.* Urbana: University of Illinois Press, 1993.

English, Peter. *Shock, Physiological Surgery, and George Washington Crile: Medical Innovation in the Progressive Era.* Westport, Conn.: Greenwood Press, 1980.

Flexner, Abraham. *I Remember: The Autobiography of Abraham Flexner.* New York: Simon & Schuster, 1940.

Hudson, Robert. "Abraham Flexner in Perspective: American Medical Education, 1865–1910." *Bulletin of the History of Medicine* 46 (1972):545–61.

Ludmerer, Kenneth. *Learning to Heal: The Development of American Medical Education.* New York: Basic Books, 1985.

Martin, Franklin. *The Joy of Living: An Autobiography,* 2 vols. Garden City, N.Y.: Doubleday, Doran, 1933.

Rosenberg, Charles. *The Care of Strangers: The Rise of America's Hospital System.* New York: Basic Books, 1987.

Sigerist, Henry. *American Medicine.* New York: W. W. Norton, 1934.

Starr, Paul. *The Social Transformation of American Medicine.* New York: Basic Books, 1982.

Stevens, Rosemary. *American Medicine and the Public Interest.* New Haven: Yale University Press, 1971.

———. *In Sickness and in Wealth: American Hospitals in the Twentieth Century.* New York: Basic Books, 1989.

1. Abraham Flexner, *I Remember: The Autobiography of Abraham Flexner* (New York: Simon & Schuster, 1940), p. 122.
2. Abraham Flexner, *Medical Education in the United States and Canada* (New York: Carnegie Foundation for the Advancement of Teaching, 1910), p. 223.
3. Ibid., p. 225.
4. Flexner, *I Remember,* p. 97.
5. Abraham Flexner, *The American College: A Criticism* (New York: Century, 1908), p. 38.
6. Flexner, *I Remember,* p. 111.
7. Ibid., p. 115.
8. Ibid., p. 131.
9. Ibid., p. 19.
10. Ibid., p. 42.
11. Ibid., p. 89.
12. Flexner, *Medical Education,* p. 16.
13. *New York Times,* Sunday, July 24, 1910, *Magazine,* p. 1.
14. Flexner, *Medical Education,* p. 142.

15. Quoted in Kenneth Ludmerer, *Learning to Heal: The Development of American Medical Education* (New York: Basic Books, 1985), pp. 180–81.
16. Flexner, *I Remember,* p. 279.
17. Samuel Chotzinoff, "Robin Hood, 1930," *New Yorker,* November 22, 1930, p. 31.
18. *New York Times,* Monday, May 28, 1928, p. 24.
19. Loyal Davis, *Fellowship of Surgeons: A History of the American College of Surgeons* (Springfield, Ill.: Charles C. Thomas, 1960), p. 444.
20. Franklin Martin, *The Joy of Living: An Autobiography,* 2 vols. (Garden City, N.Y.: Doubleday, Doran, 1933), vol. 1, p. 330.
21. Davis, *Fellowship of Surgeons,* p. 3.
22. Martin, *The Joy of,* vol. 1, p. 397.
23. Ibid., p. 404.
24. *Philadelphia Inquirer,* Saturday, November 11, 1911, p. 1.
25. Martin, *The Joy of,* vol. 1, p. 409.
26. Anon., "Editorial, The American College of Surgeons," *Journal of the Michigan State Medical Society* 12 (1913):338.
27. Martin, *The Joy of,* vol. 1, p. 414.
28. Philip Jones, "The American Royal College of Surgeons-J.B.M.," *California State Journal of Medicine* 11 (1913):176.
29. *New York Times,* Sunday, August 10, 1913, p. 11.
30. Martin, *The Joy of,* vol. 1, p. 444.
31. Ibid., p. 445.
32. "Hospital Standardization," *Bulletin of the American College of Surgeons* 6 (1922):3.
33. Ibid.
34. Ibid.
35. Martin, *The Joy of,* vol. 1, p. 446.
36. William Shepherd, "The New Control of Surgeons," *Harper's,* February 1924, pp. 303, 311.
37. Hawthorne Daniel, "Better Hospitals for Everybody," *The World's Work,* June 1920, p. 208.
38. Council on Medical Education, "Hospital Intern Year," *Journal of the American Medical Association* 73 (1919):521.
39. John Dodson, "The Fifth, or Intern, Year," *Journal of the American Medical Association* 73 (1919):471–72.
40. Council on Medical Education and Hospitals, "Hospitals Furnishing Acceptable Internships," *Journal of the American Medical Association* 75 (1920):409.
41. "Editorial: Hospital Service in the United States," *Journal of the American Medical Association* 76 (1921):1104.
42. Council on Medical Education and Hospitals, "Hospitals Approved for Advanced Internships and Residencies," *Journal of the American Medical Association* 88 (1927):828.
43. Martin, *The Joy of,* vol. 1, p. 462.
44. "Editorial: An Artist in Surgery," *New York Times,* Friday, January 8, 1943, p. 18.
45. Grace Crile, *George Crile: An Autobiography,* 2 vols. (Philadelphia: J. B. Lippincott, 1947), vol. 1, p. 248.
46. George Crile, "The Unit Plan of Organization of the Medical Reserve Corps of the U.S.A. for Service in Base Hospitals," *Surgery, Gynecology & Obstetrics* 22 (1916):68.
47. Anon., "Some Views Concerning the United States Army Medical Corps," *Boston Medical and Surgical Journal* 174 (1916):359.
48. Crile, *George Crile: An Autobiography,* vol. 1, p. 271.
49. *Philadelphia Inquirer,* Sunday, October 29, 1916, p. 2.
50. Eric Rutkow and Ira Rutkow, "George Crile, Harvey Cushing, and the Ambulance Américaine: Military Medical Preparedness in World War I," *Archives of Surgery* 139 (2004):684.

51. Crile, *George Crile: An Autobiography,* vol. 1, p. 279.
52. Ibid., pp. 301–2.
53. Martin, *The Joy of,* vol. 2, p. 200.
54. Victor Vaughan, "The Promotion of Periodic Health Examinations by the Medical Profession," *American Medical Association Bulletin* 16 (1923):297.

Seven Challenges of Success

Bordley, James III, and A. McGehee Harvey. *Two Centuries of American Medicine, 1776–1976.* Philadelphia: W. B. Saunders, 1976.

Cassedy, James. *Medicine in America: A Short History.* Baltimore: The Johns Hopkins University Press, 1991.

Duffy, John. *From Humors to Medical Science: A History of American Medicine.* Urbana: University of Illinois Press, 1993.

Fishbein, Morris. *Morris Fishbein, M.D. An Autobiography.* Garden City, N.Y.: Doubleday, 1969.

Galdston, Iago. *Progress in Medicine: A Critical Review of the Last Hundred Years.* New York: Alfred A. Knopf, 1940.

Howell, Joel. *Technology in the Hospital: Transforming Patient Care in the Early Twentieth Century.* Baltimore: The Johns Hopkins University Press, 1995.

Mueller, C. Barber. *Evarts A. Graham: The Life and Times of the Surgical Spirit of St. Louis.* Hamilton, Ontario: B. C. Decker, 2002.

Shryock, Richard. *American Medical Research, Past and Present.* New York: The Commonwealth Fund, 1947.

Starr, Paul. *The Social Transformation of American Medicine.* New York: Basic Books, 1982.

Stern, Bernhard. *American Medical Practice in the Perspectives of a Century.* New York: The Commonwealth Fund, 1945.

Stevens, Rosemary. *American Medicine and the Public Interest.* New Haven: Yale University Press, 1971.

———. *In Sickness and in Wealth: American Hospitals in the Twentieth Century.* New York: Basic Books, 1989.

1. Iago Galdston, "Recent Medical Progress," *New Republic,* June 23, 1937, p. 180.
2. Rufus Cole, "Progress of Medicine During the Past Twenty-Five Years," *Science* 71 (1930):624.
3. *New York Times,* Sunday, March 11, 1936, sec. 2, p. 1.
4. Roy Hoskins, "The Internal Secretions," in *Chemistry in Medicine,* edited by Julius Stieglitz (New York: The Chemical Foundation, 1928), p. 194.
5. I. Holmgren, "Presentation Speech on December 10, 1934," in *Nobel Lectures, Physiology or Medicine, 1922–1941* (Amsterdam: Published for the Nobel Foundation by Elsevier, 1965), p. 339.
6. *New York Times,* Friday, October 26, 1934, p. 18.
7. Editorial, *New York Times,* Saturday, October 27, 1934, p. 14.
8. William Castle, "Observations on the Etiologic Relationship of Achylia Gastrica to Pernicious Anemia," *American Journal of the Medical Sciences* 178 (1929):754.
9. Charles Truax, *The Mechanics of Surgery, Comprising Descriptions, Illustrations and Lists of the Instruments, Appliances and Furniture Necessary in Modern Surgical Art* (Chicago: Charles Truax, 1899), p. 38.
10. Cole, "Progress of Medicine," p. 622.
11. Paul White, "Angina Pectoris: Historical Background," in *Angina Pectoris,* edited by Paul Oglesby (New York: Medcom Press, 1974), p. 9.

12. Reginald H. Fitz, "Perforating Inflammation of the Vermiform Appendix; with Special Reference to Its Early Diagnosis and Treatment," *American Journal of the Medical Sciences* 92 (1886):321.

13. Samuel Hopkins Adams, "Modern Surgery," *McClure's Magazine,* March 1905, p. 484.

14. Martin Tinker, "America's Contribution to Surgery," *Johns Hopkins Hospital Bulletin* 13 (1902):212.

15. John Deaver, "Appendicitis," *Philadelphia Medical Journal* 10 (1902):21.

16. Moses Benmosché, *A Surgeon Explains to the Layman* (New York: Simon & Schuster, 1940), p. 36.

17. Ernest Smith, *The Making of a Surgeon: A Midwestern Chronicle* (Fond du Lac, Wisc.: private printing, 1942), p. 281.

18. J. B. Herbert, "Appendicitis—the Doctor's Song." Sam DeVincent Collection of Illustrated Sheet Music, Smithsonian Institution, Museum of American History, Washington, D.C.

19. Sinclair Lewis, *Arrowsmith* (New York: Harcourt, Brace, 1925), p. 210.

20. Collection of author.

21. Quoted in Kenneth Silverman, *Houdini!!! The Career of Ehrich Weiss* (New York: HarperCollins, 1996), p. 407.

22. *New York Times,* Tuesday, October 26, 1926, p. 27.

23. Astley Ashhurst, "Discussion," in Le Grand Guerry, "A Study of the Mortality in Appendicitis," *Transactions of the American Surgical Association* 54 (1926):147.

24. Quoted in Ruth Brandon, *The Life and Many Deaths of Harry Houdini* (New York: Random House, 1993), p. 291.

25. *New York Times,* Tuesday, October 26, 1926, p. 27.

26. *New York Times,* Monday, November 1, 1926, pp. 1, 6.

27. Quoted in Silverman, *Houdini!!!,* p. 412.

28. *New York Times,* Wednesday, October 27, 1926, p. 27.

29. Ibid.

30. Morris Fishbein, "Progress in Medical Science," *The Forum,* December 1923, p. 2230.

31. *New York Evening Graphic,* Monday, November 1, 1926, p. 1.

32. *New York Times,* Saturday, October 30, 1926, p. 17.

33. *New York Times,* Thursday, December 23, 1926, p. 4.

34. Bernhard Stern, *American Medical Practice in the Perspectives of a Century* (New York: The Commonwealth Fund, 1945), pp. 65, 69.

35. Michael Davis, "The American Approach to Health Insurance," *Milbank Memorial Fund Quarterly* 12 (1934):214–15.

36. Editorial, "Can We Afford Good Health?" *The New Republic,* December 7, 1932, p. 86.

37. *Time,* June 21, 1937, p. 28.

38. Morris Fishbein, *Morris Fishbein, M.D., An Autobiography* (Garden City, N.Y.: Doubleday, 1969), p. 144.

39. Quoted in Pope Brock, *Charlatan: America's Most Dangerous Huckster, the Man Who Pursued Him, and the Age of Flimflam* (New York: Crown, 2008), p. 87.

40. Morris Fishbein, *The Medical Follies* (New York: Boni & Liveright, 1925), p. 218.

41. James Rorty, "The Attack on Group Medicine," *The Nation,* July 4, 1936, p. 16.

42. Walter Bierring, "The Family Doctor and the Changing Order," *Journal of the American Medical Association* 102 (1934):1997.

43. *New York Times,* Wednesday, November 30, 1932, pp. 1, 10.

44. Morris Fishbein, Editorial, "The Report of the Committee on the Costs of Medical Care," *Journal of the American Medical Association* 99 (1932):2035.

45. Edward Bernays, *Biography of an Idea: Memoirs of Public Relations Counsel Edward L. Bernays* (New York: Simon & Schuster, 1965), pp. 477, 479.

46. Fishbein, Editorial, "The Report of," p. 2035.

47. Bernays, *Biography of an Idea,* p. 482.

48. Fishbein, *Morris Fishbein, M.D.,* p. 193.
49. *New York Times,* Wednesday, November 30, 1932, p. 10.
50. *New York Times,* Sunday, January 8, 1933, p. 31.
51. *The Nation,* February 22, 1933, p. 207.
52. *New York Times,* Sunday, January 8, 1933, p. 31.
53. *Time,* December 5, 1932, p. 45.
54. Fishbein, *Morris Fishbein, M.D.,* p. 195.
55. Bernays, *Biography of an Idea,* p. 484.
56. *Time,* June 21, 1937, cover.
57. Morris Fishbein, Editorial, "The American Foundation Proposals for Medical Care," *Journal of the American Medical Association* 109 (1937):1280.
58. Ibid., p. 1281.
59. Avis Carlson, "The Doctors Face Revolt," *Harper's,* September 1938, p. 399.
60. Morris Fishbein, *A History of the American Medical Association, 1847 to 1947* (Philadelphia: W. B. Saunders, 1947), p. 908.
61. Morris Fishbein, Editorial, "Accrediting Examining Boards in the Specialties," *Journal of the American Medical Association* 101 (1933):715.
62. Quoted in Peter Olch, "Evarts A. Graham, the American College of Surgeons, and the American Board of Surgery," *Journal of the History of Medicine and Allied Sciences* 27 (1972):252.
63. Evarts Graham, "What Is Surgery?" *Southern Medical Journal* 18 (1925):865.
64. Edward Archibald, "Address of the President—Higher Degrees in the Profession of Surgery," *Annals of Surgery* 102 (1935):481.
65. Quoted in Peter Olch, "Evarts A. Graham," p. 257.
66. "American Board of Surgery Organized," *Journal of the American Medical Association* 108 (1937):1723.

Eight Ascendancy

Bordley, James, and A. McGehee Harvey. *Two Centuries of American Medicine, 1776–1976.* Philadelphia: W. B. Saunders, 1976.
Fenster, Julie. *Mavericks, Miracles, and Medicine: The Pioneers Who Risked Their Lives to Bring Medicine into the Modern Age.* New York: Barnes & Noble Books, 2003.
Hamilton, Virginia. *Lister Hill: Statesman from the South.* Chapel Hill: University of North Carolina Press, 1987.
Johnson, Stephen. *The History of Cardiac Surgery, 1896–1955.* Baltimore: The Johns Hopkins Press, 1970.
Lederer, Susan. *Flesh and Blood: Organ Transplantation and Blood Transfusion in the 20th Century.* New York: Oxford University Press, 2008.
Love, Spencie. *One Blood: The Death and Resurrection of Charles R. Drew.* Chapel Hill: University of North Carolina Press, 1996.
Organ, Claude, and Margaret Kosiba. *A Century of Black Surgeons, the U.S.A. Experience.* Norman, Okla.: Transcript Press, 1987.
Romaine-Davis, Ada. *John Gibbon and His Heart-Lung Machine.* Philadelphia: University of Pennsylvania Press, 1991.
Shryock, Richard. *American Medical Research, Past and Present.* New York: The Commonwealth Fund, 1947.
Starr, Paul. *The Social Transformation of American Medicine.* New York: Basic Books, 1982.
Stevens, Rosemary. *American Medicine and the Public Interest.* New Haven: Yale University Press, 1971.
———. *In Sickness and in Wealth: American Hospitals in the Twentieth Century.* New York: Basic Books, 1989.

Strickland, Stephen. *Politics, Science, and Dread Disease: A Short History of United States Medical Research Policy*. Cambridge, Mass.: Harvard University Press, 1972.

1. Bernard Fantus, "The Therapy of the Cook County Hospital," *Journal of the American Medical Association* 109 (1937):128.
2. "Blood Transfusion Betterment Association," *Bulletin of the New York Academy of Medicine* 6 (1930):682.
3. *New York Times,* Monday, August 12, 1940, p. 18.
4. DeWitt Stetten, "The Blood Plasma for Great Britain Project," *Bulletin of the New York Academy of Medicine* 17 (1941):29.
5. Ibid., p. 33.
6. Ibid., p. 36.
7. Quoted in Spencie Love, *One Blood: The Death and Resurrection of Charles R. Drew* (Chapel Hill: University of North Carolina Press, 1996), p. 105.
8. Ibid., p. 143.
9. David Bull and Charles Drew, "Symposium on Fluid and Electrolyte Needs of Surgical Patients: The Preservation of Blood," *Annals of Surgery* 112 (1940):501.
10. Quoted in Love, *One Blood,* p. 149.
11. Stetten, "The Blood Plasma," p. 37.
12. Quoted in Love, *One Blood,* p. 152.
13. Quoted in Charles R(ichard) Drew, *Current Biography Yearbook* (New York: H. W. Wilson, 1944), p. 180.
14. John Rankin, "Labeling of Blood Banks," *Appendix to the Congressional Record.* Washington, D.C.: Government Printing Office, 77th Congress, 2nd session, [May 28th] 1942, 88:9, p. A1985.
15. *New York Times,* Friday, March 31, 1944, p. 23.
16. *New York Times,* Friday, August 10, 1945, p. 16.
17. Quoted in Henry Beecher, "Resuscitation of Men Severely Wounded in Battle," in *Medical Department, United States Army, Surgery in World War II,* edited by John Coates and Michael DeBakey (Washington: Office of the Surgeon General, 1955) (vol. 2), p. xiv.
18. Quoted in Chester Keefer, "Dr. Richards as Chairman of the Committee on Medical Research," *Annals of Internal Medicine* 71[supplement] (1969):61.
19. Richard Shryock, *American Medical Research, Past and Present* (New York: The Commonwealth Fund, 1947), p. 293.
20. *New York Times,* Saturday, January 15, 1944, p. 3.
21. Charles Bailey, Robert Glover, and Thomas O'Neill, "The Surgery of Mitral Stenosis," *Journal of Thoracic Surgery* 19 (1950):16.
22. John Gibbon, "The Development of the Heart-Lung Apparatus," *American Journal of Surgery* 135 (1978):608.
23. Ibid., p. 609.
24. Ibid., p. 615.
25. John Gibbon, "The Development of the Heart-Lung Apparatus," *Review of Surgery* 27 (1970):236.
26. *Time,* September 26, 1949, p. 42.
27. Quoted in Stephen Johnson, *The History of Cardiac Surgery, 1896–1955* (Baltimore: The Johns Hopkins Press, 1970), p. 149.
28. Quoted in Ada Romaine-Davis, *John Gibbon and His Heart-Lung Machine* (Philadelphia: University of Pennsylvania Press, 1991), p. 121.
29. *New York Times,* Friday, May 8, 1953, p. 31.
30. *Time,* May 18, 1953, p. 48.
31. Editorial, "Machine Hearts," *New York Times,* Sunday, May 10, 1953, section iv, p. 10.
32. Editorial, "Senator from Alabama," *New York Times,* Saturday, January 27, 1968, p. 28.

33. Morris Fishbein, *Morris Fishbein, M.D.: An Autobiography* (Garden City, N.Y.: Doubleday, 1969), p. 469.

34. Quoted in Stephen Strickland, *Politics, Science, and Dread Disease: A Short History of United States Medical Research Policy* (Cambridge, Mass.: Harvard University Press, 1972), pp. 225–26.

35. Editorial, "Money for Heart Ills," *New York Times,* Wednesday, June 16, 1948, p. 28.

36. Thomas Kennedy, "James A. Shannon and the Beginnings of the Laboratory of Kidney and Electrolyte Metabolism of the National Institutes of Health," *Kidney International* 55 (1999):329.

37. James Shannon, "The Advancement of Medical Research: A Twenty-Year View of the Role of the National Institutes of Health," *Journal of Medical Education* 42 (1967):101.

38. Elizabeth Drew, "The Health Syndicate: Washington's Noble Conspirators," *Atlantic Monthly,* December 1967, p. 80.

39. Paul Douglas, "Departments of Labor, and Health, Education, and Welfare, and Related Appropriations, 1964," *Congressional Record.* Washington, D.C.: Government Printing Office, 88th Congress, 1st session, [August 7th] 1963, 109:11, pp. 14498.

40. Kennedy, "James A. Shannon," p. 332.

41. Quoted in Patricia Kendall, *The Relationship Between Medical Educators and Medical Practitioners: Sources of Strain and Occasions for Cooperation* (Evanston, Ill.: Association of American Medical Colleges, 1965), p. 36.

42. Ibid., p. 42.

Nine Supremacy

Blumenthal, David, and James Morone. *Health and Politics in the Oval Office.* Berkeley: University of California Press, 2009.

Bordley, James, and A. McGehee Harvey. *Two Centuries of American Medicine, 1776–1976.* Philadelphia: W. B. Saunders, 1976.

Fenster, Julie. *Mavericks, Miracles, and Medicine: The Pioneers Who Risked Their Lives to Bring Medicine into the Modern Age.* New York: Barnes & Noble Books, 2003.

Krueger, Gretchen. *Hope and Suffering: Children, Cancer, and the Paradox of Experimental Medicine.* Baltimore: The Johns Hopkins University Press, 2008.

Lederer, Susan. *Flesh and Blood: Organ Transplantation and Blood Transfusion in Twentieth-Century America.* New York: Oxford University Press, 2008.

Marmor, Theodore. *The Politics of Medicare.* New York: Aldine de Gruyter, 2000.

Moore, Francis D. *Transplant: The Give and Take of Tissue Transplantation.* New York: Simon & Schuster, 1964.

———. *A Miracle and a Privilege: Recounting a Half Century of Surgical Advance.* Washington, D.C.: Joseph Henry Press, 1995.

Nuland, Sherwin. *Doctors: The Biography of Medicine.* New York: Alfred A. Knopf, 1988.

Oberlander, Jonathan. *The Political Life of Medicare.* Chicago: University of Chicago Press, 2003.

Patterson, James. *The Dread Disease: Cancer and Modern American Culture.* Cambridge, Mass.: Harvard University Press, 1987.

Retting, Richard. *Cancer Crusade: The Story of the National Cancer Act of 1971.* Princeton, N.J.: Princeton University Press, 1977.

Starr, Paul. *The Social Transformation of American Medicine.* New York: Basic Books, 1982.

Stevens, Rosemary. *American Medicine and the Public Interest.* New Haven: Yale University Press, 1971.

Strickland, Stephen. *Politics, Science, and Dread Disease: A Short History of United States Medical Research Policy.* Cambridge, Mass.: Harvard University Press, 1972.

Weisz, George. *Divide and Conquer: A Comparative History of Medical Specialization.* New York: Oxford University Press, 2005.

1. Thomas E. Starzl, *The Puzzle People: Memoirs of a Transplant Surgeon* (Pittsburgh: University of Pittsburgh Press, 1992), p. 71.
2. *Time,* May 3, 1963, cover.
3. Ibid., p. 60.
4. Francis D. Moore, *A Miracle and a Privilege: Recounting a Half Century of Surgical Advance* (Washington, D.C.: Joseph Henry Press, 1995), p. 19.
5. Ibid., p. 163.
6. S. James Adelstein, Eugene Braunwald, et al., "George Widmer Thorn," *Harvard University Gazette,* November 3, 2005, p. 8.
7. John Merrill, George Thorn, Carl Walter, et al., "The Use of an Artificial Kidney. II. Clinical Experience," *Journal of Clinical Investigation* 29 (1950):425.
8. Quoted in Francis D. Moore, *Transplant: The Give and Take of Tissue Transplantation* (New York: Simon & Schuster, 1972), p. 84.
9. *Time,* October 2, 1950, pp. 61, 62.
10. John Merrill, Joseph Murray, J. Hartwell Harrison, and Warren Guild, "Successful Homotransplantation of the Human Kidney Between Identical Twins," *Journal of the American Medical Association* 160 (1956):278.
11. Moore, *Transplant,* p. 100.
12. Quoted in Julie Fenster, *Mavericks, Miracles, and Medicine: The Pioneers Who Risked Their Lives to Bring Medicine into the Modern Age* (New York: Barnes & Noble Books, 2003), p. 277.
13. Quoted in Jürgen Thorwald, *The Patients* (New York: Harcourt Brace Jovanovich, 1971), p. 137.
14. Moore, *A Miracle,* p. 172.
15. Ibid., p. 173.
16. Carried in *New York Times,* Tuesday, December 28, 1954, p. 25.
17. Quoted in Moore, *Transplant,* p. 109.
18. Moore, *A Miracle,* p. 184.
19. A. E. Ritt, "A Tradition Well Worth Preserving," *GP* 2 (1950):123.
20. Nicholas Pisacano, "History of the Specialty," found at: https://www.theabfm.org/about/history.aspx (viewed on February 3, 2009).
21. *Stedman's Medical Dictionary* (Baltimore: Williams & Wilkins, 1972), p. 1168.
22. *New York Times,* Saturday, April 16, 1949, p. 1.
23. *New York Times,* Thursday, January 5, 1961, p. 33.
24. Quoted in Jonathan Oberlander, *The Political Life of Medicare* (Chicago: University of Chicago Press, 2003), p. 27.
25. *New York Times,* Tuesday, May 22, 1962, p. 1.
26. Ibid.
27. Statement of Donovan Ward, *Medical Care for the Aged, Executive Hearings Before the Committee on Ways and Means, House of Representatives, Eighty-ninth Congress, First Session on H.R. 1 and Other Proposals for Medical Care for the Aged, January 27, 28, February 1, 2, 3, 4, 5, 8, 9, 10, and 16, 1965 [Part one].* Washington, D.C.: Government Printing Office, 1965, p. 745.
28. Remarks of Walter Moeller, *Congressional Record,* Washington, D.C.: Government Printing Office, 89th Congress, 1st session, [April 8th] 1965, 111:6, p. 7433.
29. Quoted in the *New York Daily News,* Sunday, June 20, 1965, p. 114.
30. *New York Times,* Tuesday, June 22, 1965, p. 45.
31. Ibid.
32. *Time,* July 2, 1965, p. 36.

33. Ibid.
34. *New York Times,* Monday, June 21, 1965, p. 22.
35. *New York Daily News,* Wednesday, June 23, 1965, p. 10.
36. *New York Times,* Monday, June 21, 1965, p. 22.
37. *New York Times,* Tuesday, June 22, 1965, p. 42.
38. Quoted in *New York Times,* Thursday, December 3, 1964, p. 48.
39. Quoted in *New York Times,* Wednesday, September 2, 1981, p. A17.
40. *Time,* July 2, 1965, p. 36.
41. Quoted in *The New Republic,* July 10, 1965, p. 7.
42. *New York Times,* Monday, June 21, 1965, p. 1.
43. *AMA News,* June 28, 1965, pp. 1, 7.
44. *The New Republic,* July 10, 1965, p. 7.
45. *Time,* July 2, 1965, p. 36.
46. *New York Times,* Tuesday, June 22, 1965, p. 42.
47. Quoted in *Caring for the Country: A History and Celebration of the First 150 Years of the American Medical Association* (Chicago: American Medical Association, 1997), p. 91.
48. *AMA News,* October 11, 1965, p. 11.
49. *New York Times,* Friday, November 26, 1965, p. 39.
50. Ibid.
51. Henry Skinner, *The Origin of Medical Terms* (Baltimore: Williams & Wilkins, 1949), p. 74.
52. Sidney Farber, Louis Diamond, Robert Mercer, et al., "Temporary Remissions in Acute Leukemia in Children Produced by Folic Acid Antagonist, 4-Aminopteroyl-Glutamic Acid (Aminopterin)," *New England Journal of Medicine* 238 (1948):781, 789.
53. *Time,* October 8, 1956, p. 64.
54. Quoted in *New York Times,* Saturday, March 31, 1973, p. 38.
55. "Listen to the May 22, 1948, broadcast," found at: http://www.jimmyfund.org/abo/broad/jimmybroadcast.html (viewed on March 18, 2009).
56. Ibid.
57. *New York Times,* Saturday, November 5, 1960, p. 25.
58. *Time,* February 21, 1969, cover.
59. *New York Times,* Friday, July 11, 1969, p. 1.
60. *New York Times,* Wednesday, November 12, 1969, p. 40.
61. *New York Times,* Tuesday, December 9, 1969, p. 61.
62. Richard Nixon, "Annual Message to the Congress on the State of the Union" (January 22, 1971), found at: http://www.presidency.ucsb.edu/ws/index.php?pid=3110 (viewed on March 26, 2009).

Ten Transformation

Blumenthal, David, and James Morone. *Health and Politics in the Oval Office.* Berkeley: University of California Press, 2009.

Brownlee, Shannon. *Overtreated: Why Too Much Medicine Is Making Us Sicker and Poorer.* New York: Bloomsbury, 2007.

Cohn, Jonathan. *Sick: The Untold Story of America's Health Care Crisis—and the People Who Pay the Price.* New York: HarperCollins, 2007.

Duffy, John. *From Humors to Medical Science: A History of American Medicine,* 2nd ed. Urbana: University of Illinois Press, 1993.

Emanuel, Ezekiel. *Healthcare Guaranteed: A Simple, Secure Solution for America.* New York: Public Affairs, 2008.

Feldstein, Paul. *Health Policy Issues: An Economic Perspective.* Chicago: Health Policy Press, 2007.

Groopman, Jerome. *How Doctors Think*. Boston: Houghton Mifflin, 2007.

Kassirer, Jerome. *On the Take: How America's Complicity with Big Business Can Endanger Your Health*. New York: Oxford, 2005.

Klaidman, Stephen. *Coronary: A True Story of Medicine Gone Awry*. New York: Scribner, 2007.

Monagan, David. *Journey into the Heart: A Tale of Pioneering Doctors and Their Race to Transform Cardiovascular Medicine*. New York: Gotham Books, 2007.

Relman, Arnold. *A Second Opinion: Rescuing America's Healthcare*. New York: Public Affairs, 2007.

Rutkow, Ira, ed. *Socioeconomics of Surgery*. St. Louis, Mo.: C. V. Mosby, 1989.

Starr, Paul. *The Social Transformation of American Medicine*. New York: Basic Books, 1982.

Stevens, Rosemary, Louis Goodman, and Stephen Mick. *The Alien Doctors: Foreign Medical Graduates in American Hospitals*. New York: John Wiley & Sons, 1978.

1. Quoted in David Monagan, *Journey into the Heart: A Tale of Pioneering Doctors and Their Race to Transform Cardiovascular Medicine* (New York: Gotham Books, 2007), p. 69.
2. Quoted in Spencer King, "Angioplasty from Bench to Bedside to Bench," *Circulation* 93 (1996):1623.
3. Quoted in Monagan, *Journey into the Heart,* p. 4.
4. Andreas Grüntzig, Marko Turina, and Jakob Schneider, "Experimental Percutaneous Dilatation of Coronary Artery Stenosis," *Circulation* 54 (1976): [abstracts of the 49th scientific sessions; supplement #2] II-81.
5. Quoted in Monagan, *Journey into the Heart,* p. 112.
6. Ibid., p. 124.
7. Ibid., p. 125.
8. Quoted in Dolf Bachmann, "World's First Angioplasty Patient Now 68 Years Old and 'Happy All Around,' " found at: http://www.seconds-count.org/Details.aspx?PAGE_ID=69 (viewed on May 7, 2009).
9. Quoted in Monagan, *Journey into the Heart,* p. 129.
10. Quoted in King, "Angioplasty from Bench," p. 1625.
11. Quoted in Monagan, *Journey into the Heart,* p. 129.
12. Quoted in King: "Angioplasty from Bench," p. 1625.
13. *Time,* July 3, 1978, pp. 54–55.
14. *New York Times,* Tuesday, December 1, 1981, p. C2.
15. Quoted in Monagan, *Journey into the Heart,* p. 151.
16. Andreas Grüntzig, Åke Senning, and Walter Siegenthaler, "Nonoperative Dilatation of Coronary-Artery Stenosis: Percutaneous Transluminal Coronary Angioplasty," *New England Journal of Medicine* 301(1979):65.
17. Robert I. Levy, Michael B. Mock, Vallee L. Willman, and Peter L. Frommer, "Percutaneous Transluminal Coronary Angioplasty," *New England Journal of Medicine* 301(1979):103.
18. Arnold Relman, "The New Medical-Industrial Complex," *New England Journal of Medicine* 303(1980):963.
19. Dwight Eisenhower, "Military-Industrial Complex Speech" (January 17, 1961), found at: http://74.125.93.132/search?q=cache:abepB3lnCzsJ:avalon.law.yale.edu/20th_century/eisenhower001.asp+eisenhower+and+military+industrial+complex&cd=7&hl=en&ct=clnk&gl=us (viewed on June 19, 2009).
20. Monagan, *Journey into the Heart,* p. 171.
21. Quoted in ibid., p. 257.
22. Ronald Reagan, "Annual message to the Congress on the State of the Union" (February 6, 1985), found at: http://reagan2020.us/speeches/state_of_the_union_1985.asp (viewed on May 18, 2009).
23. Quoted in Monagan, *Journey into the Heart,* p. 101.

24. *New York Times,* Tuesday, October 29, 1985, p. D27.
25. Ibid.
26. *New York Times,* Tuesday, January 6, 2009, p. D7.
27. Bonnie Weaver, "On 30th Anniversary, Angioplasty Celebrated as Modern Medical Breakthrough in Stopping Heart Attack," found at: http://www.scai.org/pr.aspx?PAGE_ID=5186 (viewed on May 24, 2009).
28. Mark Ravitch, "Historical Perspective and Personal Viewpoint," in *Current Practice of Surgical Stapling,* edited by Mark Ravitch, Felicien Steichen, and Roger Welter (Philadelphia: Lea & Febiger, 1991), p. 3.
29. Ibid., p. 6.
30. *Time,* September 2, 1966, p. 61.
31. Ibid., p. 6.
32. Mark Ravitch, *Repair of Hernias* (Chicago: Year Book Medical Publishers, 1969), p. 7.
33. Ibid., p. 28.
34. Ibid., pp. 82–84.
35. *New York Times,* Wednesday, April 29, 2009, special report.
36. Letters to the editor (Mitchell Flaxman), *Palm Beach Post,* Sunday, April 1, 2007, p. 6E.
37. Letters to the editor (Mark Rattinger), *Palm Beach Post,* Sunday, April 1, 2007, p. 6E.
38. The Florida Masochist, "Knucklehead of the Day Award" (Monday, July 3, 2006), found at: http://thefloridamasochist.blogspot.com/2006/07/knucklehead-of-day-award_03 html (viewed on June 10, 2009).
39. *Palm Beach Post,* Thursday, March 22, 2007, p. 1.
40. *Palm Beach Post,* Tuesday, March 20, 2007, p. 1.
41. *Palm Beach Post,* Sunday, April 1, 2007, p. 19A.
42. Letters to the editor (Mark Rattinger), *Palm Beach Post,* Sunday, April 1, 2007, p. 6E.

SELECTED BIBLIOGRAPHY

Abel, John. *The Future Independence and Progress of American Medicine in the Age of Chemistry*. New York: Chemical Foundation, 1923.

Adams, George. *Doctors in Blue: The Medical History of the Union Army in the Civil War*. New York: Henry Schuman, 1962.

Allen, Arthur. *Vaccine: The Controversial Story of Medicine's Greatest Lifesaver*. New York: W. W. Norton, 2007.

Anderson, Odin. *The Uneasy Equilibrium: Private and Public Financing of Health Services in the United States, 1875–1965*. New Haven: Yale College and University Press, 1968.

Ashburn, Percy. *The Ranks of Death: A Medical History of the Conquest of America*. New York: Coward-McCann, 1947.

Atkinson, William, ed. *The Physicians and Surgeons of the United States*. Philadelphia: Charles Robson, 1878.

Austin, Robert. *Early American Medical Imprints: A Guide to Works Printed in the United States, 1668–1820*. Washington, D.C.: U.S. Department of Health, Education, and Welfare, 1961.

Barnes, Joseph, ed. *The Medical and Surgical History of the War of the Rebellion, 1861–1865*. 6 vols. Washington, D.C.: Government Printing Office, 1870–1888.

Bell, Whitfield. *The Colonial Physician and Other Essays*. New York: Science History Publications, 1975.

Berliner, Howard. *A System of Scientific Medicine: Philanthropic Foundations in the Flexner Era*. New York: Tavistock, 1985.

Blanton, Wyndham. *Medicine in Virginia in the Seventeenth Century*. Richmond, Va.: William Byrd Press, 1930.

———. *Medicine in Virginia in the Eighteenth Century*. Richmond, Va.: Garrett & Massie, 1931.

———. *Medicine in Virginia in the Nineteenth Century*. Richmond, Va.: Garrett & Massie, 1933.

Blasingame, Frank. *1846–1958, Digest of Official Actions, American Medical Association*. Chicago: American Medical Association, 1959.

Blumenthal, David, and James Morone. *Health and Politics in the Oval Office*. Berkeley: University of California Press, 2009.

Bonner, Thomas. *Medicine in Chicago, 1850–1950: A Chapter in the Social and Scien-*

tific Development of a City. Madison, Wisc.: American History Research Center, 1957.

———. *The Kansas Doctor: A Century of Pioneering*. Lawrence: University of Kansas Press, 1959.

———. *American Doctors and German Universities: A Chapter in International Intellectual Relations, 1870–1914*. Lincoln: University of Nebraska Press, 1963.

———. *Becoming a Physician: Medical Education in Britain, France, Germany, and the United States, 1750–1945*. New York: Oxford University Press, 1995.

Bordley, James, and A. McGehee Harvey. *Two Centuries of American Medicine, 1776–1976*. Philadelphia: W. B. Saunders, 1976.

Boulis, Ann, and Jerry Jacobs. *The Changing Face of Medicine: Women Doctors and the Evolution of Health Care in America*. Ithaca, N.Y.: ILR Press/Cornell University Press, 2008.

Bowers, John, and Elizabeth Purcell. *Advances in American Medicine: Essays at the Bicentennial*. 2 vols. New York: Josiah Macy, Jr., Foundation, 1976.

Brandt, Allan. *No Magic Bullet: A Social History of Venereal Disease in the United States Since 1880*. New York: Oxford University Press, 1987.

Brecher, Ruth, and Edward Brecher. *The Rays: A History of Radiology in the United States and Canada*. Baltimore: Williams & Wilkins, 1969.

Brieger, Gert. *Medical America in the Nineteenth Century*. Baltimore: The Johns Hopkins Press, 1972.

Brock, Pope. *Charlatan, America's Most Dangerous Huckster, the Man Who Pursued Him, and the Age of Flimflam*. New York: Crown Publishers, 2008.

Brown, E. Richard. *Rockefeller Medicine Men: Medicine and Capitalism in America*. Berkeley: University of California Press, 1979.

Brown, Julie. *Health and Medicine on Display: International Expositions in the United States, 1876–1904*. Cambridge, Mass.: The MIT Press, 2009.

Brownlee, Shannon. *Overtreated: Why Too Much Medicine Is Making Us Sicker and Poorer*. New York: Bloomsbury, 2007.

Bud, Robert. *Penicillin: Triumph and Tragedy*. New York: Oxford University Press, 2008.

Burns, Stanley. *Early Medical Photography in America (1839–1883)*. New York: The Burns Archive, 1983.

Burrow, James: *AMA: Voice of American Medicine*. Baltimore: The Johns Hopkins Press, 1963.

———. *Organized Medicine in the Progressive Era: The Move Toward Monopoly*. Baltimore: The Johns Hopkins University Press, 1977.

Byrd, Michael. *An American Health Dilemma: A Medical History of African Americans and the Problem of Race*. 2 vols. New York: Routledge, 2000.

Caldwell, Mark. *The Last Crusade: The War on Consumption, 1862–1954*. New York: Athenaeum, 1988.

Calhoun, Daniel: *Professional Lives in America: Structure and Aspirations, 1750–1850*. Cambridge, Mass.: Harvard University Press, 1965.

Cassedy, James. *Medicine and American Growth, 1800–1860*. Madison: University of Wisconsin Press, 1986.

———. *Medicine in America: A Short History*. Baltimore: The Johns Hopkins University Press, 1991.

Chapman, Carleton. *Order Out of Chaos: John Shaw Billings and America's Coming of Age*. Boston: Boston Medical Library in the Francis A. Countaway Library of Medicine, 1994.

Clapesattle, Helen. *The Doctors Mayo*. Minneapolis: University of Minnesota Press, 1941.

Clarke, Edward. *A Century of American Medicine, 1776–1876*. Philadelphia: Henry C. Lea, 1876.

Cleave, Edward. *Cleave's Biographical Cyclopaedia of Homoeopathic Physicians and Surgeons*. Philadelphia: Galaxy Publishing, 1873.

Cohn, Jonathan. *Sick: The Untold Story of America's Health Care Crisis—and the People Who Pay the Price*. New York: HarperCollins, 2007.

Cordasco, Francesco. *Medical Education in the United States: A Guide to Information Sources*. Detroit: Gale Research, 1980.

———. *American Medical Imprints, 1820–1910: A Checklist of Publications Illustrating the History and Progress of Medical Science, Medical Education, and the Healing Arts in the United States, a Preliminary Contribution*. 2 vols. Totowa, N.J.: Rowman & Littlefield, 1985.

———. *Medical Publishing in 19th Century America: LEA of Philadelphia; William Wood & Company of New York City; and F.E. Boericke of Philadelphia*. Fairview, N.J.: Junius-Vaughn Press, 1990.

———. *Homoeopathy in the United States: A Bibliography of Homoeopathic Medical Imprints, 1825–1925*. Fairview, N.J.: Junius-Vaughn Press, 1991.

Coulter, Harris. *Divided Legacy: A History of the Schism in Medical Thought, Science and Ethics in American Medicine, 1800–1914*. Washington, D.C.: Wehawken Books, 1973.

Cunningham, Horace. *Doctors in Gray: The Confederate Medical Service*. Baton Rouge: Louisiana State University Press, 1958.

Dary, David. *Frontier Medicine: From the Atlantic to the Pacific, 1492–1941*. New York: Alfred A. Knopf, 2008.

Davis, Nathan. *History of Medical Education and Institutions in the United States*. Chicago: S. C. Griggs, 1851.

———. *History of the American Medical Association from Its Organization Up to January, 1855*. Philadelphia: Lippincott & Grambo, 1855.

Derbyshire, Robert. *Medical Licensure and Discipline in the United States*. Baltimore: The Johns Hopkins Press, 1969.

DeVille, Kenneth. *Medical Malpractice in Nineteenth-Century America: Origins and Legacy*. New York: New York University Press, 1990.

Donegan, Jane. *Hydropathic Highway to Health: Women and Water-Cure in Antebellum America*. New York: Greenwood Press, 1986.

Duffy, John. *Epidemics in Colonial America*. Baton Rouge: Louisiana State University Press, 1953.

———. *The Sanitarians: A History of American Public Health*. Urbana: University of Illinois Press, 1990.

————. *From Humors to Medical Science: A History of American Medicine.* Urbana: University of Illinois Press, 1993.

Emanuel, Ezekiel. *Healthcare Guaranteed: A Simple, Secure Solution for America.* New York: Public Affairs, 2008.

Ettling, John: *The Germ of Laziness: Rockefeller Philanthropy and Public Health in the New South.* Cambridge, Mass.: Harvard University Press, 1981.

Feldstein, Paul. *Health Policy Issues: An Economic Perspective.* Chicago: Health Policy Press, 2007.

Fellman, Anita, and Michael Fellman. *Making Sense of Self: Medical Advice Literature in Late Nineteenth-Century America.* Philadelphia: University of Pennsylvania Press, 1981.

Fishbein, Morris. *A History of the American Medical Association, 1847 to 1947.* Philadelphia: W. B. Saunders, 1947.

Fleming, Donald. *William H. Welch and the Rise of Modern Medicine.* Boston: Little, Brown, 1954.

Flexner, James. *Doctors on Horseback: Pioneers of American Medicine.* New York: Viking, 1937.

Francis, Samuel. *Biographical Sketches of Distinguished Living New York Surgeons.* New York: John Bradburn, 1866.

————. *Biographical Sketches of Distinguished Living New York Physicians.* New York: G. P. Putnam & Son, 1867.

Fulton, John. *Harvey Cushing.* Springfield, Ill.: Charles C. Thomas, 1946.

Fye, Bruce. *The Development of American Physiology: Scientific Medicine in the Nineteenth Century.* Baltimore: The Johns Hopkins University Press, 1987.

Galishoff, Stuart. *Newark: The Nation's Unhealthiest City, 1832–1895.* New Brunswick, N.J.: Rutgers University Press, 1988.

Gamble, Vanessa. *Making a Place for Ourselves: The Black Hospital Movement, 1920–1945.* New York: Oxford University Press, 1995.

————, ed. *Germs Have No Color Lines: Blacks and American Medicine, 1900–1945.* New York: Garland Publishing, 1989.

Garrison, Fielding. *An Introduction to the History of Medicine.* Philadelphia: W. B. Saunders, 1913.

Gawande, Atul. *Complications: A Surgeon's Notes on an Imperfect Science.* New York: Metropolitan Books/Henry Holt, 2002.

————. *Better: A Surgeon's Notes on Performance.* New York: Metropolitan Books/Henry Holt, 2007.

Gerdts, William. *The Art of Healing: Medicine and Science in American Art.* Birmingham, Ala.: Birmingham Museum of Art, 1981.

Gevitz, Norman. *The DOs: Osteopathic Medicine in America.* Baltimore: The Johns Hopkins University Press, 1982.

————, ed. *Other Healers: Unorthodox Medicine in America.* Baltimore: The Johns Hopkins University Press, 1988.

Gordon, Maurice Bear. *Aesculapius Comes to the Colonies: The Story of the Early Days of Medicine in the Thirteen Original Colonies.* Ventnor, N.J.: Ventnor Publishers, 1949.

Gosling, Francis. *Before Freud: Neurasthenia and the American Medical Community, 1870–1910.* Urbana: University of Illinois Press, 1987.

Grob, Gerald. *Mental Institutions in America: Social Policy to 1875.* New York: Free Press, 1973.

———. *The Mad Among Us: A History of the Care of America's Mentally Ill.* New York: Free Press, 1994.

Groopman, Jerome. *How Doctors Think.* Boston: Houghton Mifflin, 2007.

Gross, Samuel. *Lives of Eminent American Physicians and Surgeons of the Nineteenth Century.* Philadelphia: Lindsay & Blakiston, 1861.

Guerra, Francisco. *American Medical Bibliography, 1639–1783.* New York: Lathrop C. Harper, 1962.

Hafner, Arthur, ed. *Directory of Deceased American Physicians, 1804–1929.* 2 vols. Chicago: American Medical Association, 1993.

Hall, Stephen. *A Commotion in the Blood: Life, Death, and the Immune System.* New York: Henry Holt, 1997.

Haller, John. *American Medicine in Transition, 1840–1910.* Urbana: University of Illinois Press, 1981.

———. *Medical Protestants: The Eclectics in American Medicine, 1825–1939.* Carbondale: Southern Illinois University Press, 1994.

———. *Kindly Medicine: Physio-Medicalism in America, 1836–1911.* Kent, Ohio: Kent State University Press, 1997.

———. *The People's Doctors: Samuel Thomson and the American Botanical Movement, 1790–1860.* Carbondale: Southern Illinois University Press, 2001.

———. *History of American Homeopathy: The Academic Years, 1820–1935.* Binghamton, N.Y.: Haworth Press, 2005.

Halpern, Sydney. *American Pediatrics: The Social Dynamics of Professionalism, 1880–1980.* Berkeley: University of California Press, 1988.

Hanson, William. *The Edge of Medicine: The Technology That Will Change Our Lives.* New York: Palgrave Macmillan, 2008.

Harvey, A. McGehee. *Science at the Bedside: Clinical Research in American Medicine, 1905–1945.* Baltimore: The Johns Hopkins University Press, 1981.

Hirshfield, Daniel. *The Lost Reform: The Campaign for Compulsory Health Insurance in the United States from 1932 to 1943.* Cambridge, Mass.: Harvard University Press, 1970.

Holloway, Lisbeth. *Medical Obituaries: American Physicians' Biographical Notices in Selected Medical Journals Before 1907.* New York: Garland, 1981.

Howell, Joel. *Technology and American Medical Practice, 1880–1930: An Anthology of Sources.* New York: Garland, 1988.

———. *Technology in the Hospital: Transforming Patient Care in the Early Twentieth Century.* Baltimore: The Johns Hopkins University Press, 1995.

Hurd-Mead, Kate. *Medical Women of America: A Short History of the Pioneer Medical Women of America.* New York: Froben, 1933.

Kagan, Solomon. *Jewish Contributions to Medicine in America (1656–1934).* Boston: Boston Medical Publishing, 1934.

Karolevitz, Robert. *Doctors of the Old West: A Pictorial History of Medicine on the Frontier.* New York: Bonanza Books, 1967.

Kassirer, Jerome. *On the Take: How America's Complicity with Big Business Can Endanger Your Health*. New York: Oxford University Press, 2005.

Kaufman, Martin. *Homeopathy in America: The Rise and Fall of a Medical Heresy*. Baltimore: The Johns Hopkins Press, 1971.

———. *American Medical Education: The Formative Years, 1765–1910*. Westport, Conn.: Greenwood Press, 1976.

Kaufman, Martin, Stuart Galishoff, and Todd Savitt, eds. *Dictionary of American Medical Biography*. 2 vols. Westport, Conn.: Greenwood Press, 1984.

Kelly, Howard, ed. *A Cyclopedia of American Medical Biography, Comprising the Lives of Eminent Deceased Physicians and Surgeons from 1610 to 1910*. 2 vols. Philadelphia: W. B. Saunders, 1912.

———. *Some American Medical Botanists Commemorated in Our Botanical Nomenclature*. Troy, N.Y.: Southworth Company, 1914.

Kelly, Howard, and Walter Burrage, eds. *American Medical Biographies*. Baltimore: Norman, Remington, 1920.

———, eds. *Dictionary of American Medical Biography: Lives of Eminent Physicians of the United States and Canada, from the Earliest Times*. New York: D. Appleton, 1928.

Kett, Joseph. *The Formation of the American Medical Profession: The Role of Institutions, 1780–1860*: New Haven: Yale University Press, 1968.

King, Lester. *American Medicine Comes of Age, 1840–1920*. Chicago: American Medical Association, 1984.

———. *Transformations in American Medicine*. Baltimore: The Johns Hopkins University Press, 1991.

King, William. *History of Homoeopathy and Its Institutions in America*. 4 vols. New York: Lewis Press, 1905.

Klaidman, Stephen. *Coronary: A True Story of Medicine Gone Awry*. New York: Scribner, 2007.

Kraut, Alan. *Silent Travelers: Germs, Genes, and the "Immigrant Menace."* New York: Basic Books, 1994.

Krueger, Gretchen. *Hope and Suffering: Children, Cancer, and the Paradox of Experimental Medicine*. Baltimore: The Johns Hopkins University Press, 2008.

Leavitt, Judith. *The Healthiest City: Milwaukee and the Politics of Health Reform*. Princeton, N.J.: Princeton University Press, 1982.

———, ed. *Women and Health in America: Historical Readings*. Madison: University of Wisconsin Press, 1984.

Leavitt, Judith, and Ronald Numbers. *Sickness and Health in America: Readings in the History of Medicine and Public Health*. Madison: University of Wisconsin Press, 1985.

Lederer, Susan. *Subjected to Science: Human Experimentation in America Before the Second World War*. Baltimore: The Johns Hopkins University Press, 1995.

———. *Flesh and Blood: Organ Transplantation and Blood Transfusion in Twentieth-Century America*. New York: Oxford University Press, 2008.

Lerner, Barron. *The Breast Cancer Wars: Hope, Fear, and the Pursuit of a Cure in Twentieth-Century America*. New York: Oxford University Press, 2003.

———. *When Illness Goes Public: Celebrity Patients and How We Look at Medicine*. Baltimore: The Johns Hopkins University Press, 2006.

Link, Eugene. *The Social Ideas of American Physicians (1776–1976): Studies of the Humanitarian Tradition in Medicine*. Selinsgrove, Pa.: Susquehanna University Press, 1992.

Ludmerer, Kenneth. *Learning to Heal: The Development of American Medical Education*. New York: Basic Books, 1985.

———. *Time to Heal: American Medical Education from the Turn of the Century to the Era of Managed Care*. New York: Oxford University Press, 1999.

Malmsheimer, Richard. *"Doctors Only": The Evolving Image of the American Physician*. Westport, Conn.: Greenwood Press, 1988.

Marks, Geoffrey, and William Beatty. *The Story of Medicine in America*. New York: Charles Scribner's Sons, 1973.

Marmor, Theodore. *The Politics of Medicare*. New York: Aldine de Gruyter, 2000.

Marti-Ibañez, Felix. *History of American Medicine: A Symposium*. New York: MD Publications, 1959.

Miller, Genevieve. *Bibliography of the History of Medicine of the United States and Canada, 1939–1960*. Baltimore: The Johns Hopkins Press, 1964.

Morais, Herbert. *The History of the Negro in Medicine*. New York: Publishers Company, 1967.

Morantz-Sanchez, Regina. *Sympathy and Science: Women Physicians in American Medicine*. New York: Oxford University Press, 1985.

———. *Conduct Unbecoming a Woman: Medicine on Trial in Turn-of-the-Century Brooklyn*. New York: Oxford University Press, 1999.

Mullen, Fitzhugh. *Plagues and Politics: The Story of the United States Public Health Service*. New York: Basic Books, 1989.

Mumford, James. *A Narrative of Medicine in America*. Philadelphia: J. B. Lippincott, 1903.

Norris, George. *The Early History of Medicine in Philadelphia*. Philadelphia: Collins Printing House, 1886.

Norwood, William. *Medical Education in the United States Before the Civil War*. Philadelphia: University of Pennsylvania Press, 1944.

Nuland, Sherwin. *Doctors: The Biography of Medicine*. New York: Alfred A. Knopf, 1988.

Numbers, Ronald. *Almost Persuaded: American Physicians and Compulsory Health Insurance, 1912–1920*. Baltimore: The Johns Hopkins University Press, 1978.

Oshinsky, David. *Polio: An American Story*. New York: Oxford University Press, 2005.

Packard, Francis. *History of Medicine in the United States*. 2 vols. New York: Paul B. Hoeber, 1931.

Pernick, Martin. *A Calculus of Suffering: Pain, Professionalism and Anesthesia in Nineteenth-Century America*. New York: Columbia University Press, 1985.

———. *The Black Stork: Eugenics and the Death of "Defective" Babies in American Medicine and Motion Pictures Since 1915*. New York: Oxford University Press, 1996.

Porter, Roy. *The Greatest Benefit to Mankind: A Medical History of Humanity*. New York: W. W. Norton, 1997.

Reid, T. R. *The Healing of America: A Global Quest for Better, Cheaper, and Fairer Health Care.* New York: Penguin Press, 2009.

Relman, Arnold. *A Second Opinion: Rescuing America's Healthcare.* New York: Public Affairs, 2007.

Reverby, Susan. *Ordered to Care: The Dilemma of American Nursing, 1850–1945.* New York: Cambridge University Press, 1987.

Reverby, Susan, and David Rosner. *Health Care in America: Essays in Social History.* Philadelphia: Temple University Press, 1979.

Rice, Mitchell, and Woodrow Jones. *Public Policy and the Black Hospital: From Slavery to Segregation to Integration.* Westport, Conn.: Greenwood Press, 1994.

Risse, Gunther, Ronald Numbers, and Judith Leavitt, eds. *Medicine Without Doctors, Home Health Care in American History.* New York: Science History Publications, 1977.

Roberts, Mary. *American Nursing: History and Interpretation.* New York: Macmillan, 1954.

Robins, Natalie. *Copeland's Cure: Homeopathy and the War Between Conventional and Alternative Medicine.* New York: Alfred A. Knopf, 2005.

Rosen, George. *The Specialization of Medicine.* New York: Froben Press, 1944.

———. *Fees and Fee Bills: Some Economic Aspects of Medical Practice in Nineteenth Century America.* Baltimore: The Johns Hopkins Press, 1946.

———. *The Structure of American Medical Practice, 1875–1941.* Philadelphia: University of Pennsylvania Press, 1983.

Rosenberg, Charles. *The Cholera Years: The United States in 1832, 1849, and 1866.* Chicago: University of Chicago Press, 1962.

———. *The Care of Strangers: The Rise of America's Hospital System.* New York: Basic Books, 1987.

———. *Our Present Complaint: American Medicine, Then and Now.* Baltimore: The Johns Hopkins University Press, 2007.

Rosenkrantz, Barbara: *Public Health and the State: Changing Views in Massachusetts, 1842–1936.* Cambridge, Mass.: Harvard University Press, 1972.

Rosner, David. *A Once Charitable Enterprise: Hospitals and Health Care in Brooklyn and New York, 1885–1915.* New York: Cambridge University Press, 1982.

Rothman, David. *Strangers at the Bedside: A History of How Law and Bioethics Transformed Medical Decision Making.* New York: Basic Books, 1991.

———. *Beginnings Count: The Technological Imperative in American Health Care.* New York: Oxford University Press, 1997.

Rothman, Sheila. *Living in the Shadow of Death: Tuberculosis and the Social Experience of Illness in America.* New York: Basic Books, 1994.

Rothman, Sheila, and David Rothman. *The Pursuit of Perfection: The Promise and Perils of Medical Enhancement.* New York: Pantheon Books, 2003.

Rothstein, William. *American Physicians in the 19th Century: From Sects to Science.* Baltimore: The Johns Hopkins University Press, 1972.

———. *American Medical Schools and the Practice of Medicine: A History.* New York: Oxford University Press, 1987.

Rutkow, Ira. *The History of Surgery in the United States, 1775–1900.* 2 vols. San Francisco: Norman Publishing, 1988 and 1992.

————. *Surgery: An Illustrated History.* St. Louis, Mo.: C. V. Mosby, 1993.

————. *American Surgery: An Illustrated History.* Philadelphia: Lippincott-Raven, 1998.

————. *Bleeding Blue and Gray: Civil War Surgery and the Evolution of American Medicine.* New York: Random House, 2005.

————. *James A. Garfield.* New York: Times Books/Henry Holt, 2006.

Savitt, Todd. *Medicine and Slavery.* Urbana: University of Illinois Press, 1978.

Schwartz, Seymour. *Gifted Hands: America's Most Significant Contributions to Surgery.* Amherst, N.Y.: Prometheus Books, 2009.

Shafer, Henry. *The American Medical Profession, 1783–1850.* New York: Columbia University Press, 1936.

Shryock, Richard: *American Medical Research, Past and Present.* New York: The Commonwealth Fund, 1947.

————. *Medicine and Society in America, 1660–1860.* New York: New York University Press, 1960.

————. *Medicine in America: Historical Essays.* Baltimore: The Johns Hopkins Press, 1966.

————. *Medical Licensing in America, 1650–1965.* Baltimore: The Johns Hopkins Press, 1967.

Sigerist, Henry: *American Medicine.* New York: W. W. Norton, 1934.

Starr, Douglas. *Blood: An Epic History of Medicine and Commerce.* New York: Alfred A. Knopf, 1998.

Starr, Paul. *The Social Transformation of American Medicine.* New York: Basic Books, 1982.

Steele, Velney. *Bleed, Blister, and Purge: A History of Medicine on the American Frontier.* Missoula, Mont.: Mountain Press, 2005.

Stevens, Rosemary. *American Medicine and the Public Interest.* New Haven: Yale University Press, 1971.

————. *In Sickness and in Wealth: American Hospitals in the Twentieth Century.* New York: Basic Books, 1989.

Stevens, Rosemary, Louis Goodman, and Stephen Mick. *The Alien Doctors: Foreign Medical Graduates in American Hospitals.* New York: John Wiley, 1978.

Stone, R. French. *Biography of Eminent American Physicians and Surgeons.* Indianapolis: C. E. Hollenbeck, 1894.

Strickland, Stephen. *Politics, Science, and Dread Disease: A Short History of United States Medical Research Policy.* Cambridge, Mass.: Harvard University Press, 1972.

Taylor, Lloyd. *The Medical Profession and Social Reform, 1885–1945.* New York: St. Martin's Press, 1974.

Thacher, James. *American Medical Biography, or Memoirs of Eminent Physicians Who Have Flourished in America.* Boston: Richardson & Lord and Cottons & Barnard, 1828.

Viets, Henry. *A Brief History of Medicine in Massachusetts.* Boston: Houghton Mifflin, 1930.

Vogel, Morris. *The Invention of the Modern Hospital, Boston, 1870–1930.* Chicago: University of Chicago Press, 1980.

Vogel, Morris, and Charles Rosenberg. *The Therapeutic Revolution: Essays in the Social History of American Medicine.* Philadelphia: University of Pennsylvania Press, 1970.

Vogel, Virgil. *American Indian Medicine.* Norman: University of Oklahoma Press, 1970.

Walsh, Mary. *"Doctors Wanted: No Women Need Apply": Sexual Barriers in the Medical Profession, 1835–1875.* New Haven: Yale University Press, 1977.

Warner, John. *Against the Spirit of System: The French Impulse in Nineteenth-Century American Medicine.* Princeton, N.J.: Princeton University Press, 1998.

————. *The Therapeutic Perspective: Medical Practice, Knowledge, and Identity in America, 1820–1885.* Cambridge, Mass.: Harvard University Press, 1986.

Washington, Harriet. *Medical Apartheid: The Dark History of Medical Experimentation on Black Americans from Colonial Times to the Present.* New York: Doubleday, 2006.

Watson, Irving, ed. *Physicians and Surgeons of America: A Collection of Biographical Sketches of the Regular Medical Profession.* Concord, N.H.: Republican Press Association, 1896.

Weisz, George. *Divide and Conquer: A Comparative History of Medical Specialization.* New York: Oxford University Press, 2005.

Whorton, James. *Crusaders for Fitness: The History of American Health Reformers.* Princeton, N.J.: Princeton University Press, 1982.

Williams, Stephen. *American Medical Biography: or Memoirs of Eminent Physicians.* Greenfield, Mass.: L. Merriam, 1845.

Wishart, Adam. *One in Three: A Son's Journey into the History and Science of Cancer.* New York: Grove Press, 2007.

Young, James. *The Toadstool Millionaires: A Social History of Patent Medicines in America Before Federal Regulation.* Princeton, N.J.: Princeton University Press, 1961.

————. *The Medical Messiahs: A Social History of Health Quackery in Twentieth-Century America.* Princeton, N.J.: Princeton University Press, 1967.

INDEX

Abscesses, 75–76, 78
Abolitionism, 46
Academic medicine, 123–25, 129, 131, 149,
    251, 253–54, 266, 286
  AMA and, 198, 202
  cardiology and, 279
  colonial-era, 21–24
  European, 128–29
  Flexner and, 154
  government-funded research and, 233,
    235, 245–47
  organ transplants and, 250
  proprietary medical schools versus,
    41–43, 48, 98
  sphere of influence of, 235–37
  surgery and, 204
  see also specific universities
Académie des Sciences (Paris), 51, 57, 58
Adams, John, 34
Adams, Samuel Hopkins, 151, 181
Adrenaline, 175–76
African Americans, 3, 19, 217–19
  in medical profession, 213, 218–19, 261
Agrarianism, 46
Alabama, University of, 230
Albany County (New York) Homeopathic
    Medical Society, 104
Alcott, Amos Bronson, 97
Alcott, Louisa May, 97
Allopathy, 92–95, 101, 102
Alzheimer's disease, 307
Ambulance Américaine, 167–68, 209
American Academy of General Practice,
    253–54
American Association of Orificial Surgeons,
    97, 99, 100, 104
American Board of Family Practice, 253
American Board of Internal Medicine, 203

American Board of Medical Specialties, 253
American Board of Surgery, 205, 217, 252
American Cancer Society, 269, 270
American Chamber of Commerce, 256
  in Paris, 167
American College of Cardiology, 287
American College of Physicians, 165, 202,
    203
American College of Radiology, 202
American College of Surgeons, 145, 156,
    159–69, 171, 202–5, 219, 294
American Heart Association, 248, 280, 282,
    286–87
American Homeopathic Health Resort
    Association, 97
American Hospital Association, 165
American Institute of Homeopathy, 48, 93,
    97, 101, 104
American Institute of Homeopathic Phar-
    macies, 97
American Magazine and Monthly Chronicle, 19
American Medical Association (AMA), 88,
    104, 136, 159, 189, 197–99, 231, 236
  Advisory Board for Medical Specialties,
    202
  code of ethics of, 59, 94, 103
  Committee on Railroad Practice, 111
  Council on Medical Education and Hos-
    pitals, 148, 153, 164–65, 201, 202
  declining influence of, 295–96
  founding of, 42, 47–49, 53
  journals of, 50–51, 164, 189, 193, 199, 201
  medical self-promoters opposed by,
    193–94
  national health care opposed by, 254–63
  specialism and, 106–7, 201–2, 205, 252
  of Vienna, 119
American Medical Directory, 201

American Medical Times, 85
American Orthopedic Association, 138
American Pediatric Society, 202
American Philosophical Society, 19
American Public Health Association, 86
American Roentgen Ray Society, 139
American Surgical Association, 107, 136
Amherst College, 213
Aminopterin, 265–66
Anemia
    pernicious, 175–77
    sickle-cell, 307
Anesthesia, 32, 101, 166, 173, 181
    in cardiac surgery, 224, 228, 281
    Civil War use of, 61
    discovery of, 51–59, 84, 128, 282, 305
    and Garfield's medical care, 77, 78
    Lister's support of, 65–66
    in organ transplant surgery, 246, 247
    specialized training in, 165, 190, 201, 205
    for World War I army hospitals, 169
Angina, 277, 278, 281
Angioplasty, 279–83, 286–89, 297
Animal research, 137, 226, 227, 235, 280
Antibiotics, 73, 185–88, 222, 233, 235
Antisepsis, 64–70, 85, 101, 156, 173, 230
    and decline in surgical mortality, 181
    Halsted's introduction at Bellevue of,
        127
    marketing of products for, 184, 187
    see also Listerism
Appel, James, 261–63
Appendicitis, 180–88
Apprenticeship, medical, 17–18, 20–24, 29,
    33, 40–43, 262
Arcadian Belles Lettres Society, 20
Aristotle, 36
Armory Square Hospital (Washington,
    D.C.), 74
Army, U.S., 54, 74, 124, 209, 210, 218
    base hospitals of, 169–71
    Medical Corps, 226
    Mobile Army Surgical Hospital (MASH)
        units, 110
Arrowsmith (Lewis), 183
Asclepiades, 36
Ashtabula River disaster, 108
Associated Press, 248
Association of American Physicians, 139, 180
Association of American Physicians and Sur-
    geons, 263–64
Atherosclerosis, 276–82

Atlantic Monthly, 70, 154
Austro-Hungary, 65, 150
    medical education in, 117, 118, 124
Azathioprine, 249

Bachmann, Dolf, 280–82
Bacteriology, 59, 68, 70, 80, 89, 110, 120, 124,
    173
Balloon angioplasty, 279–83, 286–89, 297
Baltimore College of Physicians and Sur-
    geons, 81
Bard, Samuel, 26
Bartlett, Josiah, 16
Bavolek, Cecilia, 228–29
Beaumont, William, 54
Beecher, Henry Ward, 97
Bellevue Hospital (New York), 85, 127
    Medical College, 65, 85, 122, 126
Bellows, George, 188
Ben Casey (television series), 238
Beriberi, 174
Bernard, Claude, 62, 70
Bernays, Edward, 196, 198
Best Doctors in America, 299
Bigelow, Henry, 3–4
Billings, John Shaw, 122–23
Black, Hugo, 230
Blacks, *see* African Americans
Bliss, Doctor Willard, 72–80
Blistering, 17, 18, 32, 35, 36, 38–39, 61, 62,
    71, 81
Blood banks, 210, 214–16
Bloodletting, 17, 35–39, 44, 46, 47, 61, 62, 70,
    81, 92
    Rush's demise from, 31–33, 68
Blood Plasma for Great Britain Project, 209,
    211–16
Blood poisoning, 69, 77, 78, 186, 223
Blood Transfusion Betterment Association,
    210–12, 214
Blood transfusions, *see* Transfusions
Blue Cross, 256
Board certification, 200–203, 205–6, 218,
    221–22, 252–54
Boston Braves baseball team, 267
Boston City Hospital, 299
Boston Gazette, 11
Boston Medical and Surgical Journal, 67,
    93–94, 169
Boston Red Sox baseball team, 268
Boston Society for the Diffusion of Useful
    Knowledge, 94

Boston University, 90, 96
Boswell, James, 21
Botanicals, 46–47
Bronchoscope, 177
Boylston, Zabdiel, 7–15, 17–18, 306
Breslau, University of, 119
Brigham Hospital (Boston), 241, 243–50
Britain, 13–15, 19, 20
   fake American physicians in, 105
   B. Franklin in, 14–15, 20
   medical education in, 18, 20, 24, 28, 44,
      117, 274
   minister-physicians in, 9
   Ministry of Health, 209
   surgery in, 270
   in World War I, 170, 172
   in World War II, 209, 211–16
British Medical Association, 112
Bypass surgery, 229, 282, 283, 285, 287–89, 292

Calomel, 38, 41, 92
Cancer, 204, 264–72, 292, 306, 307
   chemotherapy for, 238, 265–66, 268
   childhood, 268
   colonial-era treatment of, 8
   government-funded research on, 184,
      232, 234, 268–71
   microscopic images of, 135
   mortality rate for, 261
   radiation treatment of, 173, 265, 268
   X-rays of, 138, 139
Carcinomas, 265
Carnegie, Andrew, 147–49, 154
Carnegie Foundation for the Advancement
   of Teaching, 149–52
   Bulletin of, 151–55
Caroline, Princess of Wales, 13
Carrel, Alexis, 239–40
Castle, William, 176–77
Cathell, Daniel Webster, 81–84, 103–4
CBS Evening News, 283
Celsus, 36
Centennial Exhibition (Philadelphia, 1876),
   64
Centrifuge, 177–78, 182
Charity Hospital (New Orleans), 23
Charity Hospital (New York), 67
Chemotherapy, 238, 265–66, 268
Chicago, University of, Rush Medical Col-
   lege, 164
Chicago Homeopathic Medical College, 98,
   104

Children's Cancer Research Foundation, 267
Cholera, 84, 87
Citizens' Committee for the Conquest of
   Cancer, 269, 270
City That Was, The (Smith), 85
Civil War, 43, 60–63, 73, 74, 95, 136, 192
   hygienic principles in, 84
   stress-related disorders of soldiers in, 220
   surgical practices in, 85, 222
Cleveland, Grover, 86, 136
Cleveland Clinic, 167, 286
Clinical Congresses of Surgeons of North
   America, 157–58
Cloning, 306
Cocaine, 126–29
Codman, Ernest Amory, 142–45, 161, 221
Cold War, 232, 256
Columbia University, 24, 41, 126
   College of Physicians and Surgeons, 119,
      213, 214
   Law School, 230
Commerce Department, U.S., 189
Committee of American Physicians for
   Medical Preparedness, 169–70
Committee on the Costs of Medical Care,
   194–99, 255
Committee of Physicians for the Improve-
   ment of Medicine, 198–99
Community-based medicine, 236–37, 253
Computerized axial tomography (CAT), 305
Congress, U.S., 153, 218, 263, 275
   and discovery of anesthesia, 51, 54, 57–58
   cancer research funded by, 268, 270
   during Civil War, 95, 96
   health care legislation in, 256, 258–59
   hospital construction funded by, 231
   National Institutes of Health established
      by, 232
Congress of Senior Citizens of Greater New
   York, 261
Continental Army, 15–16, 27, 28, 34
Continental Congress, 16, 28, 34
Cook County Hospital (Chicago), 100, 210
Coombs, John, 157
Coronary artery disease, 276–83, 286–89,
   297, 305
Corporation for Public Broadcasting, 258
Council of National Defense, 169
Crazy Horse, 67
CR Bard Medical, 285–87
Crile, George, 166–72
Cronkite, Walter, 283

Cupping, 38–39
Custer, General George Armstrong, 67
Cyclosporine, 249
Cytoscope, 118, 177

Dartmouth College, 41
Davis, Nathan Smith, 42
Deficiency diseases, 174–77
Democracy in America (Tocqueville), 44
Democratic Party, 234, 256, 258
Dentistry, painless, 52–55
Depletion treatments, *see* Heroic therapy
Dermatology, 64, 107, 165, 201, 275
Diabetes, 174, 190, 235, 278, 307
Diagnosis-related groups (DRGs), 296, 297
Dialysis, 244, 246
Digestion, process of, 54
Diphtheria, 8, 84, 88, 89, 176, 187
Dr. Kildare (television series), 238
Doctors, The (television series), 238
"Doctors' Mob" riot, 27
Domestic Medicine (Gunn), 46
Dresden, University of, 119
Drew, Charles, 3, 213–20
Dulles, John Foster, 234
Dysentery, 8, 87

Eakins, Thomas, 64, 67
Eclecticism, 47, 83
Edinburgh, University of, 18, 20, 33, 44, 64,
    119, 225
Edison, Thomas, 139
Edwards, Ralph, 267
Einstein, Albert, 155
Eisenhower, Dwight, 234, 256, 284
Electric shock therapy, 62
Electrocardiograms, 136, 178–79
Eli Lilly & Company, 109, 287
Emerson, Ralph Waldo, 97
Emetics, 33, 38, 70
Emory University School of Medicine, 286
Endocrinology, 174
End results system, 143–45, 161
Engels, Friedrich, 117
England, *see* Britain
Epidemics, 17, 84, 194
    influenza, 162
    smallpox, 7–12, 14
Erlangen, University of, 91
Ether, 51–52, 55–58, 61, 69, 128
Evanston Century Club, 99
Ewell, James, 46

Family practice, 253–54, 262, 274, 298
Farber, Sidney, 265–71
Fascism, 274
Female doctors, 112, 275–76, 297–98
Fishbein, Morris, 192–94, 196–99, 201, 202,
    205
Fitz, Reginald, 180–81
Flexner, Abraham, 147–55, 164, 252
Flexner, James, 22
Flexner, Simon, 150
Florida Board of Medicine, 301–2
Florida Vascular Society, 299
Fluoroscope, 139
Food, Drug, and Cosmetic Act (1938), 189
Food and Drugs Act (1906), 153
Food and Drug Administration (FDA),
    260
Foreign medical graduates, 274–76, 297–98
Fort Wayne College of Medicine, 109
France, 59, 60
    American Chamber of Commerce in,
        167
    anesthesia use in, 51, 57
    eighteenth-century, 20, 21
    medical education in, 44–45, 117, 274
    in World War I, 167–70, 172, 209
Franklin, Benjamin, 11, 14–16, 20, 22, 23
Franklin, James, 11
Freedmen's Hospital (Washington, D.C.),
    218
Freiberg, University of, 118
French and Indian War, 20
Freud, Sigmund, 127–28, 196

Galen, 36
Garfield, James A., 71–80, 125, 306
Gas gangrene, 120, 168
Gastroenterology, 107, 203, 275
General Education Board, 154
General Hospital (television series), 238
Generalists, 106, 113, 199, 251–54, 259
    AMA support for, 201, 202
    in apprenticeship system, 18
    income of, 189
    licensing standards and, 160
    surgery by, 156–59
    during World War II, 220, 221, 235
Genetics, 173, 235, 245, 248, 278, 307
George I, King of England, 13
George II, King of England, 13
Georgetown University School of Medicine,
    299

Germany, 65, 150
  medical education in, 117, 118–24, 126,
    127, 133, 142, 150–51, 158, 274, 278
  in World War I, 167, 168, 172
  in World War II, 209, 215, 223
  X-rays discovered in, 137
Germ theory, 66, 68, 79, 80, 89, 173
Gibbon, John, 225–26, 235, 240, 244
Gilbreth, Frank, 142
Glomerulonephritis, 244, 245, 248
Goldwater, Barry, 258, 259
Goodell, William, 61–62
Good Housekeeping magazine, 161
Göttingen, University of, 118
GP (journal), 253
Grace Hospital (Detroit), 185
Graham, Evarts, 204–5
Graham, Sylvester, 47
Grant, Ulysses S., 74–75
Great Depression, 191, 221, 255
Great Society, 258
Greeks, ancient, 36, 37, 264, 304
Gross, Samuel, 67
Gross Clinic, The (Eakins), 64, 67
Grüntzig, Andreas, 276, 278–88
Guadalcanal, Battle of, 226–27
*Guide to American Medical Students in
    Europe, A* (Hun), 118
Guiteau, Charles, 72
Gunn, John, 46
Gustafson, Einar ("Jimmy"), 268–69
Gynecology, 106, 107, 112, 201, 298, 299

Hahnemann, Samuel, 90–94, 103–5
Hahnemann Medical College of Chicago, 98
Hahnemann University Hospital (Philadel-
    phia), 105
Halle, University of, 118
Halsted, William Stewart, 126–34, 136, 137,
    142, 150, 156, 221, 293
Hamilton, Alexander, 27
Hamilton, Frank Hastings, 65, 67–69, 71,
    74–81, 85–86, 117
Hand-book of Surgical Operations (Smith), 85
Harper's Magazine, 163, 199
Harrison, Benjamin, 112
Harrison's Principles of Internal Medicine
    (textbook), 244
Hartford, John A., Foundation, 248
Harvard University, 9, 142, 149–50, 168, 242,
    253
  Children's Hospital, 265–68

Dana-Farber Cancer Institute, 268
Medical School, 3, 41, 53–55, 70, 96,
    133, 138, 142, 144, 145, 176, 180, 225,
    242–44, 286
Hawthorne, Nathaniel, 97
Hayes, Rutherford B., 86
Head Start, 258
Health, Education, and Welfare, U.S.
    Department of, 230
Health insurance, 195, 197, 296–97
  government-sponsored, 192, 198, 236,
    255, 256 (*see also* Medicaid; Medicare)
Health Maintenance Organizations
    (HMOs), 296
Heart disease, 179, 190, 223, 270, 271, 276,
    278
  government-funded research on, 232–34
  treatment of, 279–83, 286–89, 297
Heart-lung machine, 223–29, 282
Heidelberg, University of, 119, 278
Henry, Patrick, 16
Herbal medicine, 39, 90–92
Hernia repair, 292–94
Heroic therapy, 32–33, 35–40, 49, 60–62, 91,
    97
  decline of, 44–46, 70, 80–81, 93
Herrick, Richard, 245–48
Herrick, Ronald, 246–48
Higher Education Act, Title IX Education
    Amendments (1972), 275
High Museum of Art (Atlanta), 286
Hill, Joseph Lister, 230–34, 248, 268
Hill-Burton Act (1946), 231, 236
Hippocrates, 36
*Historical Account of the Small-Pox Inoculated
    in New England, A* (Boylston), 13
Holmes, Oliver Wendell, 94
Homeopathic Intercollegiate Congress of the
    United States, 97
Homeopathy, 47, 48, 50, 83, 89–105, 148
Hoover, Herbert, 120–21
Hormones, 174–75, 238, 265
Hospital for Joint Diseases (New York), 212
Hospitals, 1, 63–65, 89, 107, 126–27, 187–89,
    198
  accreditation of, 165
  colonial-era, 17, 20, 23–24, 28–29
  community, 236, 253
  cost of care in, 190–91
  end result system of record-keeping in,
    143–45
  government funding of, 231, 234

group practice based in, 195, 198
homeopathic, 90, 97, 100, 114
military, 166–72, 220, 226
modern, 140–42
railroad, 110–11
segregated, 219
standardization of, 161–66, 188
surgery in, 160–61, 180–84, 190
teaching, 117–18, 133–35, 148–49 (*see also* Internships; Residency programs)
see also specific hospitals
Houdini, Harry, 185–88
House of Representatives, U.S., 58, 230, 234, 262
Howard University Medical School, 218
Howe, Julia Ward, 16
Humors, bodily, 32, 37, 174
Hun, Henry, 118
Hydropathic medicine, 47, 83
Hygiene, public, 65, 85–88
Hypertension, 238, 277, 278

Illinois Homeopathic Association, 100
Immunology, 49, 242, 245, 246
Immunosuppressant drugs, 249–50
Independent Practice Associations (IPAs), 296
Infantile paralysis, *see* Polio
Infant mortality, 87, 190
Infectious diseases, 3, 87, 220
see also specific diseases
Influenza, 8, 162, 190, 271
Inoculation, 17, 23
smallpox, 1, 7–16, 306
Insulin, 190
Insurance
health, *see* Health insurance
malpractice, 299
Intermittent claudication, 277
Internal medicine, 170, 203, 243–44
International Business Machines (IBM), 227
International Hahnemannian Association, 104
International Homeopathic Congress (Chicago, 1893), 100
International Medical Congress (Philadelphia, 1876), 64–67, 71, 86
International Sanitary Conference (Paris, 1894), 86
Internships, 132–33, 156, 164–65, 201, 252, 261, 274
Interstate Commerce Commission, 108

Intrinsic factor, 177
Iowa, University of, 90
Irregular practitioners, 46, 48–49, 81, 83, 93, 103, 113

Jackson, Andrew, 45, 105
Jackson, Charles, 53–55, 57–59
Jay, John, 27
Jefferson Medical College, 51, 136, 225, 227
Hospital, 228
Jimmy Fund, 267–68
Jo's Boys (Alcott), 97
Johns Hopkins University, 121, 123, 149, 253–54
Hospital, 29–30, 123–25, 130–32, 134, 139, 243, 290
School of Medicine, 29–30, 119, 121, 123–26, 129–31, 133, 148, 150–51, 164
Johnson, Lyndon, 258, 263
Johnson & Johnson, 109
Joint Commission on Accreditation of Hospitals, 165
Journal of the American Medical Association, 164, 189, 193, 199, 201
Journal of Orificial Surgery, 99, 104
Journals, medical, 11, 49–51, 70, 76, 108, 128, 168, 189
homeopathic, 90, 93, 95
specialization and, 155, 157
see also specific journals
Jungle, The (Sinclair), 151

Keen, William Williams, 136–40, 142
Kennedy, John, 256–58
Kidney transplants, 240–50, 307
King's College, 24, 26, 41

Lafayette, Marquis de, 44
Laparoscopy, 290–94, 297
Laryngology, 97, 107
Laryngoscope, 118, 177
Leipzig, University of, 119
Lenox Hill Hospital (New York), 212
Leukemias, 265
Lewis, Sinclair, 183
Library of Congress, 71
Licensing, 2, 81, 105–6, 113, 141
colonial-era, 26–27, 29, 30
opposition of proprietary medical schools to, 42, 43, 48
state board standards for, 153, 160, 164, 188

Liebman, Paul, 299–302
Life expectancy, 189–90
Lincoln, Abraham, 72, 95
Lincoln Park Sanitarium, 100
Lincoln Park Training School for Nurses, 100
Lister, Joseph, 62, 64–71, 76, 78–80, 86, 127, 136, 230, 305
Listerism, 68–70, 81, 127, 136
    Garfield's death due to failure to implement, 74, 76–80, 306
    homeopathy and, 101
    in railway medicine, 110
Little Bighorn River, battle of, 67
Long Island College Hospital (Brooklyn), 65, 81, 212
Lymphomas, 265

Magnetic resonance imaging (MRI), 305
Malaria, 91, 220, 233
Malpractice, 11, 79, 85, 297–301
Managed care, 111, 296–97
Manual of the Principles and Practice of Operative Surgery (Smith), 85
March of Dimes, 183, 267
Martin, Franklin, 155–63, 166, 169–71, 203, 221
Massachusetts General Hospital (Boston), 51, 53, 56, 59, 70, 142, 144, 243
Mather, Cotton, 9–12
Mayo, Charles, 156
Mayo, William, 156, 184
McGill University, 213
McKessin & Robbins, 109
McKinley, William, 103
McLean Insane Asylum (Charlestown, Massachusetts), 59
Measles, 8
Medicaid, 269, 284, 296
Medical education
    colonial-era, 17–24, 29
    and doctor shortage, 273–76
    European, 18, 20, 24, 28, 44–45, 69, 117–24, 126, 127, 133, 150–51, 158, 274
    Flexner's investigation of, 147–55
    government grants for, 234–35
    homeopathic, 93, 104
    philanthropic funding of, 154–55
    reform of, 122–26, 166, 188
    scientific medicine and, 83
    specialization in, 252
    see also Academic medicine; Apprentice-

ship, medical; Proprietary medical schools; *specific medical schools*
Medical-industrial complex, 284–91, 295, 305
Medical Repository, The (journal), 50
Medical Society of the County of New York, 93
Medicare, 258–64, 269, 296, 306
Memorial Hospital (New York), 212, 284
Meningitis, 36, 223
Mesenteric insufficiency, chronic, 277
Metropolitan Health Bill (New York, 1866), 86, 87
Michigan, University of, 90
Microbiology, 81, 85, 148, 173, 237
Military medicine, 63, 95, 166–72
Minnesota, University of, 90, 164
Missouri Pacific Hospital, 110
Moore, Francis, 242–48, 250, 253, 306–7
Morgan, John, 20–30, 33, 49, 106, 117, 120
Mormonism, 46
Morphine, 70, 129
Morse, Samuel, 54
Morton, William Thomas Green, 51, 53–60, 305
Mount Sinai Hospital (New York), 212

Nation, The, 194
National Association for the Advancement of Colored People (NAACP), 219
National Association of Railway Surgeons, 108, 110, 112
National Association of Superintendents and Managers of Homeopathic Hospitals for the Insane, 97
National Board of Health, 86
National Broadcasting Corporation (NBC), 257
National Cancer Act (1971), 269–71
National Cancer Institute, 183, 268, 270, 271
National Endowment for the Arts, 258
National Endowment for the Humanities, 258
National Farm and Home Radio Hour, 196
National health care, 254–60
    see also Medicaid; Medicare
National Heart Institute, 233, 235
National Institutes of Health (NIH), 232–35, 260, 270
National Research Council, 216
Navy, U.S., 73, 169, 209, 219
Neurology, 61, 107, 127, 169, 201
Neuropsychiatry, 165

New Deal, 192, 229, 255
New England Courant, 11
New England Journal of Medicine, 283, 284
New Jersey, College of, 33
New Republic, The, 173, 191
New York Daily Tribune, 89
New Yorker, 154
New York Evening Graphic, 187
New York Hospital, 51, 182, 212
New York Journal of Medicine, 58
New York Medico-Legal Society, 65, 111
New York Public Library, 123
New York State Medical Society, 65
New York Times, 59, 75, 95, 137, 155, 159, 167,
    176, 187, 195, 197, 212, 219, 221, 231,
    257, 260, 270, 283
    Magazine, 153
New York University, 233
Nietzsche, Friedrich, 117
Nitrous oxide, 52–53, 55, 58
Nixon, Richard, 256, 269–71, 305
Nobel Prize in Physiology or Medicine,
    176–77, 209, 229, 235, 239
Northwestern University, 168

Obstetrics, 50, 64, 106, 112, 119, 165, 254, 275,
    298, 299
Ohio State University, 243
Oklahoma, University of, 290
Open-heart surgery, 239, 283, 285, 305
Ophthalmology, 64, 97, 107, 118, 160, 165,
    200
Ophthalmoscope, 118, 177
Opium, 70
Organ transplantation, 239–50, 305, 307
Orificial surgery, 98–100, 104
Orthopedics, 107, 134, 165, 171, 201, 203,
    220, 291
Osler, William, 130–31
Otolaryngology, 134, 165
Otology, 64, 97
Otoscope, 118, 177

Palm Beach Post, 302
Paris Medical Society, 59
Parke-Davis Company, 109, 187
Pasteur, Louis, 62, 66, 70
Pasteur Vaccine Company, 109
Pathology, 23, 48, 49, 81, 129, 162, 173, 176,
    213, 225, 237
    in medical education, 45, 122–24, 147,
    148, 150

microscopic, 83
resistance to, 70
specialization in, 160, 165, 169, 190, 201,
    246, 265, 266, 275
Peace Corps, 258
Pediatrics, 33, 201, 202, 251, 254, 265
    homeopathic, 97, 107, 160
    residencies in, 165, 274
    women in, 275, 298
Pellagra, 174
Penicillin, 3, 222–23
Penn, Thomas, 21–22, 26
Pennsylvania, University of, 20, 35, 41, 51,
    65, 168
    School of Medicine, 261
Pennsylvania Assembly, 14
Pennsylvania Gazette, 14, 22
Pennsylvania Hospital (Philadelphia), 20,
    23–24, 34
Pennsylvania Railroad Company, 109
Peritonitis, 186–88
Pernicious anemia, 175–77
Pfizer, 287
Pharmaceutical companies, 109, 128, 174,
    184, 187–89, 209, 223, 264
Philadelphia, College of, 20, 22, 26
Philadelphia Academy of Fine Arts, 136
Philadelphia Athletics baseball team, 157
Philadelphia Bible Society, 33
Philosophical Transactions (Royal Society of
    London), 10
Physician Himself, The (Cathell), 81–82, 103
Physiology, 23, 48, 49, 70, 147, 148, 176, 177,
    225, 233, 237
Pittsburgh, Fort Wayne and Chicago Rail-
    way, 109, 110
*Planter's and Mariner's Medical Companion,
    The* (Ewell), 46
Plasma, 211–17, 219, 220
Pneumonia, 187, 190, 223, 271
Point of Service (POS) plans, 296–97
Polio, 136, 184, 191, 232
Popular Science Monthly, 137
Prague, University of, 119
Pratt, Edwin Hartley, 98–101, 104
Preferred Provider Organizations (PPOs),
    296
Presbyterian Hospital (New York), 212–14
Princeton University, 33
    Institute for Advanced Study, 155
Proctology, 107
Proctoscope, 118, 177

Progressive Era, 141–42, 151
Proprietary medical schools, 40–44, 49, 81,
    98, 148, 152
    homeopathic, 93, 98
    licensing opposed by, 42, 43, 48
    for railway medicine, 109
Psychiatrists, 107, 171, 201, 274, 275
Psychological medicine, 97
Public health, 84–89, 120, 173, 194, 235, 275
    homeopathy and, 97
    nutrition and, 174
    railway medicine and, 108
Public Health Service, U.S., 230, 232, 233,
    248
Pulitzer Prize, 183
Purdue University, 112
Purging, 17, 32, 35, 36, 38, 45, 46, 61, 70, 71,
    81
Puritans, 9

Radiation therapy, 173, 265, 268
Radiology, 139, 165, 169, 201, 202, 281
Railway medicine, 107–12, 155
Railway Surgeon, The (Stemen), 110, 112
Ravitch, Mark, 289–93
Reagan, Ronald, 257, 287
Red Cross, 168–70, 212, 214–16
Red Scare, 196
Reed, Walter, 124, 176, 188
Remington, Frederic, 188
Renal artery atherosclerosis, 277
Republican Party, 71, 234, 256, 258, 259
Residency programs, 134, 165, 202, 222, 251,
    253, 274, 298
    surgical, 133–34, 165, 203, 290
Resource-Based Relative Value Scale
    (RBRVS), 296, 297
Revolutionary War, 15–16, 23, 26, 28–29,
    34, 44
Rhode Island Medical Society, 94
Rickets, 174
Rockefeller, John D., 154, 210, 211
Rockefeller Institute for Medical Research,
    150, 179, 239
Roentgen, William, 137, 138
Romans, ancient, 37, 264, 304
Roosevelt, Franklin, 136, 189, 192, 198, 230,
    255
Rostock, University of, 118
Royal Air Force, 214–15
Royal College of Physicians, 13, 20
Royal College of Surgeons, 166–67

Royal Society of London, 10, 13, 20
Rush, Benjamin, 30–40, 45–47, 49, 58, 70,
    103, 117

Sanitation, 63, 84–89, 108, 220
Sarcomas, 265
Scarlet fever, 8
Schick, Béla, 176
Schopenhauer, Arthur, 117
Scientific medicine, 63, 68–70, 80, 110, 140,
    144, 238, 306
    in Germany, 121–24
    licensing standards and, 105
    public acceptance of, 84, 89
    specialization and, 107
    unification of medical profession by, 83, 102
Scurvy, 174
Searle & Hereth, 109
Segregation
    gender, 275
    racial, 3, 213, 217–19
Self-help medicine, 45–46
Senate, U.S., 58, 230–31, 234, 262, 269
Septicemia, see Blood poisoning
Shannon, James, 233–35, 248
Sherman Anti-Trust Act (1890), 263
Sickle-cell anemia, 307
Sigerist, Henry, 24, 41
Sinclair, Upton, 151
Sitting Bull, 67
6-mercaptopurine, 249
Smallpox, 1, 7–16, 187, 306
Smith, Stephen, 84–88, 220
Social Security, 192, 198, 257
Southworth, Billy, 267
Soviet Union, 232, 289–90
Spahn, Warren, 267
Spanish-American War, 103
Specialization, 83–84, 89, 106–7, 113, 142,
    172, 235
    certification of, 200–203, 205–6, 218,
        221–22, 252–54
    colonial-era origins of, 25–27
    earnings and, 189
    growth in, 199–200, 251
    homeopathy and, 97, 99, 103–4
    interdisciplinary teams and, 243, 251
    medical education and, 132–34, 155, 165,
        252
    in railway medicine, 107–10
    surgery and, 18, 63, 120, 155–61, 183,
        203–5

during World War I, 170, 171
during World War II, 220–22
see also specific specialties
Sphygmomanometer, 190–91
Squibb Institute for Medical Research, 233
Stanford University Medical School, 286
Stapler, surgical, 289–91
Stem cells, 306
Stemen, Christian, 109–12
Stents, 288–89, 297, 305
Sternberg, George, 124
Stethoscope, 45, 118, 178
Steuben, Baron von, 27
Stimulants, alcoholic, 70–71
Strasbourg, University of, 119
Streptococci, 186–88
Streptomycin, 233, 249
Stroke, 224, 277, 278
Sulfa drugs, 173, 190
Supreme Court, U.S., 230, 295
Surgeon General of the United States, Office
    of, 248
    Library of, 123
Surgery, 3, 85
    abdominal, 181, 187–88, 241, 291–94
    antiseptic, *see* Antisepsis
    appendectomy, 180–86, 190
    cancer, 265, 268
    cardiac, 1, 223–29, 239, 281–83, 285,
        287–89, 292, 305, 307
    colonial-era, 8, 18, 20–22, 25, 26, 28, 30
    during Civil War, 62–63, 73, 74
    Halsted's innovations in, 126–28, 130–32
    heroic therapies and, 32–33
    homeopathy and, 97, 101, 103
    laparoscopic, 290–94, 297
    organ transplant, 239–50, 305
    orificial, 98–101, 104
    pain-free, *see* Anesthesia
    in railway medicine, 108–13
    residency programs in, 133–34, 165, 203,
        290
    robotic, 307, 308
    specialization in, 18, 63, 120, 155–61, 183,
        201, 203–5, 221–22, 251–53
    standards for, 142–45, 161–63
    staples versus sutures for, 289–91
    technology and, 136–37, 140, 291
    unnecessary, 270
    vascular, 299–302
    during World War I, 166–71
    during World War II, 218, 220

Surgery, Gynecology & Obstetrics (journal),
    157
Syphilis, 3, 8, 98, 140, 214
System of Surgery (Keen), 136

Taylor University, 112
Thomsonianism, 46–47
Thoreau, Henry David, 97
Thorn, George, 243–46, 248, 250, 253, 306–7
Thyroxine, 176
Time magazine, 120, 197, 198, 227–29, 242,
    244–45, 248, 269, 283, 290
Tocqueville, Alexis de, 44
Tombs Prison (New York), 58
Tonics, 70–71, 128
Torgeson, Earl, 267
*Transactions of the American Medical Associa-
    tion* (journal), 50–51
Transcendentalism, 97
Transfusions, 73, 175, 177, 209–10, 220, 223
    plasma for, 211–17, 219, 220
Transient ischemic attack, 277
Transplants, *see* Organ transplantation
Trocars, 291
Truman, Harry, 233, 255, 256, 263
Truth or Consequences (radio show), 267
Tuberculosis, 31, 80, 89, 98, 139, 164, 165, 187,
    190, 238
Tuskagee syphilis study, 3
Typhoid, 84, 87, 89

Union College, 65
United Press International, 288
United States Mint, 33
United States Surgical Corporation, 291, 293
Unorthodox medicine, 46–49, 93, 94
    see also Homeopathy; Irregular practi-
        tioners
Urinalysis, 178
Urology, 107, 165, 201, 203

Vaccination, 10, 12, 187, 235, 238
Varicose veins, surgery for, 299–302
Variety Club of New England, 266–67
Vascular surgery, 299–302
Vegetarianism, 47
Vienna, University of, 119, 122, 126
Virginia, Medical College of, 299
Vitamins, 174–75, 177
Volunteers in Service to America (VISTA),
    258
Voting Rights Act (1965), 258

Wabash, St. Louis and Pacific Railway East of the Mississippi River, Surgical Society of, 109–10
Ward, Samuel, 16
War of 1812, 44
Warren, John Collins, 53, 55, 56
Warren, John Collins, II, 69–70, 79
Washington, George, 15–16, 34
Washington Post, 270
Washington University, 168, 204
Water cure, 47
Watson, Thomas, 227
Watts Hospital (Durham, North Carolina), 182–83
Welch, William Henry, 119–26, 129–33, 135, 150
Wells, Horace, 52–55, 57–59
Western Reserve University
    Lakeside Hospital, 167
    Medical School, 166
Who Is Insane? (Smith), 85
Wilson, Henry, 74
Wilson, Woodrow, 169, 172
Woman's Christian Temperance Union, 71
World's Columbian Exposition (Chicago, 1893), 100

World's Work, 163
World War I, 104, 120, 166–73, 180, 209, 220, 222, 226–27
    Red Scare following, 196
World War II, 209, 211, 220–23, 255
    Blood for Britain program in, 209, 211–16
    racism during, 3, 217–18
    research during, 222–23, 229, 233, 248
    specialists in, 220–22
    stress-related disorders of soldiers in, 220
Würzburg, University of, 118

X-rays, 73, 135, 137–41, 143, 166, 173, 177, 179, 204
    for cardiac catherization, 281, 283
    in defensive medical practice, 299
    in hospitals, 162, 190
    for kidney transplant patients, 249
    for World War I casualties, 170

Yale, Elihu, 9
Yale University, 9, 119, 126, 132, 253
Yellow fever, 8, 176, 220
Young, Brigham, 188

Zurich University Hospital, 278–83

ABOUT THE AUTHOR

Ira Rutkow is a general surgeon and historian of American medicine. He also holds a doctorate of public health from Johns Hopkins University. Among Dr. Rutkow's books on medical history, his *Surgery: An Illustrated History* was selected as a *New York Times* Notable Book of the Year. Dr. Rutkow's recent works include *Bleeding Blue and Gray*, a narrative history of Civil War medicine, and *James A. Garfield*, a political biography and reappraisal of the medical aspects of Garfield's assassination. Dr. Rutkow and his wife divide their time between New York City and their farm in the Hudson Valley.